# THIRD EDITION

# CASE FILES®
## Biochemistry

D1593196

**Eugene C. Toy, MD**
Vice Chair of Academic Affairs and
   Residency Program Director
Obstetrics and Gynecology
The Methodist Hospital, Houston
Clinical Professor and Clerkship Director
Department of Obstetrics/Gynecology
University of Texas Medical School at
   Houston
Houston, Texas
John S. Dunn Senior Academic Chair
Department of Obstetrics and Gynecology
St Joseph Medical Center
Houston, Texas

**William E. Seifert Jr., PhD**
Adjunct Associate Professor
McGovern Center for Humanities and
   Ethics
Former Medical Biochemistry Course
   Director
University of Texas Medical School at
   Houston
Houston, Texas

**Henry W. Strobel, PhD**
Professor
Department of Biochemistry and
   Molecular Biology
Distinguished Teaching Professor
Associate Dean for Faculty Affairs
University of Texas Medical School at
   Houston
Houston, Texas

**Konrad P. Harms, MD**
Clinical Assistant Professor
Weill Cornell College of Medicine
Associate Program Director
Obstetrics and Gynecology Residency
The Methodist Hospital, Houston
Houston, Texas

Medical

New York   Chicago   San Francisco   Athens   London   Madrid
Mexico City   Milan   New Delhi   Singapore   Sydney   Toronto

Case Files®: Biochemistry, Third Edition

1 2 3 4 5 6 7 8 9 0   DOC/DOC   19 18 17 16 15 14

ISBN 978-0-07-179488-6
MHID 0-07-179488-3

---

**Notice**

Medicine is an ever-changing science. As new research and clinical experience broaden our knowledge, changes in treatment and drug therapy are required. The authors and the publisher of this work have checked with sources believed to be reliable in their efforts to provide information that is complete and generally in accord with the standard accepted at the time of publication. However, in view of the possibility of human error or changes in medical sciences, neither the editors nor the publisher nor any other party who has been involved in the preparation or publication of this work warrants that the information contained herein is in every respect accurate or complete, and they disclaim all responsibility for any errors or omissions or for the results obtained from use of the information contained in this work. Readers are encouraged to confirm the information contained herein with other sources. For example and in particular, readers are advised to check the product information sheet included in the package of each drug they plan to administer to be certain that the information contained in this work is accurate and that changes have not been made in the recommended dose or in the contraindications for administration. This recommendation is of particular importance in connection with new or infrequently used drugs.

---

This book was set in Goudy by Cenveo® Publisher Services.
The editors were Catherine A. Johnson and Cindy Yoo.
The production supervisor was Catherine Saggese.
Project management was provided by Hardik Popli, Cenveo Publisher Services.
The designer was Janice Bielawa.
The cover designer was Thomas De Pierro.
RR Donnelley was printer and binder.

This book is printed on acid-free paper.

**Library of Congress Cataloging-in-Publication Data**

Toy, Eugene C., author.
    Case files. Biochemistry / Eugene C. Toy, William E. Seifert Jr., Henry W. Strobel, Konrad P. Harms. —Third edition.
        p. ; cm.
    Biochemistry
    Preceded by Case files. Biochemistry / Eugene C. Toy ... [et al.]. 2nd ed. c2008.
    Includes bibliographical references and index.
    ISBN 978-0-07-179488-6 (pbk. : alk. paper)—ISBN 0-07-179488-3 (pbk. : alk. paper)
    I. Seifert, William E., Jr., author.   II. Strobel, Henry W., author.   III. Harms, Konrad P., author.   IV. Title.
V. Title: Biochemistry.
    [DNLM: 1. Metabolism—Case Reports.   2. Metabolism—Examination Questions.   3. Biochemical Phenomena—Case Reports.   4. Biochemical Phenomena—Examination Questions.   QU 18.2]
    QP171
    572'.4—dc23                                                                                    2014007206

McGraw-Hill Education books are available at special quantity discounts to use as premiums and sales promotions or for use in corporate training programs. To contact a representative, please visit the Contact Us pages at www.mhprofessional.com.

*To my friend, mentor, and role model, Dr. Benton Baker III, who taught me by his example the importance of integrity, unselfishness, and teamwork.*

*—ECT*

*To my wife, Heidi, and to Koen and Kort, for their unwavering love and support and for reminding me daily of what is really important in life.*

*—KPH*

*To Dr. John A. DeMoss, Founding Chair of the Department of Biochemistry and Molecular Biology of the University of Texas Medical School at Houston. Dr. DeMoss served as Department Chair from 1971 until he stepped down from that office in 1992, serving as Professor until 2001 when he became Emeritus Professor, his present position. Dr. DeMoss is that unique kind of scholar who excels at both research and teaching. He loves teaching and he is gifted at it. Dr. DeMoss not only has taught and continues to teach generations of students, but he also teaches faculty, especially young faculty, how to teach and to love teaching. Therefore, it is in gratitude for his teaching of us that we dedicate this book to Dr. John A. DeMoss.*

*—WES & HWS*

# CONTENTS

**Sayeepriyadarshini Anakk, PhD**
Assistant Professor
Department of Biology
University of Illinois
Urbana, Illinois
*β-Thalassemia*
*HIV*

**Leposava Antonovic, PhD**
Assistant Professor
Department of Molecular & Integrative Physiology
University of Illinois, Urbana-Champaign
Urbana, Illinois
*β-Thalassemia*
*HIV*

**Michael R. Blackburn, PhD**
Professor and Vice-Chair
Department of Biochemistry, Medical School
Dean, Graduate School of Biomedical Sciences
University of Texas Health Science Center at Houston
Houston, Texas
*Adenosine Deaminase Deficiency*
*Gout*
*Vegetarian–Essential Amino Acids*

**Phillip B. Carpenter, PhD**
Associate Professor
Department of Biochemistry and Molecular Biology
University of Texas Medical School at Houston
Houston, Texas
*Tumor Suppressor Genes and Cancer*

**Raegan D. Hunt, MD, PhD**
Assistant Professor of Dermatology and Pediatrics
Baylor College of Medicine
Texas Children's Clinical Care Center
Houston, Texas
*Cholestasis of Pregnancy*
*Folate Deficiency*

**Auinash Kalsotra, PhD**
Assistant Professor
Departments of Biochemistry and Medical Biochemistry
Affiliate, Institute of Genomic Biology
University of Illinois, Urbana-Champaign
Urbana, Illinois
*Erythromycin and Lyme Disease*
*Quinolones*

**Richard J. Kulmacz, PhD**
Professor
Departments of Internal Medicine and Biochemistry and
    Molecular Biology
University of Texas Medical School at Houston
Houston, Texas
*NSAIDs*

**Julia E. Lever, PhD**
Professor Emerita
Department of Biochemistry and Molecular Biology
University of Texas Medical School at Houston
Houston, Texas
*Addison Disease*
*Diabetes Insipidus*
*Hyperparathyroid Disease*
*Hypothyroidism*
*Menopause*

**Alan E. Levine, PhD, MEd**
Associate Professor, Deceased
Department of Diagnostics and Biomedical Sciences
University of Texas School of Dentistry at Houston
Houston, Texas
*Hypercholesterolemia*
*Methotrexate*
*Statin Medications*
*Tay-Sachs Disease*

**John A. Putkey, PhD**
Professor
Department of Biochemistry and Molecular Biology
University of Texas Medical School at Houston
Houston, Texas
*Sickle Cell Disease*

**Daniel J. Ryder, PhD, MPH**
Postdoctoral Associate
Department of Physical Therapy
University of Florida
Gainesville, Florida
*Cushing Syndrome*

**Jennifer L. Seifert, PhD**
Faculty Associate Researcher
Department of Bioengineering
The University of Texas at Dallas and The University of
    Texas Southwestern Medical Center
Dallas, Texas
*Maple Syrup Urine Disease*
*Pheochromocytoma*

**Nathaniel H.P. Strobel, MD**
Assistant Professor
Division of Critical Care Medicine
Department of Pediatrics
University of Texas Medical School at Houston
Houston, Texas
*Anaerobic Metabolism-Metabolic Acidosis/Septic Shock*

**Jade M. Teakell, MD, PhD**
Resident
Department of Internal Medicine
University of Texas Medical School at Houston
Houston, Texas
*Porphyria*

**Allison L. Toy**
Senior Nursing Student
Scott & White Nursing School
Belton, Texas
Primary manuscript reviewer

**Cheri M. Turman, PhD**
Coats Aloe International, Inc.
Dallas, Texas
*Fragile X Syndrome*
*Gallstones*

**Martin E. Young, DPhil**
Associate Professor
Department of Medicine
University of Alabama at Birmingham School of Medicine
Birmingham, Alabama
*Anorexia Nervosa*
*Somogyi Effect*
*Type 2 Diabetes*

We appreciate all the kind remarks and suggestions from the many medical students during the last 5 years. Your positive reception has been an incredible encouragement, especially in light of the short life of the *Case Files* series. In this third edition of *Case Files: Biochemistry*, the basic format of the book has been retained. Improvements were made in updating many of the chapters. New cases include adenosine deaminase deficiency, maple syrup urine disease, alcoholic ketoacidosis, glucose-6-phosphate dehydrogenase deficiency, medium chain fatty acyl dehydrogenase deficiency, pheochromocytoma, and pediatric methomoglobinemia. We reviewed the clinical scenarios with the intent of improving them; however, their "real-life" presentations patterned after actual clinical experience were accurate and instructive. The multiple-choice questions have been carefully reviewed and rewritten to ensure that they comply with the National Board and USMLE format. Through this third edition, we hope that the reader will continue to enjoy learn diagnosis and management through the simulated clinical cases. It certainly is a privilege to be teachers for so many students, and it is with humility that we present this edition.

The Authors

# ACKNOWLEDGMENTS

The inspiration for this basic science series occurred at an educational retreat led by Dr. Maximilian Buja, who, at the time, was the dean of the medical school. It has been such a joy to work together with Drs. William Seifert and Henry Strobel, who are both accomplished scientists and teachers, as well as the other excellent authors and contributors. It has been rewarding to collaborate with Dr. Konrad Harms, whom I have watched mature from a medical student to resident and now a brilliant faculty member. I would like to thank McGraw-Hill for believing in the concept of teaching by clinical cases. I owe a great debt to Catherine Johnson, who has been a fantastically encouraging and enthusiastic editor. It has been amazing to work together with my daughter Allison, who is a senior nursing student at the Scott and White School of Nursing. She is an astute manuscript reviewer and already in her early career she has a good clinical acumen and a clear writing style.

At the University of Texas Medical School at Houston, we would like to recognize Dr. Rodney E. Kellems, Chair of the Department of Biochemistry and Molecular Biology, for his encouragement and delight in this project; Johnna Kincaid, former Director of Management Operations for her support; Nina Smith and Bonnie Martinez for their help in preparing the manuscript; and Amy Gilbert for her assistance with the figures. We also would like to thank the many students who have allowed us to teach them over the years and who have in the process taught us. Dr. Seifert thanks his wife Margie for her encouragement, patience, and support.

At Methodist Hospital, I appreciate Drs. Mark Boom, Alan Kaplan, and Judy Paukert. At St. Joseph Medical Center, I would like to recognize our outstanding administrators: Pat Mathews and Paula Efird. I appreciate Linda Bergstrom's advice and assistance. Without the help from my colleagues, Drs. Konrad Harms, Priti Schachel, Gizelle Brooks-Carter, and Russell Edwards, this book could not have been written. Most important, I am humbled by the love, affection, and encouragement from my lovely wife, Terri and our 4 children, Andy and his wife Anna, Michael, Allison, and Christina.

Eugene C. Toy

Drs. Seifert and Strobel want to recognize Alan Levine, who joined our Department of Biochemistry and Molecular Biology when the basic faculties of the Dental Branch and the Medical School were combined in 2005, as he was a gifted and innovative teacher. He plunged into our teaching programs with great enthusiasm for the material he taught, for seeking ways in which the material could be better communicated, but especially for the students who would use the biochemical principles to become excellent physicians, dentists, and researchers. An enormously generous and selfless man, teaching came naturally to Alan and that gift was widely recognized in our institution. We miss his presence.

Often, the medical student will cringe at the "drudgery" of the basic science courses and see little connection between a field such as biochemistry and clinical problems. However, clinicians often wish they knew more about the basic sciences, because it is through the science that we can begin to understand the complexities of the human body and, thus, have rational methods of diagnosis and treatment.

Mastering the knowledge in a discipline such as biochemistry is a formidable task. It is even more difficult to retain this information and to recall it when the clinical setting is encountered. To accomplish this synthesis, biochemistry is optimally taught in the context of medical situations, and this is reinforced later during the clinical rotations. The gulf between the basic sciences and the patient arena is wide. Perhaps one way to bridge this gulf is with carefully constructed clinical cases that ask basic science-oriented questions. In an attempt to achieve this goal, we have designed a collection of patient cases to teach biochemistry related points. More importantly, the explanations for these cases emphasize the underlying mechanisms and relate the clinical setting to the basic science data. We explore the principles rather than emphasize rote memorization.

This book is organized for versatility: to allow the student "in a rush" to go quickly through the scenarios and check the corresponding answers and to provide more detailed information for the student who wants thought-provoking explanations. The answers are arranged from simple to complex: a summary of the pertinent points, the bare answers, a clinical correlation, an approach to the biochemistry topic, a comprehension test at the end to reinforcement or emphasis, and a list of references for further reading. The clinical cases are arranged by system to better reflect the organization within the basic science. Finally, to encourage thinking about mechanisms and relationships, we intentionally did not primarily use a multiple-choice format. Nevertheless, several multiple-choice questions are included at the end of each scenario to reinforce concepts or introduce related topics.

## HOW TO GET THE MOST OUT OF THIS BOOK

Each case is designed to introduce a clinically related issue and includes open-ended questions usually asking a basic science question, but at times, to break up the monotony, there will be a clinical question. The answers are organized into 4 different parts:

## PART I

1. **Summary**
2. A **straightforward answer** is given for each open-ended question.
3. Clinical Correlation—A discussion of the relevant points relating the basic science to the clinical manifestations, and perhaps introducing the student to issues such as diagnosis and treatment.

## PART II

An **approach to the basic science concept** consisting of 3 parts:

1. **Objectives**—A listing of the 2 to 4 main principles critical for understanding the underlying biochemistry to answer the question and relate to the clinical situation.
2. **Definitions of basic terminology**
3. **Discussion of topic**

## PART III

**Comprehension Questions**—Each case includes several multiple-choice questions that reinforce the material or introduces new and related concepts. Questions about the material not found in the text are explained in the answers.

## PART IV

**Biochemistry Pearls**—A listing of several important points, many clinically relevant reiterated as a summation of the text and to allow for easy review, such as before an examination.

# Applying the Basic Sciences to Clinical Medicine

## Part 1. Approach to Learning Biochemistry

Biochemistry is best learned by a systematic approach, first by learning the **language** of the discipline and then by understanding the **function** of the various processes. Increasingly, cellular and molecular biology play an important role in the understanding of disease processes and also in the treatment of disease. Initially, some of the terminology must be memorized in the same way that the alphabet must be learned by rote; however, the appreciation of the way that the biochemical words are constructed requires an understanding of mechanisms and a manipulation of the information.

## Part 2. Approach to Disease

Physicians usually tackle clinical situations by taking a history (asking questions), performing a physical examination, obtaining selective laboratory and imaging tests, and then formulating a diagnosis. The conglomeration of the history, physician examination, and laboratory tests is called the **clinical database.** After reaching a diagnosis, a treatment plan is usually initiated, and the patient is followed for a clinical response. Rational understanding of disease and plans for treatment are best acquired by learning about the normal human processes on a basic science level; likewise, being aware of how disease alters the normal physiologic processes is understood on a basic science level.

## Part 3. Approach to Reading

There are 6 key questions that help to stimulate the application of basic science information to the clinical setting. These are:

1. *What is the most likely biochemical mechanism for the disease causing the patient's symptom or physical examination finding?*

2. *Which biochemical marker will be affected by treating a certain disease, and why?*

3. *Looking at graphical data, what is the most likely biochemical explanation for the results?*

4. *Based on the deoxyribonucleic acid (DNA) sequence, what is the most likely amino acid or protein result, and how will it be manifest in a clinical setting?*

5. *What hormone–receptor interaction is likely?*

6. *How does the presence or absence of enzyme activity affect the biochemical (molecular) conditions, and how does that in turn affect the patient's symptoms?*

1. **What is the most likely biochemical mechanism for the disease causing the patient's symptom or physical examination finding?**
   This is the fundamental question that basic scientists strive to answer—the underlying cause of a certain disease or symptom. Once this underlying mechanism is discovered, then progress can be made regarding methods of diagnosis and treatment. Otherwise, our attempts are only *empiric*—in other words, only by trial and error and observation of association. Students are encouraged to think about the mechanisms and underlying cause rather than just memorizing by rote.

   For example, in sickle cell disease, students should connect the various facts together, setting the foundation for understanding disease throughout their life. In sickle cell disease, valine (a hydrophobic amino acid) is substituted for glutamate (a charged, hydrophilic amino acid) in the sixth position in the β-globin chain of hemoglobin. This decreases the solubility of hemoglobin when it is in the deoxygenated state, resulting in its precipitation into elongated fibers in the red blood cell.

   This causes the red blood cell to have less distensibility and, thus, to *sickle*, leading to rupture of the red blood cell (hemolysis) and blockage in small capillaries. The *sludging* in small capillaries leads to poor oxygen delivery, ischemia, and pain.

2. **Which biochemical marker will be affected by therapy?**
   After a diagnosis has been made and therapy initiated, then the patient response should be monitored to assure improvement. Ideally, the patient response should be obtained in a scientific manner: unbiased, precise, and consistent. Although more than one physician or nurse may be measuring the response, it should be as carefully performed with little intervariation (one person to the next) or intravariation (one person measuring) as possible. One of the therapeutic measures includes serum or imaging markers; for example, in diabetic ketoacidosis, the serum glucose and pH levels would be measured to confirm improvement with therapy. Another example would be to follow the volume of a pulmonary mass imaged by computed tomography following chemotherapy. The student must know enough about the disease process to know which marker to measure and the expected response over time.

3. **Looking at graphic data, what is the most likely biochemical explanation for the results?**
   Medicine is art and science. The **art** aspect consists of the way that the physician deals with the human aspect of the patient, expressing empathy, compassion, establishing a therapeutic relationship, and dealing with uncertainty; the **science** is the attempts to understand disease processes, making rational treatment plans, and being objective in observations. The physician as scientist must be precise about how to elicit data and then carefully make sense of the information, using up-to-date evidence. Exercises to develop the skills of data analysis require interpretation of data in various representations, such as in tables or on graphs.

4. **Based on the DNA sequence, what amino acid or protein would be produced, and how would the protein be manifested in a clinical setting?**

   The clinician–basic scientist collaboration requires each party to "speak the same language" and translate forward and backward from science to clinical, and vice versa. Biochemical thinking is very stepwise, for example, the relationship among DNA, RNA, proteins, and clinical findings. Because the genomic information (DNA) codes for proteins that affect physiologic or pathologic changes, it is of fundamental importance that the student becomes very comfortable thinking about these relationships:

   Forward: DNA → Proteins → Clinical Manifestations
   Backward: Clinical Findings → Effects of Protein → DNA

5. **What hormone–receptor interaction is likely?**

   A **hormone** is a substance, usually a peptide or steroid, produced by one tissue and conveyed by the bloodstream to another part of the body to affect physiologic activity, such as growth or metabolism. A **receptor** is a cellular structure that mediates between a chemical agent (hormone) and the physiologic response. The way that the hormone causes its effect is vital to understand, because many diseases occur as a result of abnormal hormone production, abnormal hormone receptor interaction, or abnormal cellular response to the hormone–receptor complex. For example, diabetes mellitus is manifest clinically by high blood glucose levels. However, in type 1 diabetes (usually juvenile onset), the etiology is insufficient insulin secreted by the pancreas. (Insulin acts to put serum glucose into cells or store it as glycogen.) By contrast, the mechanism in type 2 diabetes (usually adult onset) is a defect of the insulin receptor messenger; in fact, the insulin levels in these individuals are usually higher than normal. Understanding the difference between the two mechanisms allows the scientist to approach individualized therapy, and it allows the clinician to understand the differences in these patients, such as the reason that people with type 1 diabetes are much more prone to diabetic ketoacidosis (because of insulin deficiency).

6. **How does the presence or absence of enzyme activity affect the biochemical (molecular) conditions, and how does that in turn affect patient symptoms?**

   Enzymes are proteins that act as catalysts, speeding the rate at which biochemical reactions proceed but not altering the direction or nature of the reactions. The presence or absence of these important substances affects the biochemical conditions, which then influence the other physiologic processes in the body. Enzyme deficiencies are often inherited as autosomal recessive conditions and may be passed from parent to child. Clearly, when students begin to understand the role of the enzyme and the chemical reaction that it governs, they begin to understand the intricacies of the human biologic processes.

## BIOCHEMISTRY PEARLS

▶ There are 6 key questions to stimulate the application of basic science information to the clinical arena.

▶ Medicine consists of both art and science.

▶ The scientific aspect of medicine seeks to gather data in an objective manner, understand physiologic and pathologic processes in light of scientific information, and propose rational explanations.

▶ The skilled clinician must be able to translate back and forth between the basic sciences and the clinical sciences.

## REFERENCE

Longo D, Fauci AS, Kasper KL, et al., eds. *Harrison's Principles of Internal Medicine.* 18th ed. New York: McGraw-Hill; 2011.

# Clinical Cases

A 15-year-old African-American girl presents to the emergency department with complaints of bilateral thigh and hip pain. The pain has been present for 1 day and is steadily increasing in severity. Acetaminophen and ibuprofen have not relieved her symptoms. She denies any recent trauma or excessive exercise. She does report feeling fatigued and has been having burning with urination along with urinating frequently. She reports having similar pain episodes in the past, sometimes requiring hospitalization. On examination, she is afebrile (without fever) and in no acute distress. No one in her family has similar episodes. Her conjunctiva and mucosal membranes are slightly pale in coloration. She has nonspecific bilateral anterior thigh pain with no abnormalities appreciated. The remainder of her examination is normal. Her white blood cell count is elevated at 17,000/mm$^3$, and her hemoglobin level is decreased at 7.1 g/dL. Urinalysis demonstrated an abnormal number of numerous bacteria.

▶ What is the most likely diagnosis?
▶ What is the molecular genetics behind this disorder?
▶ What is the pathophysiologic mechanism of her symptoms?

# ANSWERS TO CASE 1:
## Sickle Cell Disease

*Summary:* A 15-year-old African-American girl with recurrent bilateral thigh and hip pain, anemia, and symptoms and laboratory evidence of a urinary tract infection.

- **Most likely diagnosis:** Sickle cell disease (pain crisis).

- **Biochemical mechanism of disease:** Single amino acid substitution on hemoglobin β chain, inherited in an autosomal recessive fashion (1 in 12 African Americans in United States are carriers of the trait).

- **Pathophysiologic mechanism of symptoms:** The sickled red blood cells cause infarction of the bone, lung, kidney, and other tissue from vasoocclusion.

## CLINICAL CORRELATION

This 15-year-old girl's description of her pain is typical of a sickle cell pain crisis. Many times, infection is a trigger, most commonly pneumonia or urinary tract infection. This case is consistent with urinary tract infection, indicated by her symptoms of urinary frequency and burning with urination (dysuria). Her white blood cell count is elevated in response to the infection. The low hemoglobin level is consistent with sickle cell anemia. Because she is homozygous (both genes coding for sickle hemoglobin), both her parents have sickle cell trait (heterozygous) and, thus, do not have symptoms. The diagnosis can be established with hemoglobin electrophoresis. Treatment includes searching for an underlying cause of crisis (infection, hypoxia, fever, excessive exercise, and extreme changes in temperature), administration of oxygen, intravenous fluids for hydration, pain management, and consideration of blood transfusion.

# APPROACH TO:
## Sickle Cell Disease

## OBJECTIVES

1. Understand the primary, secondary, tertiary, and quaternary levels of protein structure.

2. Describe the structure of hemoglobin and its role in oxygen binding and dissociation.

3. Describe the mechanism that amino acid substitution results in sickle cell hemoglobin.

## DEFINITIONS

**ALLOSTERIC EFFECTORS:** Molecules that bind to enzymes or protein carriers at sites other than the active- or ligand-binding site. On binding, allosteric effectors either positively or negatively affect the enzymatic activity or capability of the protein to bind its ligand.

**GLOBIN:** The globular proteins that are the polypeptide components of myoglobin and hemoglobin. They contain a hydrophobic pocket that holds the heme prosthetic group.

**GLOBIN FOLD:** The 3-dimensional (3D) structure of the proteins that is common to myoglobin and the subunits of hemoglobin.

**HEME:** A porphyrin ring that has a $Fe^{+2}$ ion coordinately bound in the center of the molecule. Heme binds oxygen in hemoglobin and myoglobin and serves as an electron carrier in the cytochromes.

**HEMOGLOBIN:** The tetrameric protein in high concentration in red blood cells that binds oxygen in the capillaries of the lungs and delivers it to peripheral tissues. Each globin subunit contains a heme group that binds oxygen when the iron atom is in the ferrous (+2) oxidation state.

**MYOGLOBIN:** A protein having a single globin polypeptide with a bound heme group. It is primarily located in muscle cells and stores oxygen for times when a high demand exists for energy.

**PROTEIN PRIMARY (I°) STRUCTURE:** The amino acid sequence of the protein, listed from the amino-terminal amino acid to the carboxy-terminal amino acid.

**PROTEIN SECONDARY (II°) STRUCTURE:** The local 3D spatial arrangement of amino acids close to one another in the primary sequence. α-Helices and β-sheets are the predominant secondary structures in proteins.

**PROTEIN TERTIARY (III°) STRUCTURE:** The overall 3D structure of a single polypeptide chain, including positions of disulfide bonds. Noncovalent forces such as hydrogen bonding, electrostatic forces, and hydrophobic effects are also important.

**PROTEIN QUATERNARY (IV°) STRUCTURE:** The overall 3D arrangement of polypeptide subunits in a multisubunit protein.

## DISCUSSION

The **activity** of a given protein is dependent on **proper folding** of its polypeptide chain to assume a defined **3D structure.** The importance of protein folding to molecular medicine is emphasized by the fact that many disease-causing mutations do not directly affect the active- or ligand-binding site of proteins, but instead cause **local or global alterations in protein structure** or **disrupt the folding pathway** such that the native protein fold is not achieved, or undesirable interactions with other proteins are promoted. The molecular defect that changes adult hemoglobin (HbA) to sickle hemoglobin (HbS), leading to sickle cell anemia, is a classic example of mutations that affect protein structure.

Protein structure is typically classified as consisting of 4 levels: **primary (I°)**, **secondary (II°)**, **tertiary (III°)**, and **quaternary (IV°)**. **Primary structure** is the **sequence of amino acids in the protein. Secondary structure** is the **local 3D spatial arrangement of amino acids that are close to one another** in the primary sequence. **α-Helices and β-sheets** compose the majority of secondary structures in all known proteins. **Tertiary structure** is the **spatial arrangement of amino acid residues that are far apart** in the linear primary sequence of a single polypeptide chain, and it includes **disulfide bonds** and **noncovalent forces.** These noncovalent forces include **hydrogen bonding,** which is also the primary stabilization force for the formation of α-helices and β-sheets, **electrostatic interactions, van der Waals forces,** and **hydrophobic effects. Quaternary structure** is the manner in which **subunits of a multisubunit protein are arranged** with respect to one another.

Normal **hemoglobin has 4 subunits called globins.** HbA has **2 β ($\alpha_1$ and $\alpha_2$) and 2 β ($\beta_1$ and $\beta_2$) globin chains.** Each globin chain has an associated heme prosthetic group, which is the site of oxygen binding and release. All globin chains have similar primary sequences. The secondary structure of globin chains consists of approximately **75%** α-helix. The similar primary sequence promotes a similar tertiary structure in all globins that is called the **globin fold,** which is compact and globular in overall conformation. The **quaternary structure of HbA can be described as a dimer of $\alpha_1\beta_1$ and $\alpha_2\beta_2$ dimers.** The **αβ** dimers move relative to one another during the binding and release of oxygen.

**Hemoglobin must remain soluble** at high concentrations within the red blood cell to support normal oxygen binding and release properties. This is made possible by a distribution of **amino acid side chains** in which **hydrophobic residues are sequestered in the interior core** of the folded globin subunits, while **hydrophilic residues** dominate the **water-exposed surface** of the globin fold. The disk-shaped heme prosthetic group is inserted into a hydrophobic pocket formed by the globin.

Hemoglobin and the homologous monomeric protein myoglobin (Mb) both bind and release oxygen as a function of the surrounding concentration, or partial pressure of oxygen. A plot of percent saturation of hemoglobin or Mb with oxygen versus the partial pressure of oxygen is called the oxygen dissociation curve. Unlike Mb, which has a simple hyperbolic **oxygen dissociation curve** typical of ligand binding to a monomeric protein, the **quaternary structure of HbA** allows it to bind oxygen with **positive cooperativity,** giving a **sigmoidal** oxygen dissociation curve (Figure 1-1). Essentially, binding of oxygen to one HbA subunit increases the affinity of binding to other subunits in the tetramer, thereby shifting the equilibrium between oxy and deoxy forms. The net effect of this cooperativity is that HbA releases oxygen, whereas Mb globin would be most saturated with oxygen at the partial pressure of oxygen normally found in resting peripheral tissues. The quaternary structure of HbA also allows it to respond to **2,3-bisphosphoglycerate, carbon dioxide, and hydrogen ion, all of which are heterotropic negative allosteric effectors of oxygen binding.**

**Sickle cell anemia** is due to a particular defect in the *HBB* gene. The *HBB* gene, located on the short arm of chromosome 11, codes for the formation of the *globin-β* gene product of 146 amino acids. A single base mutation in the coding region at amino acid position 6 in the protein results in the conversion of a GAG codon to GTG, leading to the **nonconservative substitution of a hydrophobic valine residue for a hydrophilic glutamate in the protein,** which is now called **HbS.** This conversion brings about the profound structural changes in the deoxygenated HbS described below. Because sickle cell anemia is an **autosomal recessive disease,** an individual must carry 2 copies of the HbS variant to develop the symptoms of the disease. Individuals with 1 variant (HbS) and 1 normal (HbA) allele are carriers and are generally free of symptoms. If one parent has sickle cell trait (HbAS) and the other parent is homozygous for HbA, then no offspring will have sickle cell disease, but some may be carriers (HbAS) and some homozygous for hemoglobin A (HbAA). By contrast, if both parents have sickle trait, there is a 1 out of 4 chance that the child will be homozygous for HbA (HbAA), a 2 out of 4 chance that the offspring will be heterozygous (HbAS) and carry sickle cell trait, and a 1 out of 4 chance that the offspring will have sickle cell disease (HbSS), as illustrated in Figure 1-1.

The intrinsic oxygen-binding properties of HbA and HbS are the same; however, the **solubility of deoxy HbS is reduced** because exposure of **Val-6** at the **surface of the β-chain** leads to a hydrophobic interaction with hydrophobic residues on another β-chain. Because hemoglobin is present at very high concentrations in the red blood cell, **deoxy HbS will polymerize and precipitate inside the cell.** The precipitate takes the form of elongated fibers because of the association of complementary hydrophobic surfaces on the β- and α-chains of deoxy HbS. At oxygen saturations found in arterial blood, the oxy HbS predominates and HbS does not precipitate because Val-6 of the β-chain is not exposed to the surface.

The tendency for deoxy HbS to precipitate is why clinical manifestations of sickle cell anemia are brought on by **exertion** and why **treatment includes oxygen administration.** The stiff fibrous precipitate causes the red blood cell to deform into the characteristic sickle shape and makes the normally malleable cell susceptible to hemolysis.

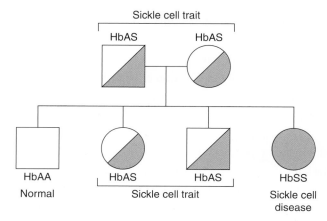

**Figure 1-1.** Genetics of the sickle cell disease when both parents are heterozygous for HbS (sickle cell trait).

Although sickle cell disease may be the most widely known condition resulting from a variant in the *HBB* gene, other conditions are also recognized. Hemoglobin C is produced when the glutamate at position 6 is changed to a lysine residue. Hemoglobin SC disease occurs when an individual has 1 HbS and 1 HbC allele, resulting in symptoms similar to sickle cell anemia, and the severity of the condition may range from mild to equivalent to sickle cell disease. However, 2 hemoglobin C alleles have a milder resultant disease that causes anemia (hemoglobin C disease). Hemoglobin E results when amino acid position 26 of the *β-globin* gene is changed from glutamic acid to lysine. When an individual carries both HbS and HbE, symptoms may be as severe as in sickle cell disease. Hemoglobin S and hemoglobin C variants are more common in West African lineages, while hemoglobin E variants are more common in those with Southeast Asian lineages.

## COMPREHENSION QUESTIONS

1.1  A newly married African-American couple, both from families having histories of good health, is about to have a child. If the incidence of the sickle cell trait is approximately 1 in 12 among persons of African descent in the United States, then what is the chance that the woman will give birth to a child affected by sickle cell disease?

    A.  1 in 12

    B.  1 in 24

    C.  1 in 96

    D.  1 in 288

    E.  1 in 576

1.2  A 25-year-old African-American man with sickle cell anemia, who has been hospitalized several times for painful sickle cell crises, has successfully been free of these crises since he has been on hydroxyurea therapy. Treatment with hydroxyurea results in which of the following?

    A.  An increase in the oxygen affinity of HbS

    B.  An increase in the levels of hemoglobin F (HbF) in red blood cells

    C.  A decreased cooperativity in oxygen binding by HbS

    D.  A post-translational modification of HbS that prevents polymerization

    E.  A decreased ability of HbS to bind 2,3-bisphosphoglycerate (2,3-BPG)

1.3  A pregnant woman is able to transfer oxygen to her fetus because fetal hemoglobin has a greater affinity for oxygen than does HbA. Why is the affinity of fetal hemoglobin for oxygen higher?

    A.  The tense form of hemoglobin is more prevalent in the circulation of the fetus.

    B.  There is less 2,3-BPG in the fetal circulation compared with maternal circulation.

    C.  Fetal hemoglobin binds 2,3-BPG with fewer ionic bonds than HbA.

    D.  The Bohr effect is enhanced in the fetus.

    E.  The oxygen-binding curve of fetal hemoglobin is shifted to the right.

# ANSWERS

1.1 **E.** Because sickle cell anemia has an autosomal recessive inheritance pattern and the incidence in the United States to persons of African descent is approximately 1 in 12, each parent has a 1 in 12 chance of being a carrier. Because it is an autosomal recessive gene, the couple's offspring would have a 1 in 4 chance of being homozygous if both parents were also carriers. Thus, the chance of having a child with the sickle cell trait is 1 in 576 (or [1/12][1/12][1/4]).

1.2 **B.** By inhibiting the enzyme ribonucleotide reductase, hydroxyurea has been shown to increase the levels of fetal hemoglobin (HbF, $\alpha_2\gamma_2$) by mechanisms not fully understood. The increase in HbF concentrations has the effect of decreasing HbS levels in the red blood cell. The increased concentration of HbF disrupts the polymerization of HbS and decreases the incidence of sickle cell crises. Hydroxyurea does not affect the oxygen affinity or cooperativity of oxygen binding of HbS, nor does it react with HbS to cause a post-translational modification or affect 2,3-BPG binding.

1.3 **C.** In HbA 2,3-BPG binds to ionized residues in the interface between the 2 $\beta$-chains, thus decreasing the oxygen affinity. The $\gamma$-chains of fetal hemoglobin have fewer ionized residues in the corresponding interface and bind 2,3-BPG with less affinity, which allows for a greater binding affinity for oxygen.

## BIOCHEMISTRY PEARLS

▶ The quaternary structure of HbA allows it to bind oxygen with positive cooperativity, giving a sigmoidal oxygen dissociation curve.

▶ Sickle cell anemia results from the nonconservative substitution of valine for glutamate at the sixth residue of the $\beta$ chain of hemoglobin.

▶ Precipitation of HbS is more likely to occur from exertion and deoxygenation. Therefore, treatment consists of oxygen and hydration.

▶ The stiff fibrous precipitate of HbS causes the red blood cell to deform into the characteristic sickle shape and makes the normally malleable cell susceptible to hemolysis.

# REFERENCES

Schultz RM, Liebman MN. Proteins II: structure-function relationships in protein families. In: Devlin TM, ed. *Textbook of Biochemistry with Clinical Correlations.* 5th ed. New York: Wiley-Liss; 2002.

Weatherall DJ, Beaudet AL, Vogelstein B, et al. The hemoglobinopathies. In: Scriver CR, Beaudet AL, Sly W, et al, eds. *The Metabolic & Molecular Basis of Inherited Disease.* 8th ed. New York: McGraw-Hill; 2001.

# CASE 2

A 1-month-old baby girl is brought to the emergency department (ED) by her mom with concerns over her baby's decreased activity level, lack of appetite, and worsening diaper rash that has not resolved with usual antifungal treatment. The baby was born at term and mother denies any pregnancy or delivery complications. The baby was seen by the pediatrician at 2 wks and was doing okay but has had frequent upper respiratory infection symptoms. The mother denies any fever or nausea/vomiting in her newborn. On examination, the baby is afebrile but is noted to be lethargic with no lymphadenopathy. Mild hepatosplenomegaly and hypotonia are noted on physical examination. Chest radiography demonstrates an absent thymic shadow but normal heart silhouette. Laboratory values revealed elevated levels of adenosine and deoxyadenosine in the urine and blood.

▶ What is the likely diagnosis?
▶ What is the biochemical basis for this disorder?
▶ What are potential treatment options for this baby?

# ANSWERS TO CASE 2:
## Adenosine Deaminase Deficiency

*Summary:* A 1-month-old baby with a recent history of upper respiratory infection symptoms with an absent thymic shadow on chest radiography and elevated adenosine and deoxyadenosine levels in the urine and blood.

- **Likely diagnosis:** Adenosine deaminase (ADA) deficiency

- **Biochemical basis for this disorder:** ADA is an enzyme involved in the breakdown of purines. Specifically, it is responsible for the deamination of adenosine and deoxyadenosine to inosine and deoxyinosine. Individuals with mutations in the *ADA* gene, typically inherited in an autosomal recessive manner, exhibit decreased ADA enzymatic activity together with elevations in adenosine and deoxyadenosine. Deoxyadenosine is highly cytotoxic, particularly to lymphocytes. Thus, ADA-deficient individuals exhibit a severe combined immunodeficiency and suffer from secondary complications associated with a compromised immune system.

- **Potential treatment options:** Haploidentical bone marrow transplantation, ADA enzyme replacement therapy, *ADA* gene therapy.

## CLINICAL CORRELATION

ADA deficiency is a rare autosomal recessive genetic disorder that results in severe combined immunodeficiency disease (SCID) characterized by decreased levels and function of T and B lymphocytes as well as decreased levels of Natural Killer (NK) T cells. The most severe form of the disease, typically associated with near complete lack of ADA enzymatic activity, is seen in infants where secondary infections resultant from a compromised immune system appear in the first 6 months of life. However, there are less severe forms of the disease-associated mutations in ADA that still provide low levels of enzyme activity. These partially ADA-deficient individuals present later in childhood. Although the SCID associated with ADA deficiency is clearly the phenotype that leads to the most severe complications in these patients, there are other nonimmune phenotypes found in these patients. Most notable are neurologic problems and hearing loss. Other noted but less common phenotypes include lung disease, hepatocellular damage, kidney disease, and bone disorders. These nonimmune phenotypes are thought to be associated with accumulation of the ADA substrate adenosine, which is a potent cell-signaling molecule. It is clear that both the immune and nonimmune phenotypes in ADA deficiency are resultant from the accumulation of the ADA substrates deoxyadenosine (immunotoxic) and adenosine (abnormal cell signaling). The monogenetic nature of this disorder together with the relatively well-defined biochemical basis of the disorder have led to effective therapies that target the restoration of ADA enzymatic activity and the lowering of ADA substrates.

## APPROACH TO:

# Adenosine Deaminase Metabolism and Association With Severe Combined Immunodeficiency Disease

## OBJECTIVES

1. Describe the metabolic basis of the immunodeficiency associated with ADA deficiency.

2. Explain the treatment options that are based on the ability to reverse the metabolic effects of ADA deficiency.

## DEFINITIONS

**ADENOSINE DEAMINASE (ADA):** An important enzyme involved in the breakdown of purines. It is responsible for the deamination of adenosine and 2′-deoxyadenosine to inosine and 2′-deoxyinosine. This enzyme is found in the cytoplasm of most cells; however, it is expressed at particularly high levels in developing T lymphocytes, which accounts for the sensitivity of this cell population to loss of this enzyme.

**ADENOSINE:** Adenosine is a purine nucleoside that serves as a potent extracellular signal. It signals in an autocrine and paracrine manner by engaging cell surface adenosine receptors. Adenosine signaling has numerous physiologic and pathologic functions, and abnormal adenosine signaling may account for many of the nonimmune phenotypes seen in ADA deficiency.

**DEOXYADENOSINE:** 2′-Deoxyadenosine is generated as a breakdown product of DNA catabolism. In its further metabolism, deoxyadenosine is deaminated by ADA. If it is allowed to accumulate, as in the case of ADA deficiency, deoxyadenosine is cytotoxic to cells through a mechanism that involves its phosphorylation to deoxyadenosine triphosphate (dATP), which can promote a cell death process known as apoptosis. This is the mechanism by which lymphocytes are killed in ADA deficiency.

**ADA ENZYME REPLACEMENT THERAPY:** ADA enzyme replacement therapy is an effective treatment for ADA deficiency. It involves the injection of purified ADA protein that has been modified with polyethylene glycol (PEG-ADA). PEG-ADA injections effectively lower the levels of ADA substrates and alleviate the symptoms of ADA deficiency.

**ADA GENE THERAPY:** The monogenetic nature of this disorder lends itself to effective gene-replacement strategies. ADA deficiency was the first case of gene therapy in humans. The approach involves removal of the patient's bone marrow followed by the stable transfer of a "good" *ADA* gene into the bone marrow cells that are then transferred back into patients, where they expand and populate the immune system. The metabolic disturbances are corrected, as are many of the other phenotypes seen.

## DISCUSSION

Nucleotides play an essential role in a number of different metabolic processes, including RNA and DNA synthesis and transmittal of genetic information as energy stores, as structural components of coenzymes, and as signaling molecules. Because of their importance to overall metabolism, nucleotides are continuously turned over. Although the metabolism of the purine nucleotides, adenylate (AMP), 2′deoxy-adenylate (dAMP), guanylate (GMP), and 2′-deoxyguanylate (dGMP) can occur throughout the body, the primary site of their degradation is the liver.

The first step in catabolism of the purine mononucleotides is the hydrolysis of the phosphate by a nucleotidase to give the corresponding nucleoside. Guanosine and deoxyguanosine are converted to the purine base, guanine, by removal of the pentose sugar by a phosphorolytic cleavage catalyzed by purine nucleoside phosphorylase. Guanine deaminase hydrolytically removes the amino group to convert guanine to xanthine. Xanthine oxidase converts xanthine to uric acid. The catabolic pathway for adenosine and deoxyadenosine is similar in strategy but has more enzymatic steps (Figure 2-1). Adenosine and deoxyadenosine are first deaminated by adenosine deaminase to yield the nucleosides inosine and deoxyinosine. Purine nucleoside phosphorylase then removes the pentose sugars from the nucleosides, releasing the purine base hypoxanthine. Hypoxanthine is sequentially converted to xanthine and then uric acid by the enzyme xanthine oxidase. Uric acid, the end product of purine catabolism, is not very soluble in blood and is excreted. If uric acid levels in blood are excessive, then sodium urate can crystallize (usually in the joints) to cause gout.

ADA, the enzyme that catalyzes the deamination of adenosine and deoxyadenosine to inosine and deoxyinosine, respectively, has been shown to be deficient in some patients with heritable immunodeficiency. Autosomal recessive mutations in ADA lead to reduction or complete loss of ADA enzymatic activity in cells (Figure 2-2, A), which in turn leads to elevations in adenosine and deoxyadenosine. Elevations in deoxyadenosine that occur in response to ADA deficiency are cytotoxic to cells by a pathway that involves the phosphorylation of deoxyadenosine to dATP. Elevations in intracellular dATP can activate pathways that lead to apoptosis, a form of cell death. This is the mechanism that accounts for the loss of lymphocytes in ADA deficiency (Figure 2-2B). Accumulation of extracellular adenosine leads to activation of adenosine receptors on numerous cells that can impact the development of non-immune phenotypes associated with ADA deficiency (Figure 2-3C). These phenotypes include neurological problems and hearing loss, as well as liver, kidney, and lung disorders.

ADA deficiency was the first immunodeficiency disease for which the molecular defect was identified, making possible both prenatal and a postnatal molecular diagnosis. In addition, understanding the metabolic basis of this disease underscored the importance of normal purine metabolism for the development of the immune system. This disorder has also allowed for the development of novel treatment strategies. PEG-ADA became the first PEG-modified protein to be used in a therapeutic setting and opened the door for the development of additional PEG-modified proteins that are in wide clinical use today. In addition, ADA deficiency was the first inherited disease to be treated with gene therapy.

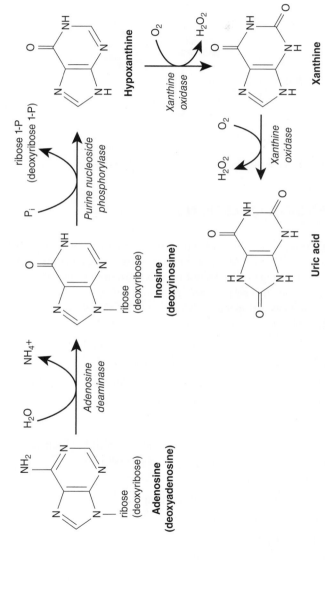

**Figure 2-1.** Degradation pathway of adenosine and deoxyadenosine.

**Figure 2-2.** Metabolic basis of phenotypes associated with ADA deficiency.

## COMPREHENSION QUESTIONS

2.1 A 6-month-old infant presents with an oral yeast infection and the patient history reveals that there have been persistent infections since approximately 1 month of age. Blood work reveals decreased numbers of T and B lymphocytes, and you thus suspect an immunodeficiency. Which of the following laboratory results would specifically implicate ADA deficiency as the molecular basis for the immunodeficiency seen in this patient?

A. Increased adenosine and deoxyadenosine in the blood

B. Elevated inosine and deoxyinosine in the blood

C. Decreased levels of adenosine and deoxyadenosine in the blood

D. Increased glucose levels in the blood

E. Increased creatinine levels in the blood

2.2 With a patient diagnosed with ADA-deficient SCID, which of the following treatment approaches is most likely to be successful?

A. Kidney transplantation

B. Liver transplantation together with immunoglobulin therapy

C. ADA enzyme replacement therapy

D. Immunoglobulin therapy

E. Dietary restriction of adenine

2.3 Which of the following clinical parameters should be followed in an ADA-deficient patient following the use of ADA enzyme replacement therapy to assess the efficacy of the therapy?

A. Blood urea nitrogen

B. Erythrocyte cell counts

C. Ferritin levels

D. Hemoglobin levels

E. Immunoglobulin levels

2.4 A deficiency of ADA can lead to lymphopenia and immune dysfunction. The accumulation of which substance is most likely to result in these lymphotoxic effects?

A. Adenosine

B. Deoxyadenosine

C. Hypoxanthine

D. Inosine

E. Uric acid

# ANSWERS

2.1 **A.** ADA is responsible for deaminating adenosine and deoxyadenosine, hence, elevations in adenosine and deoxyadenosine are specifically diagnostic for ADA deficiency.

2.2 **C.** ADA enzyme replacement therapy is an approach that can increase ADA enzymatic activity in patients that will lead to a lowering of ADA substrates and an attenuation of the associated phenotypes.

2.3 **E.** Diminished immunoglobulin levels are indicative of decreased immune function and are a prominent feature of ADA deficiency. Thus, monitoring immunoglobulin levels is a way of assessing the efficacy of ADA enzyme replacement therapy. An increase in immunoglobulin levels is a positive result.

2.4 **B.** Deoxyadenosine is the primary lymphotoxic substance that accumulates as a result of adenosine deaminase deficiency. It can be phosphorylated to dATP, an accumulation of which leads to programmed cell death (apoptosis) of lymphoid cells. An accumulation of adenosine also occurs due to ADA deficiency, but it is not lymphotoxic. A buildup of adenosine can lead to neurologic as well as liver, kidney, and lung disorders. Inosine, hypoxanthine, and uric acid are downstream metabolites of ADA and would not be expected to accumulate with a deficiency in the enzyme.

## BIOCHEMISTRY PEARLS

▶ ADA deficiency was the first immunodeficiency disease for which the molecular defect was identified.

▶ ADA catalyzes the deamination of adenosine and deoxyadenosine to inosine and deoxyinosine, respectively.

▶ Elevations in deoxyadenosine that occur in response to ADA deficiency are cytotoxic to cells and lead to apoptosis, a form of cell death (in this case loss of lymphocytes).

## REFERENCE

Hershfield MS, Mitchell BS. Immunodeficiency diseases caused by adenosine deaminase deficiency and purine nucleoside phosphorylase deficiency. In: Valle D, Vogelstein B, Kinzler KW, et al, eds. *The Online Metabolic & Molecular Basis of Inherited Disease.* New York: McGraw-Hill, pp 2586-2588; http://dx.doi.org/10.1036/ommbid.137.

# CASE 3

A 32-year-old woman is being treated with methotrexate for a recently diagnosed choriocarcinoma of the ovary and presents with complaints of oral mucosal ulcers. The patient recalls being advised not to take folate-containing vitamins during therapy. An uncomplicated surgical exploration was performed 5 weeks ago with removal of the affected ovary. The patient has been taking methotrexate for 2 weeks and has never had any of the above symptoms before. On examination, patient was afebrile and appeared ill. Several mucosal ulcers were seen in her mouth. The patient also had some upper abdominal tenderness. Her platelet count is decreased at 60,000/mm$^3$ (normal, 150,000–450,000/mm$^3$).

- ▶ What is the most likely etiology of her symptoms?
- ▶ What is the biochemical explanation of her symptoms?
- ▶ What part of the cell cycle does methotrexate act on?

# ANSWERS TO CASE 3:

## Methotrexate and Folate Metabolism

*Summary:* A 32-year-old woman has oral ulcerations and thrombocytopenia (low platelet count) after beginning methotrexate initiated for recently diagnosed ovarian cancer. She recalls being instructed to avoid folate during therapy.

- **Likely cause of her symptoms:** Adverse events of methotrexate (antimetabolite chemotherapy) affecting rapidly dividing cells such as oral mucosa.

- **Biochemical explanation of her symptoms:** Related to effects of methotrexate on cell cycle of all cells (particularly rapidly dividing cells). Folate antagonists inhibit dihydrofolate reductase (tetrahydrofolate needed for purine synthesis).

- **Cell cycle affected by methotrexate:** DNA synthesis (S) phase.

## CLINICAL CORRELATION

Chemotherapeutic agents are used to treat various types of cancers. Although some are specific for cancer cells, most chemotherapeutic agents are toxic for both normal and cancer cells. Methotrexate acts as a folate antagonist, affecting DNA synthesis. Because cancer cells divide faster than normal cells, a higher proportion of these neoplastic cells will die. Nevertheless, normal cells that also are rapidly dividing, such as the gastrointestinal mucosa, the oral mucosa, and the bone marrow cells, may be affected. The patient was advised to avoid folate during therapy, since folate would be an "antidote," and would allow the cancer cells to escape cell kill.

# APPROACH TO:

## Cell Cycle

## OBJECTIVES

1. Understand the components of the cell cycle.

2. Know how folate is involved in DNA synthesis.

3. Be familiar with the terminology of nucleoside and nucleotide.

## DEFINITIONS

**CELL CYCLE:** The time interval between cell divisions in proliferating cells. The cell cycle is divided into 4 phases: M phase, in which mitosis takes place; $G_1$ phase, prior to synthesis of DNA; S phase, in which DNA and histones are synthesized to duplicate the chromosomes; and $G_2$ phase, during which there is cell growth and synthesis of macromolecules. Under certain conditions, the cell can enter a quiescent, or $G_0$ phase, which is not part of the regular cell cycle.

**DIHYDROFOLATE REDUCTASE (DHFR):** The enzyme required to convert folic acid to its active form, tetrahydrofolate. It requires the cofactor NADPH as a source of reducing equivalents to reduce folate first to dihydrofolate (DHF) and then to tetrahydrofolate.

**METHOTREXATE:** A drug that has a similar structure to DHFR. It binds to DHFR reductase and competitively inhibits it, thus decreasing the levels of tetrahydrofolate in the cells. It effectively stops DNA synthesis in rapidly dividing cells such as cancer cells.

**TETRAHYDROFOLATE (THF):** The active form of the vitamin folic acid. THF is one of the major carriers of one-carbon units at various oxidation states for biosynthetic reactions. It is required for the synthesis of the nucleotide thymidylate (dTMP). Although bacteria can synthesize folic acid, eukaryotes must obtain folate from the diet. Dietary sources of folate include leafy green vegetables (eg, spinach and turnip greens), citrus fruits, and legumes. Many breakfast cereals, breads, and other grain products are fortified with folate.

**DNA:** Two large molecules composed of deoxynucleotides attached by hydrogen bonds in a helical, antiparallel relationship.

**NUCLEOSIDES:** Nitrogenous base plus a sugar (bases in DNA are adenine [A], thymine [T], cytosine [C], and guanine [G]; bases in RNA are A, C, G, but uracil [U] instead of T; sugar moiety in DNA is deoxyribose, and in RNA is ribose).

**NUCLEOTIDE:** Nucleoside plus phosphate group (Table 3-1).

**DEOXYTHYMIDYLATE (DTMP):** DNA nucleotide consisting of the deoxyribose sugar, thymidine as nitrogenous base, and 1 phosphate.

## DISCUSSION

The **cell cycle** is defined as the time interval between cell divisions in proliferating cells. It is important to note that the cell cycle is not a simple "clock." Movement through the cell cycle is controlled by a variety of proteins that allow the cell to respond to various stimuli. The eukaryote cell cycle is composed of the following **4 phases** (Figure 3-1):

1. M phase: Mitosis
2. $G_1$ phase (gap 1): Between mitosis and initiation of DNA synthesis

| Table 3-1 • TERMINOLOGY OF NUCLEIC ACIDS | |
|---|---|
| Bases | Purine (adenine [A], guanine [G]); Pyrimidine (uracil [U], cytosine [C], thymine [T]) |
| Sugar x | Deoxyribose (DNA), Ribose (RNA) |
| Base + Sugar | Nucleoside |
| Base + Sugar + phosphate | Nucleotide |

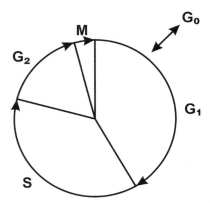

**Figure 3-1.** Cell cycle. G0 = rest phase, G1 = cell growth, G2 = proteins made in preparation for cell division, M = mitosis, S = DNA synthesis and replication.

3. S phase: When DNA synthesis occurs

4. $G_2$ phase (gap 2): Cell growth and macromolecule synthesis

Although great variation exists in the length of the mammalian cell cycle (hours to days), as a generalization, mammalian cells divide once every 24 hours. The M and S phases of the cell cycle are relatively constant. Therefore, the length of the mammalian cell cycle is determined by length of the $G_1$ and $G_2$ phases. **Cell division** occurs during **M phase, and the mitotic interphase** is composed of $(G_1 + S + G_2)$. **M phase, or mitosis,** is divided into 4 subphases: **prophase, metaphase, anaphase,** and **telophase.** In **prophase,** the nuclear membrane breaks down while the replicated chromosomes condense and are released into the cytoplasm. The chromosomes become aligned on the equatorial plate of the cell during **metaphase,** and they move from the equatorial plate to the poles during **anaphase.** The final step in M phase, **telophase,** is reformation of the nuclear membrane around the chromosomes followed by cytokinesis, or formation of two daughter cells. During the $G_1$ phase, the cell "monitors" itself and its environment. The cell is metabolically active and undergoes continuous growth, but no DNA synthesis occurs during this phase. During $G_1$ the cell makes a "decision" either to continue in the cell cycle and divide or to "withdraw" from the cell cycle and differentiate. The synthesis of DNA and histones to form two sets of chromosomes occurs during S phase. The key event of the $G_2$ phase is for the cell to "make sure that its entire DNA has replicated." Continued cell growth and the synthesis of cellular macromolecules also occur during the $G_2$ phase, preparing for cell division.

Under certain conditions cells can leave $G_1$ and enter into the $G_0$ **phase** of the cell cycle. This phase is not part of the regular cell cycle and represents a specialized state, which can be temporary or permanent. Entry into the $G_0$ phase can be triggered by growth factor withdrawal, negative growth factors, or limited protein synthesis. The cells in $G_0$ are in a **nonproliferative or quiescent state,** which can vary tremendously in length. Some cells differentiate and never divide again. Others can resume proliferation to replace lost cells as a result of injury or cell death. An important point is that cancer cells do not generally have a $G_0$ phase.

   **Key regulatory proteins that govern the cell cycle** are the **cyclin-dependent kinases (CDKs),** which are **serine/threonine protein kinases,** and the **cyclins,** which are regulatory proteins that bind to the CDKs. Proteins that inhibit the kinase activity (cyclin-dependent kinase inhibitors [CDIs]) are also present in the cell. The CDKs are regulated by the levels of cyclins and the CDK/cyclin complex phosphorylates proteins on serine or threonine residues. The cyclins bind to and activate CDKs via protein–protein interactions. Cyclins act as regulatory subunits controlling activity and specificity of the CDK activity. These cyclins can themselves be phosphorylated and dephosphorylated. **Cyclin accumulation and degradation controls normal cell cycle** activity. For example, the degradation of specific cyclins by proteolysis at the metaphase-anaphase transition ends mitosis.

   **THF is the major source of 1-carbon units** used in the biosynthesis of many important biologic molecules. This **cofactor** is derived from the **vitamin folic acid** and is a carrier of activated 1-carbon units at various **oxidation levels (methyl, methylene, formyl, formimino, and methenyl).** These compounds can be interconverted as required by the cellular process. The major donor of the 1-carbon unit is **serine** in the following reaction:

$$\text{Serine} + \text{THF} \rightarrow \text{Glycine} + N^5, N^{10}\text{-methylene-THF}$$

   All cells, especially rapidly growing cells, must synthesize thymidylate (dTMP) for DNA synthesis. The difference between (T) and (U) is one methyl group at the carbon-5 position. **Thymidylate is synthesized by the methylation of uridylate (dUMP)** in a reaction catalyzed by the enzyme **thymidylate synthase.** This reaction requires a methyl donor and a source of reducing equivalents, which are both provided by $N^5, N^{10}$-methylene THF (Figure 3-2). For this reaction to continue, the regeneration of THF from dihydrofolate (DHF) must occur.

$$\text{DHF} + \text{NADPH} + H^+ \rightarrow \text{THF} + \text{NADPH}^+$$

   The enzyme **dihydrofolate reductase (DHFR)** catalyzes this reaction, which is a target of the **anticancer drugs aminopterin and methotrexate.** These drugs are analogs of DHF and act as **competitive inhibitors of DHFR.** Inhibition of this enzyme prevents the regeneration of THF and **blocks dTMP synthesis** because of the lack of the methyl donor required for the reaction of thymidylate synthase.

   **THF is also required as a donor of 2 carbon atoms in the synthesis of the purine ring structure required for adenine and guanine.** The carbon atoms donated by THF are indicated in Figure 3-3. Therefore, a lack of THF blocks the synthesis of the purine ring structure because of the lack of the ability of the cell to synthesize $N^{10}$-formyl-THF.

   In summary, **DNA synthesis requires synthesis of dTMP and the purines adenine and guanine.** THF, derived from the **vitamin folic acid,** is required for the biosynthesis of these nucleotides. Treatment with methotrexate blocks the ability of the cell to regenerate THF, leading to inhibition of these biosynthetic pathways. The lack of nucleotides prevents DNA synthesis, and these cancer cells cannot divide without DNA synthesis. Unfortunately, the effects of methotrexate are nonspecific and other rapidly dividing cells, such as epithelial cells in the oral cavity, intestine, skin, and blood cells, are also inhibited. This leads to the adverse

**Figure 3-2.** Thymidylate synthesized by the methylation of uridylate (dUMP) in a reaction catalyzed by the enzyme thymidylate synthase.

**Figure 3-3.** Origin of the atoms of the purine base ring system. RP = pentose phosphate.

events associated with methotrexate (and other cancer chemotherapy drugs) such as mouth sores, low white blood cell counts, stomach upset, hair loss, skin rashes, and itching.

## COMPREHENSION QUESTIONS

3.1 A 44-year-old woman who recently lost her job because of absenteeism presents to her physician complaining of loss of appetite, fatigue, muscle weakness, and emotional depression. The physical examination reveals a somewhat enlarged liver that feels firm and nodular, and there is a hint of jaundice in the sclerae and a hint of alcohol on her breath. The initial laboratory profile included a hematologic analysis that showed that she had an anemia with enlarged red blood cells (macrocytic). A bone marrow aspirate confirmed the suspicion that she has a megaloblastic anemia because it showed a greater than normal number of red and white blood cell precursors, most of which were larger than normal. Further analyses revealed that her serum folic acid level was 2.9 ng/mL (normal = 6 to 15), her serum $B_{12}$ level was 153 pg/mL (normal = 150 to 750), and her serum iron level was normal. Megaloblastic anemia in this patient is most likely caused by which of the following?

A. Decreased synthesis of methionine

B. Decreased conversion of dUMP to dTMP

C. Decrease in the synthesis of phosphatidyl choline

D. Decrease in the levels of succinyl CoA

E. Decreased synthesis of dUTP

3.2 A patient presents with a urinary tract infection and is prescribed a combination drug containing trimethoprim and sulfamethoxazole. These drugs are effective because they do which of the following?

A. Bind to operons to prevent synthesis of bacterial messenger RNA

B. Block transport across bacterial cell walls

C. Inhibit bacterial synthesis of cobalamin ($B_{12}$)

D. Inhibit bacterial synthesis of THF

E. Inhibit synthesis of phospholipids in bacteria

3.3 Methotrexate is often used as a chemotherapeutic agent to treat patients with leukemia. This drug is effective because it inhibits cells in which part of the cell cycle?

A. $G_1$ phase

B. S phase

C. M phase

D. $G_2$ phase

E. $G_0$ phase

3.4 Leukemia patients are often given the compound leucovorin ($N^5$-formyl THF) following treatment with the drug methotrexate. What is the mechanism whereby Leucovorin is useful as part of this treatment protocol?

A.   It facilitates the uptake of methotrexate by cells.

B.   It can be converted to THF by bypassing DHFR.

C.   It acts as an activator of thymidylate synthase.

D.   It prevents the uptake of methotrexate by normal cells.

E.   It stimulates cells of the immune system.

## ANSWERS

3.1   **B.** Megaloblastic anemia is caused by a decrease in the synthesis of deoxythymidylate and the purine bases usually caused by a deficiency in either THF or cobalamin or both. This results in decreased DNA synthesis, which results in abnormally large hematopoietic cells created by perturbed cell division and DNA replication and repair. This patient exhibits signs of chronic alcoholism, which often leads to a folate deficiency. This can occur due to poor dietary intake, decreased absorption of folate due to damage of the intestinal brush border cells and resulting conjugase deficiency, and poor renal resorption of folate.

3.2   **D.** Bacteria must synthesize the folate required for their biosynthetic processes; they do not have a transporter to bring folate into the cell. Trimethoprim inhibits prokaryotic DHFR (eukaryotic is not affected) and sulfamethoxazole is an analog of p-aminobenzoic acid (PABA), a precursor to folic acid. Bacteria will use this analog instead of PABA and produce a nonfunctional folate.

3.3   **B.** Methotrexate inhibits the synthesis of deoxythymidine by preventing the regeneration of THF by inhibiting the enzyme DHFR. Inhibiting the synthesis of deoxythymidylate prevents the cell from synthesizing its DNA. DNA synthesis occurs exclusively during S phase of the cell cycle.

3.4   **B.** Leucovorin ($N^5$-formyl THF, folinic acid) is used as an antidote for cells that have decreased levels of folic acid. Treatment of leukemia patients with methotrexate kills not only the tumor cells but also other normal rapidly dividing cells. $N^5$-formyl THF is normally administered 24 hours following treatment with methotrexate; it can be converted to THF by these normal cells by bypassing the block caused by methotrexate. Therefore, these normal cells can synthesize deoxythymidine and carry out DNA synthesis.

## BIOCHEMISTRY PEARLS

▶ The eukaryote cell cycle is composed of the following 4 phases: M phase, mitosis; $G_1$ phase (gap 1), between mitosis and initiation of DNA synthesis; S phase, DNA synthesis; and $G_2$ phase (gap 2), cell growth and macromolecule synthesis.

▶ The cells in $G_0$ are in a nonproliferative or quiescent state that can vary tremendously in length.

▶ DNA synthesis requires the formation of dTMP and the purines adenine and guanine. THF, derived from the vitamin folic acid, is required for the biosynthesis of these nucleotides.

▶ The cell cycle is regulated by the specific proteins CDKs, which are serine/threonine protein kinases, and the cyclins, which are regulatory proteins that bind to the CDKs.

▶ Treatment with methotrexate blocks the ability of the cell to regenerate THF, leading to inhibition of these biosynthetic pathways. Thus, methotrexate affects DNA synthesis.

## REFERENCES

Alberts B, Johnson A, Lewis J, et al. The cell cycle and programmed cell death. *Molecular Biology of the Cell.* 5th ed. New York: Garland; 2007.

Cory JG. Purine and pyrimidine nucleotide metabolism. In: Devlin TM, ed. *Textbook of Biochemistry with Clinical Correlations.* 7th ed. New York: Wiley-Liss; 2010.

# CASE 4

A 47-year-old woman is brought to the emergency department with complaints of malaise, nausea, vomiting, and fatigue. The patient reveals a long history of alcohol abuse for the last 10 years and requires drinks daily, especially in the morning as an "eye opener." She has been to rehabilitation on several occasions for alcoholism but has not been able to stop drinking. She is currently homeless and jobless. She denies cough, fever, chills, upper respiratory symptoms, sick contacts, recent travel, hematemesis, or abdominal pain. She reports feeling hungry and has not eaten very well in a long time. On physical examination, she appears malnourished but in no distress. Other findings on physical exam are normal. Her blood count reveals a normal white blood cell count but does show an anemia with large red blood cells. Her amylase, lipase, and liver function tests were normal.

▶ What is the most likely cause of her anemia?
▶ What is the molecular basis for the large erythrocytes?

# ANSWERS TO CASE 4:
## Folic Acid Deficiency

*Summary*: 47-year-old alcoholic white woman has fatigue, malaise, nausea, vomiting, and poor nutritional intake with macrocytic anemia and no evidence of pancreatitis, liver disease, or peptic ulcer disease.

- **Cause of anemia:** Folic acid deficiency.

- **Molecular basis of macrocytosis:** Abnormal proliferation of erythroid precursors in the bone marrow, because folate deficiency encumbers the maturation of these cells by inhibition of DNA synthesis.

## CLINICAL CORRELATION

Folate is an essential vitamin, found in green leafy vegetables. It is essential for many biochemical processes in the body, including DNA synthesis and red blood cell synthesis. Recently, folate supplementation has been found to be important in the prevention of fetal neural tube defects, such as anencephaly (absence of brain cerebral cortex and no skull or skin covering the brain) and spina bifida (spinal cord malformation, whereby the meninges are exposed leading to neurologic deficits). In particular, people who abuse alcohol are at risk for folate deficiency because of impaired gastrointestinal absorption and poor nutrition. Macrocytic anemia (large red blood cells) may be seen with folate deficiency. Treatment consists of folic acid replacement (usually 1 mg/day) by mouth with correction of anemia over the following 1 to 2 months. The diet usually requires adjustment, and correctable causes addressed (malnutrition in this case). Notably, folate deficiency in pregnancy has been associated with neural tube defects (NTDs) in fetuses. It is recommended that mothers take at least 400 µg of folic acid 3 months prior to conception to reduce the risk of NTD. At times, more than 400 µg of folic acid per day is recommended prior to conception. Some specific examples include a history of previous NTD, sickle cell disease, multiple gestations, and Crohn disease.

# APPROACH TO:
## Folate and DNA Synthesis

## OBJECTIVES

1. Understand the important metabolic roles of folic acid with production of thymine, purine synthesis, and methionine.

2. Be aware of how folate deficiency causes megaloblastic anemia.

# DEFINITIONS

**S-ADENOSYL METHIONINE:** An important carrier of activated methyl groups. It is formed by the condensation of ATP with the amino acid methionine catalyzed by the enzyme methionine adenosyltransferase in a reaction that releases triphosphate.

**DIHYDROFOLATE REDUCTASE:** The enzyme that reduces folic acid (folate) first to dihydrofolate and then to the active tetrahydrofolate. Dihydrofolate reductase uses NADPH as the source of the reducing equivalents for the reaction.

**FOLIC ACID:** An essential vitamin composed of a pteridine ring bound to p-aminobenzoate, which is in an amide linkage to one or more glutamate residues. The active form of the enzyme is tetrahydrofolate (THF; $FH_4$), which is an important carrier of 1-carbon units in a variety of oxidation states.

**MEGALOBLASTIC ANEMIA:** An anemia characterized by macrocytic (large) erythrocytes produced by abnormal proliferation of erythroid precursors in the bone marrow due to a limitation in normal DNA synthesis. The cytoplasm continues to grow, even though the nucleus cannot due to DNA synthesis problems.

**METHOTREXATE:** One of a number of antifolate drugs, methotrexate, is an analog of folate that competitively inhibits dihydrofolate reductase. Because a plentiful supply of THF is required for ongoing synthesis of the pyrimidine nucleotide thymidylate, synthesis of this nucleotide is inhibited, resulting in decreased DNA synthesis.

**METHYL TRAP:** The sequestering of tetrahydrofolate as $N^5$-methyl THF because of decreased conversion of homocysteine to methionine as a result of a deficiency of methionine synthase or its cofactor, cobalamin (vitamin $B_{12}$).

# DISCUSSION

**Folate (folic acid) is an essential vitamin,** which, in its **active form of THF** (Figure 4-1), **transfers 1-carbon groups to intermediates in metabolism.** Folate plays an important role in **DNA synthesis.** It is required for the de novo synthesis of **purines** and for the **conversion of deoxyuridine 5-monophosphate (dUMP) to deoxythymidine**

**Figure 4-1.** Structure of tetrahydrofolate, the active form of folic acid.

**5′-monophosphate (dTMP).** In addition, folate derivatives participate in the biosynthesis of choline, serine, glycine, and methionine. However, in situations of folate deficiency, symptoms are not observed from the lack of these products, as adequate levels of choline and amino acids are obtained from the diet (see also Case 3).

**Folate deficiency** results in **megaloblastic anemia.** Megaloblastic anemia is characterized by **macrocytic erythrocytes** produced by **abnormal proliferation of erythroid precursors in the bone marrow.** Folate deficiency encumbers the maturation of these cells by **inhibition of DNA synthesis.** Without an adequate supply of folate, DNA synthesis is limited by **decreased purine and dTMP levels.**

Folate exists in a pool of interconvertible intermediates, each carrying a 1-carbon fragment in several different oxidation states (Figure 4-2). The total body stores of folate is approximately 110 mg/70 kg, and approximately 420 μg/70 kg is lost each day via the urine and feces. **A total of 2 different forms of folate are required for different aspects of nucleotide biosynthesis.** $N^{10}$-**formyl THF** provides the **C-2 and C-8 carbons** for the de novo synthesis of **purine rings** and, thus, is critical for DNA metabolism.

**Figure 4-2.** Structures of the various 1-carbon carriers of tetrahydrofolate (THF). THF can carry 1-carbon units in the oxidation states of methanol ($N^5$-methyl THF), formaldehyde ($N^5$, $N^{10}$-methylene THF) or formic acid (remaining structures).

The **methylene form, $N^5$, $N^{10}$-methylene THF,** is required for the production of **dTMP from dUMP.** This reaction involves the transfer of a $CH_2$ group and a hydrogen from $N^5$, $N^{10}$-methylene THF. In this process, THF is oxidized to dihydrofolate (DHF). For subsequent dTMP production, THF must be regenerated. THF is produced from DHF by the enzyme DHF reductase (DHFR) in a reaction requiring NADPH. DHFR is the target of methotrexate, an antifolate cancer chemotherapeutic, which, by limiting the available pool of $N^5$, $N^{10}$-methylene THF inhibits DNA synthesis in rapidly dividing cancer cells. Methotrexate therapy can produce adverse events resembling folate deficiency. In addition, bacterial DHFR is a target for antimicrobials.

Outside of DNA synthesis, **folate plays a role in methylation metabolism.** The major **methyl donor is S-adenosyl methionine (SAM),** which is required for many reactions. For example, SAM is needed for the **production of norepinephrine from epinephrine and for DNA methylation,** which can influence **gene transcription.** After methyl group transfer, SAM is converted to **S-adenosyl homocysteine (SAH),** which is hydrolyzed to **homocysteine and adenosine.** To restore the levels of methionine (an essential amino acid), homocysteine must be methylated (Figure 4-3). This reaction is dependent on $N^5$-methyl THF and vitamin $B_{12}$. **Methionine levels can be limiting,** making the availability of $N^5$-methyl THF for conversion of homocysteine to methionine critical. Further, in the absence of $B_{12}$, THF can be trapped in the $N^5$-methyl THF form and thus be removed from the THF pool. This is referred to as the **"methyl trap,"** which can impact other areas of 1-carbon metabolism, such as dTMP production.

Folate deficiency perturbs DNA metabolism and methylation reactions. **Leafy green vegetables are good sources of folate;** however, folate is labile and may be

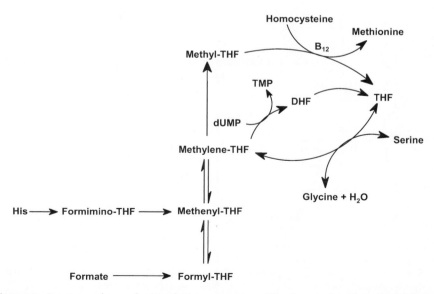

**Figure 4-3.** Reaction pathways showing the interconversion of 1-carbon carriers of tetrahydrofolate (THF). Note that all interconversions are reversible, except for the conversion of $N^5$, $N^{10}$-methylene THF to $N^5$-methyl THF.

damaged during food preparation. Another dietary source of folate is cereal products, especially breads and breakfast cereals that have been fortified with folic acid. Folate is also produced within the gut lumen by certain intestinal bacteria; however, the amount of folate absorbed from this source is minor in humans. In its simplest form, folate consists of 3 connected chemical moieties: a pteridine ring (6-methylpterin), p-aminobenzoic acid (PABA), and glutamate. In nature, folate is generally polyglutamated (decorated by two to seven additional glutamic acid residues). Conjugases (γ-glutamyl carboxypeptidases) in the intestinal lumen cleave off extra glutamic acid residue, and folate is absorbed by the mucosa of the small intestine (Figure 4-4).

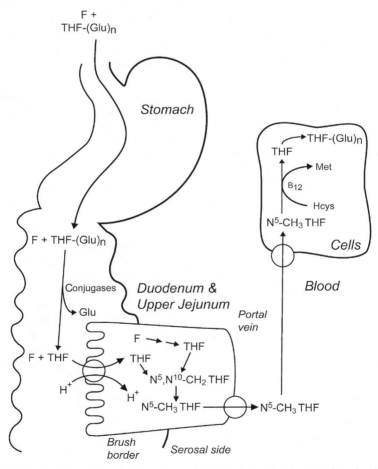

**Figure 4-4.** Intestinal absorption of dietary folates (THF-[Glu]n) and folic acid (F) from fortified cereal products and vitamin supplements. In the duodenum and upper jejunum, extra glutamate residue is cleaved by conjugases (γ-glutamyl carboxypeptidases). Both folate (F) and reduced folate (THF) are absorbed by a proton-coupled, high-affinity, folate transporter into the mucosal cell, converted to $N^5$-methyl THF, and then exported into the portal circulation. N5-methyl THF is taken up into cells by facilitative diffusion, converted to THF by the $B_{12}$-requiring methionine synthase, and then converted to a polyglutamate.

In cases of chronic alcoholism, folate deficiency may result from poor nutrition or from poor absorption of folate secondary to a conjugase deficiency. Once folate deficiency occurs, abnormal megaloblastic replication of epithelial mucosa can occur, which further impairs folate uptake.

After absorption, folate is reduced to THF by dihydrofolate reductase. The majority of circulating folate is in the form of $N^5$-methyl THF. Cells use specific transporters for THF uptake, and cellular machinery polyglutamates the folate to aid in cellular retention.

In summary, **folate** is a vitamin acquired from the diet **essential for 1-carbon metabolism.** Inadequate folate levels inhibit **DNA synthesis** by limiting **purine nucleotide and dTMP levels,** which results in the abnormal cellular proliferation observed in **megaloblastic anemia.** Folate is also required to replenish the **methionine pool for SAM-dependent methylation reactions.**

## COMPREHENSION QUESTIONS

4.1 A 35-year-old woman is noted to have a hemoglobin level of 9 g/dL (normal range: 12-14 g/dL). The red cell size is enlarged. Which of the following tests would best help distinguish between a folate and vitamin $B_{12}$ deficiency?

    A.  Activity of methionine synthase

    B.  Blood level of cystathionine

    C.  Blood level of homocysteine

    D.  Blood level of methionine

    E.  Blood level of methylmalonate

4.2 A muscular 25-year-old man presents with dermatitis and an inflamed tongue. A history reveals that he has been consuming raw eggs as part of his training regimen for the past 6 months. Which of the following vitamins is most likely to be deficient in this patient?

    A.  Ascorbic acid (vitamin C)

    B.  Biotin

    C.  Cobalamin (vitamin $B_{12}$)

    D.  Folic acid

    E.  Niacin (vitamin $B_3$)

    F.  Pantothenic acid

    G.  Riboflavin (vitamin $B_2$)

    H.  Thiamine (vitamin $B_1$)

4.3  A 30-year-old man goes to his dentist complaining of loosening teeth. Examination also reveals his gums are swollen, purple, and spongy. The dentist also notes that the patient's fingers have multiple splinter hemorrhages near the distal ends of the nail and that a wound on the patient's forearm has failed to heal properly. Which of the following vitamins is most likely to be deficient in this patient?

A.  Ascorbic acid (vitamin C)

B.  Biotin

C.  Cobalamin (vitamin $B_{12}$)

D.  Folic acid

E.  Niacin (vitamin $B_3$)

F.  Pantothenic acid

G.  Riboflavin (vitamin $B_2$)

H.  Thiamine (vitamin $B_1$)

4.4  A female neonate is found to have a small spina bifida in her lower spinal column that could affect bladder and lower limb function. Which of the following vitamins is most likely to be deficient in this patient?

A.  Ascorbic acid (vitamin C)

B.  Biotin

C.  Cobalamin (vitamin $B_{12}$)

D.  Folic acid

E.  Niacin (vitamin $B_3$)

F.  Pantothenic acid

G.  Riboflavin (vitamin $B_2$)

H.  Thiamine (vitamin $B_1$)

## ANSWERS

4.1  **E.** Vitamin $B_{12}$ is a cofactor in 2 biochemical reactions, the conversion of homocysteine to methionine by the enzyme methionine synthase and the conversion of L-methylmalonyl-CoA to succinyl-CoA by methylmalonyl-CoA mutase. $N^5$-methyl THF is a methyl donor in the methionine synthase reaction. Folate deficiency would result in decreased methionine synthase activity and decreases in methionine and cystathionine concentrations, while homocysteine levels would be increased. A vitamin $B_{12}$ deficiency would also yield these same results, but, in addition, methylmalonate levels would increase as a consequence of a decrease in the activity of methylmalonyl-CoA mutase activity.

4.2  **B.** Raw eggs contain avidin, a protein that strongly binds biotin. Because native avidin is resistant to hydrolysis by digestive proteases, when it binds biotin it prevents its absorption. Avidin that has been denatured by cooking will be broken down during the digestive process. Biotin deficiency manifests itself as an erythematous, scaly skin eruption, and can also cause hair loss and conjunctivitis. Biotin deficiency can also occur following prolonged total parenteral nutrition if biotin is not supplemented.

4.3  **A.** The patient exhibits the classic symptoms of scurvy, a deficiency in vitamin C. In addition to being an important biologic antioxidant, ascorbic acid is required for the hydroxylation of proline and lysine residues of procollagen in the synthesis of collagen. A deficiency leads to defects in collagen synthesis, which adversely affects the intercellular cement substances in connective tissue, bones, and dentin.

4.4  **D.** The fetus needs a constant supply of cofactors for normal development. Folic acid supplements of 400 μg/day prior to conception have been shown to decrease the incidence of neural tube defects such as spina bifida.

## BIOCHEMISTRY PEARLS

▶ Folate (folic acid) is an essential vitamin that, in its active form of tetrahydrofolate, transfers 1-carbon groups to intermediates in metabolism and plays an important role in DNA synthesis.

▶ THF is necessary for the de novo synthesis of purines and the conversion of dUMP to dTMP.

▶ The major metabolic perturbation in folate deficiency occurs in megaloblastic anemia.

## REFERENCES

Devlin TM, ed. *Textbook of Biochemistry with Clinical Correlations*. 7th ed. New York: Wiley-Liss; 2010.

Frenkel EP, Yardley DA. Clinical and laboratory features and sequelae of deficiency of folic acid (folate) and vitamin $B_{12}$ (cobalamin) in pregnancy and gynecology. *Hematol Oncol Clin North Am.* 2000;14(5):1079-1100.

Lin Y, Dueker SR, Jones AD, et al. Quantitation of in vivo human folate metabolism. *Am J Clin Nutr.* 2004;80(3):680-691.

Que A, et al. Identification of an intestinal folate transporter and the molecular basis for hereditary folate malabsorption. *Cell.* 2006;127(5):917-928.

Murray RK, Bender DA, Botham KM, et al, eds. *Harper's Illustrated Biochemistry*. 29th ed. New York: Lange Medical Books/McGraw-Hill; 2012.

A 32-year-old man presents to your clinic with complaints of a sore throat. He reports numerous upper respiratory infections during the last 3 months. The patient also states that he required antibiotics for some of these infections. The patient's sore throat has been present for 4 days and is progressively worsening. He is no longer able to eat solid foods because of the pain. No one else in contact with him has been ill. Patient gives a history of previous intravenous (IV) drug use, but no other significant medical history is given. On examination, the patient is found to have a temperature of 100.0°F (37.8°C) and is in minimal distress from the sore throat. His pharynx is erythematous and has numerous white plaques coating the throat. There is also prominent cervical lymph node enlargement. His chest is clear to auscultation and heart is regular rate and rhythm. A CD4 T-lymphocyte cell count is performed and is less than 200 cells/mm³ (normal > 500 cells/mm³). The responsible organism is composed of the ribonucleic acid (RNA) genome.

▶ What is the most likely diagnosis?
▶ What is the biochemical mechanism that the pathogen uses to affect the patient's cells?
▶ What enzyme is required for this pathogen to affect the host genome?

# ANSWERS TO CASE 5:
## HIV

*Summary:* A 32-year-old man with history of IV drug use has numerous upper respiratory symptoms and adenopathy, and he presents now with sore throat with numerous white plaques. He also has a low CD4 count. The pathogen has an RNA genome.

- **Most likely diagnosis:** Candida esophagitis secondary to HIV infection.

- **Biochemical mechanism of disease:** The HIV genome is composed of single-stranded RNA. Reverse transcription of the viral RNA is required to infect the host cells. HIV causes immunosuppression because it has a propensity for attaching to helper T cells (CD4 cells), the cells that support cell mediated immunity.

- **Enzyme necessary:** Reverse transcriptase.

## CLINICAL CORRELATION

This 32-year-old man likely acquired HIV infection by sharing needles with an infected individual. Initially, HIV infection may cause systemic, flulike symptoms, adenopathy, and fatigue. During this phase, the patient experiences viremia. The next phase is largely asymptomatic as the virus slowly causes attrition of the CD4 helper T cells. When the levels of these important cells drop to low levels, the patient cannot fend off organisms commonly colonizing the skin, gastrointestinal tract, or in the air. Treatment for HIV infection includes agents that attack the unique aspects of the virus, such as nucleoside analogue reverse transcriptase inhibitors and protease inhibitors.

# APPROACH TO:
## HIV

### OBJECTIVES

1. Understand normal transcription/translation.

2. Be familiar with reverse transcriptase and mechanism by which HIV works.

3. Know the mechanism of action of HIV medications.

### DEFINITIONS

**DNA REPLICATION:** The process by which DNA is duplicated in the cell takes place during the S-phase of the cell cycle. DNA is duplicated in a semiconservative manner; that is, each new DNA double-strand contains one of the original strands (parent strands) and one of the newly synthesized strands (daughter strands).

**HIV:** Human immunodeficiency virus; a retrovirus that causes AIDS.

**RETROVIRUS:** A virus in which the genetic material located in the virus is RNA. The genetic information in the retrovirus must be converted to DNA in the host by the process of reverse transcription.

**REVERSE TRANSCRIPTION:** The synthesis of DNA from an RNA template.

**TRANSCRIPTION:** The process by which the information contained in the nuclear DNA is converted to cytosolic messenger RNA (mRNA). This is accomplished by RNA polymerases that synthesize an mRNA that has a complementary sequence to the DNA strand that was used as the template.

**TRANSLATION:** The synthesis of proteins from mRNA. This is a process that takes place on ribosomes and requires the participation of aminoacyl-charged transfer RNA (tRNA), mRNA, and various initiation and elongation factors.

**EXONS:** Sequence of nucleotides that appear in mature RNA.

**INTRONS:** Sequences of nucleotides that do not appear in mature RNA but are excised and do not appear in messenger RNA.

**SPLICEOSOME:** A complex of small nuclear ribonucleoprotein particles (snRNPs) that catalyze the splicing, or removal of introns, of mRNA precursors.

## DISCUSSION

**DNA is the biologic blueprint material,** which authentically carries all the necessary cellular information and passes it from generation to generation. Thus, it is essential for the cells to preserve the integrity of the DNA and keep it as error free as possible. One is amazed with the versatile DNA molecule, which dictates both the unique and the similar features of the offspring from its parents. What are the processes that take place in a cell to duplicate and interpret this genetic code into functional signals? DNA is duplicated in a **semiconservative fashion** in a process called **DNA replication.**

DNA **interpretation** follows the central dogma (Figure 5-1): first, the DNA is **decoded to form mRNA** in the nucleus by a process called **transcription.** Transcription is a complex process involving an **enzyme RNA polymerase and several transcription factors.** The DNA strand that directs RNA synthesis via **complementary base pairing** is called the **template. RNA synthesis is always unidirectional from 5′ (phosphate) to 3′ (hydroxyl).** One can organize transcription in a stepwise fashion:

1. **Binding of RNA polymerase** to the DNA

2. Formation of the **transcription bubble** (separation of the DNA strands)

3. **Addition of the first RNA residue**

4. Addition of the **second residue,** formation of a **phosphodiester bond** between the ribonucleic acid residues, and **release of pyrophosphate**

Figure 5-1. The central dogma.

The addition process continues until the **termination signal** is encountered. Once the **nascent RNA chain emerges, it is capped with methylguanylate at the 5′ end and polyadenylated in the 3′ end.** This primary RNA transcript is processed further by splicing machinery to yield the mature functional mRNA. **Heterogenous nuclear RNA (hnRNA) contains exons and introns.** The introns are excised and **mature RNA enters the cytoplasm.**

The **mRNA** is then processed in the cytoplasm by a process called **translation.** Translation involves the **ribosomes** along with a battery of **initiating (IF), elongation (EF), and release (RF) factors.** An important rule to remember in translation is that each **triplet nucleotide codon codes for a specific amino acid (the 3-letter genetic code).** Maintaining the order of amino acids is important to obtain a functional protein. mRNA is translated into protein with the help of **tRNA,** which **brings an amino acid along with it (aminoacyl tRNA) and ribosomes.** Ribosomes are in turn composed of numerous proteins and several rRNA molecules. The step-wise process of **translation** is as follows:

1. The ribosomal unit along with the **initiation factors and formyl-methionine (fMet)-tRNA bind close to the initiating codon AUG in the 5′ region** of the mRNA.

2. The **ribosomal complex consists of 3 sites, namely, A, P, and E.** The **aminoacyl tRNA binds the triplet codon at the A site.** The **formyl-methionyl group** forms a peptide bond with the amino group of the aminoacyl tRNA in **the P site,** releasing the now **uncharged tRNA$_{fMet}$,** which exits the ribosome assembly through the **E site.**

3. **Elongation** continues until the ribosome encounters one of the **stop codons UAA, UAG, and UGA.**

4. **Termination of protein synthesis** occurs with the help of release factors that cleave the peptide chain from the tRNA and dissolve the ribosomal complex.

In **retroviruses such as HIV** in which the genetic material is **RNA** rather than DNA, **reverse transcription** occurs. The life cycle of HIV begins when the virion binds to cell surface receptors (CD4 receptors) on helper T lymphocytes. This results in a conformational change that enables the viral coat to fuse with the lymphocyte membrane, thus releasing the viral RNA and viral proteins into the cytosol, including reverse transcriptase and integrase. The **RNA genome (Figure 5-2) is reverse**

| LTR | gag | pol | env | LTR |
|-----|-----|-----|-----|-----|

**Figure 5-2.** Simplified HIV genome.

transcribed into a double-stranded DNA molecule by utilizing the **reverse transcriptase enzyme**. This enzyme is an unusual **DNA polymerase, because it uses both DNA and RNA as template.** It makes DNA from the RNA and uses this in turn to make the second strand of DNA. This double-stranded DNA is transported into the nucleus and is recognized by the **viral enzyme integrase**, which catalyzes the insertion of the viral DNA into the host genome, thus establishing a permanent infection. The final step is the transcription of the integrated viral DNA producing a large amount of **viral RNA, which is packaged in a capsid** along with the other essential proteins and can bud from the plasma membrane. Based on the pathogenesis of HIV, it is very important to understand the transcription mechanism of this virus. The HIV life cycle can be simplified and drawn out as shown in Figure 5-3.

The **long terminal repeat (LTR) contains the enhancer and the promoter** regions of HIV. The *gag* encodes the structural proteins, which help in packaging the RNA of the virus to generate new virus particles. The *pol* gene encodes both the critical enzymes **reverse transcriptase and integrase.** The *env* **codes for envelope proteins** of the virus that along with the host plasma membrane help the complete

**Figure 5-3.** Life cycle of HIV.

virus particle to bud off from the cell. Apart from these proteins, the **3 regulatory proteins,** namely, the negative factor **Nef,** transactivator of transcription **Tat,** and the regulator of viral gene expression, **Rev,** can affect viral transcription output. Tat specifically promotes transcriptional activity, while Rev is responsible for switching from early to late HIV gene expression and is located in the 3′ end of the *env* gene. With the latest research identifying new proteins in addition to the pre-existing knowledge, one wonders what would be the most effective antiretroviral therapy. The available drugs in the market include **nucleoside reverse transcription inhibitors and protease inhibitors.**

**Nucleoside reverse transcriptase inhibitors** act as substrates for the reverse transcriptase enzyme and require a phosphorylation event to be activated. The **nucleoside drugs lack the 3′-hydroxyl group;** therefore, their incorporation into viral DNA will effectively **terminate the elongation process.** This class includes zidovudine, didanosine, stavudine, lamivudine, and abacavir. As these agents affect very early events in pathogenesis of HIV, they prevent acute infection of susceptible cells but have little effect on already infected cells. The common adverse events of these drugs are lactic acidosis, hepatomegaly, anemia, anorexia, fatigue, nausea, and insomnia. A subcategory to this class of drugs is the nonnucleoside inhibitors, which act by binding close to the active site, inducing a conformation change and thereby inhibiting enzyme function. Some of the members of the class are delavirdine, nevirapine, and efavirenz. A major drawback with these nonnucleoside drugs is that they are effectively metabolized by the cytochrome P450 system and are prone to drug interaction. The most common adverse effects are rash, elevated liver function, and impaired concentration.

**Protease inhibitors** are targeted toward the **HIV proteases, which are essential to activate precursors of gag-pol. HIV protease is essential for infectivity** and cleaves the viral polyprotein (*gag-pol*) into active viral enzymes and structural proteins. The mechanism of action of these drugs is binding reversibly to the active site of HIV protease and blocking subsequent viral maturation. This major class includes saquinavir, ritonavir, indinavir, and nelfinavir. Toxicities of protease inhibitors include nausea, vomiting, and diarrhea.

HIV inhibitor treatment eventually leads to the selection of resistant mutations, one key reason being that the reverse transcriptase is error prone because it lacks the 3′ exonuclease activity. Currently, combinatorial inhibitors with different protein targets; for example, 2 reverse transcriptase nucleoside inhibitors and 1 protease inhibitor, are used in highly active antiretroviral therapy (HAART). To overcome drug resistance and find a definitive cure for HIV infection, several efforts are being made to develop vaccines and also use ribozymes to target HIV mRNA. Because of the molecular understanding of HIV, the future of anti-HIV therapy seems bright and promises an effective cure for patients with AIDS.

## COMPREHENSION QUESTIONS

5.1 The current therapeutic strategy for patients who have been infected with HIV is a multidrug regimen known as HAART. One type of drug used in this therapy is a nucleoside/nucleotide analog (eg, didanosine). Which of the following best describes the mechanism of action of these drugs?

A. They inhibit the synthesis of viral proteins.

B. They directly bind to and inhibit reverse transcriptase.

C. They prevent the hydrolysis of the viral polyprotein.

D. They prematurely terminate the DNA synthesized by reverse transcriptase.

E. They inhibit the viral enzyme integrase.

5.2 Enzyme-linked immunosorbent assay is used for routine screening of HIV infection, and the Western blot test has been successfully used as a confirmatory test. Which of the following best describes the strategy used to confirm the presence of an HIV infection by Western blot analysis?

| | Gel Electrophoresis and Blot Performed On | Blot Incubation With | Blot Detects |
|---|---|---|---|
| A. | HIV protein standards | Patient serum | Presence of anti-HIV antibodies in serum |
| B. | Patient serum | Anti-HIV antibodies | Presence of HIV proteins in serum |
| C. | Anti-HIV antibody standards | Patient serum | Presence of HIV proteins in serum |
| D. | Patient serum | Labeled oligonucle- otides | Presence of HIV RNA in serum |

5.3 The following diagram schematically represents the life cycle of HIV. Which of the labeled steps best indicates the site at which an HIV protease inhibitor disrupts the cycle?

5.4 Given the mRNA nucleotide sequence, choose the best protein sequence that will likely result. (Hint: Use the amino acid table in questions 13.2 and 13.3 in Case 13, keeping in mind that [T] and [U] are analogous). mRNA 5′ AUCG-GAUGUCUCGGGUUCUGUAAAGGUAAUC 3′

   A.  Met-Ser-Arg-Val-Leu

   B.  Ser-Arg-Val-Leu

   C.  Met-Leu-Ser-Val

   D.  Ser-Arg-Val-Phe-Phe

   E.  Pro-Ser-Val-Gly

# ANSWERS

5.1 **D.** The nucleoside/nucleotide analogs like azidothymidine and didanosine are incorporated into the DNA synthesized by HIV reverse transcriptase. Because they do not have a 3′-hydroxyl group, they cannot form a bond with the next nucleotide and the chain is terminated. Host-cell DNA synthesis is not affected because of the nuclear DNA repair mechanisms.

5.2 **A.** In the Western blot confirmatory test, standard HIV proteins (*gag, pol,* and *env*) are separated by gel electrophoresis and then blotted onto a nitrocellulose membrane. The membrane is then incubated with the patient's serum. Any anti-HIV antibodies will bind to the respective HIV protein on the membrane. Finally, a labeled antihuman antibody is added to indicate the presence of any anti-HIV antibody binding. The test is highly specific; that is, a positive result is highly indicative of HIV infection.

5.3 **E.** The HIV proteins synthesized by the host cell are produced as a long polyprotein that must be cleaved to the active HIV enzymes and structural proteins. HIV protease inhibitors bind to and inhibit the aspartic protease that hydrolyzes the polyprotein, thus preventing the assembly of infective viral particles.

5.4 **A.** The initiator codon is AUG and codes for Met; UCU = Ser; CGG = Arg; GUU = Val; CUG = Leu; UAA = stop codon. The mRNA is read in the 5′→ 3′ direction.

## BIOCHEMISTRY PEARLS

▶ DNA is decoded to form mRNA in the nucleus by a process called transcription. RNA synthesis is always unidirectional from 5′ (phosphate) to 3′ (hydroxyl), and begins at the 3′ end of the DNA chain toward the 5′ end.

▶ The mRNA is processed in the cytoplasm (translation) involving the ribosomes. Each triplet nucleotide codon codes for a specific amino acid (the 3-letter genetic code).

▶ Messenger RNA is translated into protein with the help of tRNA, which brings an amino acid along with it (aminoacyl tRNA) and ribosomes.

▶ Some viruses, such as HIV, have RNA genomes, and they usually are reverse transcribed into a double-stranded DNA molecule by utilizing the reverse-transcriptase enzyme.

## REFERENCES

Levy JA. *HIV and the Pathogenesis of AIDS.* 2nd ed. Washington DC: ASM Press;1998.

Lodish H, Berk A, Kaiser CA, et al. *Molecular Cell Biology.* 7th ed. New York: Freeman; 2012.

Raffanti S, Haas DW. Anti-bacterial agents. In: Brunton L, Chabner B, Bjorn Knollman, eds. *Goodman and Gilman's The Pharmacological Basis of Therapeutics.* 12th ed. New York: McGraw-Hill; 2010.

A 21-year-old woman presents to the physician's office with complaints of very painful vulvar ulcers. The patient states she has had the symptoms for approximately 3 days, and they are worsening. She says that prior to the ulcerations, there was a burning and tingling sensation of the skin in the same area. She has noted similar symptoms like this before and has been told it is sexually transmitted. On examination you see multiple extremely tender, vesicular (blister-like) lesions on an erythematous (red) base on both labia majora of the vulva. She has a moderate amount of tender inguinal lymph nodes bilaterally. The physician uses a swab to sample the ulcer and send it off for diagnostic analysis.

► What is the most likely diagnosis?
► If the test is for DNA, then what method would be used to amplify the fragments of DNA sampled?

## ANSWERS TO CASE 6:

## Herpes Simplex Virus/Polymerase Chain Reaction

*Summary:* A 21-year-old woman presents with recurrent episodes of painful ulcerations on vulva. The physician uses a swab to sample the ulcer for diagnosis. She also has some neurologic symptoms at the vulva prior to appearance of lesions.

- **Most likely diagnosis:** Herpes simplex virus (HSV) type 2 outbreak.

- **Biochemical Technique:** Polymerase chain reaction (PCR) to amplify the small amount of HSV DNA. This is a very sensitive diagnostic technique that is able to detect small amounts of HSV DNA, and through in vitro techniques, it is able to rapidly produce large quantities of DNA.

### CLINICAL CORRELATION

This 21-year-old woman has a recurrent episode of vulvar ulcers accompanied by burning and tingling in the same region. These symptoms are caused by the HSV affecting the afferent nerve. After a primary infection, the herpes virus lays dormant in the dorsal ganglia of the nerve root. Then, in times of stress or for unknown reasons, the virus becomes active and travels down the nerve to the skin. Thus, the patient often has neurologic symptoms even before the outbreak on the skin. Viral culture is an accurate method of diagnosis. Perhaps even better is PCR, which can also be used for detection of numerous infectious organisms, genetic mutations, and forensic testing.

## APPROACH TO:

## Polymerase Chain Reaction

### OBJECTIVES

1. Describe the life cycle of HSVs.

2. Describe the process of PCR.

3. Know the definitions and purpose of restriction endonucleases and oligonucleotides.

4. Be familiar with how PCR may be used for identifying infections and mutations.

5. Cite the advantages of PCR over other biotechnology involving recombinant DNA.

## DEFINITIONS

**ANNEALING:** The process of allowing single-stranded lengths of DNA to base pair to form double-stranded DNA. It is used most frequently when referring to the process of binding an oligonucleotide primer or probe to a longer DNA fragment.

**DENATURATION:** The process by which the secondary and tertiary structure of proteins and nucleic acids is broken down to form random chains. In the case of DNA, it specifically refers to the separation of double-stranded DNA into single strands by the breaking of the hydrogen bonds that form the complementary base pairing, usually by increasing the temperature.

**POLYMERASE CHAIN REACTION (PCR):** PCR is a method by which DNA or DNA fragments can be amplified through several steps of denaturation, annealing, and elongation. Through this process, the amount of target DNA can be increased by a factor of $10^6$ to $10^9$.

**RESTRICTION ENZYMES:** Endonucleases isolated from bacteria that will selectively cleave DNA having specific nucleotide sequences. The enzyme recognizes particular palindromic nucleotide sequences and will hydrolyze both strands within that sequence. Molecular biologists use these enzymes in various recombinant DNA techniques.

**TAQ DNA POLYMERASE:** A DNA polymerase isolated from the thermophilic bacteria *Thermus aquaticus*. It has the advantage that it remains active during the denaturation steps of PCR in which the temperature is increased to separate the DNA strands.

**PALINDROME:** Having the same sequence in the complimentary strand as the original strand of DNA or RNA when read from the 5′ to the 3′ direction.

**ACYCLOVIR (ACYCLOGUANOSINE):** Acycloguanosine, a prodrug that is activated to the active acycloguanosine triphosphate (acyclo-GTP), which inhibits viral DNA polymerase by acting as a DNA chain terminator.

## DISCUSSION

HSVs are members of Herpesviridae, which also includes Epstein-Barr virus (infectious mononucleosis), varicella-zoster virus (chicken pox), and cytomegalovirus (CMV). Herpesviruses are large (150 nm in diameter) enveloped linear double-stranded DNA viruses. Because of the phospholipid envelope, herpesviruses are sensitive to acids, detergents, solvents, and drying. In general, herpesvirus replication begins with the attachment of the viral particle to the host cell surface, followed by the fusion of the viral envelope and cell membrane and release of the viral nucleocapsid into the cell cytoplasm. The nucleocapsid attaches to the nuclear envelope and then the viral genome is released into the cellular nucleus. The herpesvirus genome is transcribed and translated by host factors but is replicated by a viral encoded DNA polymerase. This HSV DNA polymerase is an important target for drug therapy. The viral nucleocapsids are formed in the nucleus, and the envelope is acquired from the nuclear or Golgi membrane. Mature viral particles are released from the host cell by exocytosis or cell lysis. Depending on the herpesvirus and type of host cell that is infected, a lytic, persistent (macrophages and lymphocytes), or latent (nerve cells) infection can be established.

HSV can infect many cell types (including macrophages, lymphocytes, and neurons), causing lytic, persistent, and latent infections. Because of nerve cell involvement in latent infections, a recurrence of the disease is often preceded by a prodrome (sensations such as burning or tingling). Initial HSV-1 and HSV-2 infections are usually established on mucous membranes. Although HSV-1 and HSV-2 are respectively referred to as oral herpes and genital herpes based on their typical site of infection, HSV-1 and HSV-2 can be found on both oral and genital tissue.

Diagnosis can be made by examining infected tissue or cells for characteristic cytopathologic effects, virus isolation and culture, or serology. Molecular methods (such as DNA in situ hybridization and PCR of vesicle fluid or scrapings) are also used for diagnosis. The molecular methods are gaining favor because they yield rapid results and identify the viral type or strain. Because of these diagnostic advantages, PCR is the preferred method for diagnosis of HSV encephalitis.

The **PCR** is an in vitro method for the **exponential amplification of a specific DNA region.** Today, PCR is one of the most important biochemical techniques and is applied in virtually all fields of modern molecular biology. The ingredients for PCR reactions are very simple: the **target DNA to be amplified, a heat-stable DNA polymerase, the 4 deoxyribonucleotides, 2 oligonucleotide primers, and a reaction buffer.** The entire PCR reaction is carried out in a single tube containing all these necessary components. The **target DNA segment is amplified** with a high degree of specificity by using **2 DNA oligonucleotide primers** that are complementary to sequences on the 3′-flanking regions of opposite strands of the target segment. The PCR amplification occurs by repeated cycles of **three temperature-dependent steps** called **denaturation, annealing, and elongation** (Figure 6-1). Native DNA exists as a double helix; therefore, the first step, denaturation, of the process separates the 2 DNA chains by **heating** the reaction mixture to 194 to 203°F (90–95°C). In the second step, **annealing,** the reaction mixture is **cooled** to 113 to 140°F (45–60°C) so that the **oligonucleotide primers can bind or anneal** to the separated strands of the target DNA. In the final step of the process, **elongation,** the **DNA polymerase adds nucleotides to the 3′ ends of the primers to complete a copy of the target DNA template.** A heat-stable DNA polymerase obtained from the thermophilic bacterium **T. aquaticus** is used to synthesize the new strands in most PCRs. Since this Taq DNA polymerase works best at around 161.6°F (72°C), the temperature of the PCR mixture is raised to that temperature for elongation to proceed efficiently. At the end of a three-step cycle, each target region of DNA in the vial has been duplicated. This 3-step cycle is then repeated multiple times. Each new DNA strand can then act as a new template in the next cycle, yielding approximately **1 million copies of a target DNA after 20 cycles.** Therefore, PCR is a method able to amplify any DNA sequence virtually without limit and allows the separation of the nucleic acid of interest from its context.

PCR is also becoming the leading method for detection of the continuously increasing number of human pathogens. Examples include HSV, human

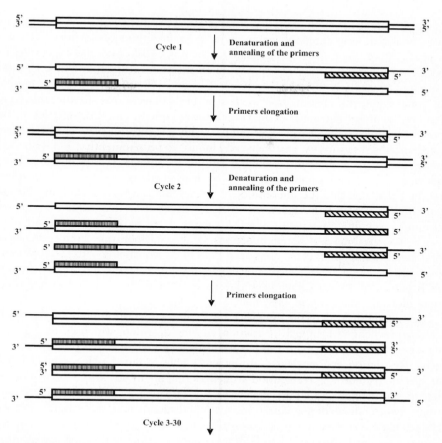

**Figure 6-1.** Polymerase chain reaction diagram.

papillomavirus, HIV, human *T. lymphotropic* virus types 1 and 2, CMV, Epstein-Barr virus, human herpesvirus-6 (HHV-6), hepatitis B virus, B16 parvovirus, JC and BK viruses, rubella virus, mycobacteria, *Toxoplasmosis gondii*, *Trypanosoma cruzi*, and malaria, with many more to follow. PCR can be applied as a detection method for virtually any pathogen for which even limited nucleotide sequence information is known and for which a specimen of infected tissue can be readily obtained. In most cases, PCR assays are more discriminative than conventional serology. For example, it is difficult to distinguish HSV-1 from HSV-2 or HIV-1 from HIV-2 by serology, yet such distinctions can be readily made on the basis of PCR amplification of type-specific genetic sequences. PCR yields rapid results, typically in 1 to 2 days in a clinical setting. It is applicable to a wide variety of clinical, pathologic, or forensic specimens, as well as to formalin-fixed tissue, inactivated bacterial cultures, and archaeological specimens. However, since **PCR detects nucleic acids from both living and dead microbes,** this must be taken into account if PCR is used to monitor response to therapy.

Prior to the PCR method for detection of HSV-1 and HSV-2, clinical specimens were analyzed using immunologic methods to confirm the virus identity following a viral culture. Such methods are time consuming (3-12 days) and expensive. In addition, cultivation of the virus is not always successful. Turnaround time for viral culture averaged 108 hours for positive results and 154 hours for negative results. In comparison, the present PCR method of HSV detection is specific, relatively fast and accurate. The method allows detection of one to ten virus particles in the presence of microgram quantities of cellular or heterogeneous DNA. The PCR assay offers increased sensitivity, specificity, and improved turnaround time (24-48 hours) when compared with traditional viral culture techniques. These methods have allowed a better understanding of the physiopathogeny of the disease. In particular, PCR has revealed the importance of asymptomatic viral shedding in infected patients. PCR also helps diagnosis in many situations where viral isolation by culture proves difficult or impossible, for example, in treated or atypical lesions, or in newborn central nervous system infections. PCR has demonstrated the existence of prolonged viremia in infected newborns. PCR helps sequencing of the viral genome for further epidemiologic studies or analysis of resistance to antiviral drugs. Recently, PCR-derived techniques have been developed to quantify viral load in real time, thus allowing a diagnosis in a few hours.

After **amplification of the samples** using PCR, the identification of the virus species can be achieved through **restriction enzyme digestion,** which yields a unique pattern of **different fragment sizes** characteristic for each herpesvirus (or other pathogen). **Restriction endonucleases are enzymes able to cut double-stranded DNA at specific palindromic recognition sequences** that are mostly 4 to 6 nucleotides in length. Furthermore, a well-designed restriction enzyme panel allows the discrimination between human herpes virus 6 variant A and variant B. In this way, this method can readily detect human herpesviruses, including occasional multiple infections, in a variety of clinical samples. When PCR assay was compared to isolation and electron microscopy for the detection of HSV in clinical samples, all specimens positive by conventional methods were also positive by PCR. However, in a number of clinical specimens in which HSV could not be detected by conventional methods, PCR was able to demonstrate the presence of the virus.

Treatment of HSV typically involves the use of nucleoside analog prodrugs that when activated specifically inhibit the viral DNA polymerase, thereby preventing replication of the viral genome. Acyclovir is a guanosine analog (Figure 6-2) that has been shown to be effective against HSV. It is first phosphorylated to the mono-phosphate derivative by viral thymidine kinase. Cellular kinases then convert it to the triphosphate. The now activated drug, acyclo-GTP, inhibits replication of the viral genome. The viral DNA polymerase will incorporate the acycloguanine nucleotide into the viral DNA in the replication process, but because there is no 3'-hydroxyl to form the next phosphodiester, the chain terminates and replication stops.

Acyclovir has a relatively poor oral bioavailability. Valacyclovir is a modified version of acyclovir that has been esterified with the amino acid valine. Its oral bioavailability is about 3 to 5 times that of acyclovir. When it is absorbed, it is converted to acyclovir by cellular esterases and then further phosphorylated to the active acyclo-GTP (see Figure 6-2).

**Figure 6-2.** Conversion of the prodrug valacyclovir to the active acycloguanosine triphosphate.

## COMPREHENSION QUESTIONS

6.1 One of the steps in the PCR amplification of DNA fragments is the denaturation step in which the temperature is raised to break the hydrogen bonds that make up the base pairing. Which of the following DNA fragments would most likely require the greatest increase in temperature to cause complete denaturation?

A. 5′–C-A-A-T-G-T-A-A-T-T-G-C-A-T-3′
   3′–G-T-T- A-C-A-T-T-A-A-C-G-T-A-5′

B. 5′–A-T-A-T-A-T-A-T-A-T-A-T-A-T-3′
   3′–T- A-T- A-T-A-T-A-T- A-T-A-T-A-5′

C. 5′–A-A-C-C-G-G-A-C-C-G-C-G-A-T-3′
   3′–T- T-G-G-C-C-T-G-G-C-G-C-T-A-5′

D. 5′–A-G-A-G-A-G-A-G-A-G-A-G-A-G-3′
   3′–T-C-T-C-T-C-T-C-T- C-T-C-T-C-5′

E. 5′–G-A-C-T-G-T-A-A-T-A-C-G-A-T-3′
   3′–C-T-G-A-C-A-T-T-A-T-G-C-T-A-5′

6.2 Restriction enzymes are used to cleave genomic DNA into smaller fragments. Which of the following single-strand DNA sequences has the best potential to be a site of action for a restriction endonuclease?

A. T–A–G–C–T–T

B. C–T–G–C–A–G

C. A–A–C–C–A–A

D. G–T–G–T–G–T

E. A–A–A–C–C–C

6.3 A 21-year-old woman was abducted when she went to the local convenience store. Her body was found the next morning in a wooded area behind the store. The autopsy revealed that she had been sexually assaulted and strangled. Crime scene investigators were able to collect a semen sample from vaginal fluid as well as tissue samples from underneath the victim's fingernails. DNA samples were obtained from three suspects besides the victim. A variable number of tandem repeats (VNTR) analysis was performed on the DNA samples from the evidence collected, the victim, and the suspect, and the results were compared. Which of the following techniques is the most appropriately applied for this analysis?

A. Allele-specific oligonucleotide probes

B. DNA sequencing

C. Northern blot

D. Southern blot

E. Western blot

6.4  A 40-year-old man presents to his primary care physician due to a painful lesion on his scrotum. On examination, the physician observed what appeared to be herpetic vesicles on the left underside of the scrotum. He prescribed a course of valacyclovir. Valacyclovir treats outbreaks of HSV infection by which of the following?

A.  Acting as a protease inhibitor

B.  Inhibiting protein translation

C.  Inhibiting reverse transcriptase

D.  Inhibiting packaging of new viral particles

E.  Inhibiting replication of the viral genome

## ANSWERS

6.1  **C.** The temperature at which the DNA strands separate is dependent on the number of hydrogen bonds that make up the base pairing. Because G-C pairs have three hydrogen bonds while A-T pairs only have 2, then the strand that has the greatest number of G-C pairs will have the higher melting temperature, Tm, which is the temperature at which one-half of the base pairs are broken. Interestingly, the TATA box, the starting point of transcription in eukaryotes, has weaker bonding.

6.2  **B.** Most of the sequences recognized by restriction endonucleases are palindromes; that is, they have the same nucleotide sequence on both strands when read in the 5′ to 3′ direction. Because answer B has the only sequence that will be a palindrome when paired with its complementary strand, it is the most likely to be a site recognized by a restriction endonuclease (it is the site recognized by the restriction endonuclease *Pst*1).

6.3  **D.** A VNTR analysis examines the hypervariable regions of the human genome. These contain sequences that are repeated in tandem a variable number of times and the length is unique for each individual. Because it is DNA fragments that are being analyzed, the Southern blot is the most appropriate technique to use to separate and detect these regions. DNA sequencing is too time consuming to be practical for forensic analyses. The Northern blot is used to separate and detect RNA, whereas the Western blot is used for proteins. Allele-specific oligonucleotide probes are used when testing for the presence of a genetic mutation that either introduces or removes a restriction site.

6.4  **E.** Valacyclovir is a prodrug that is metabolized to an analog of GTP. The nucleotide analog is incorporated into viral DNA as it is replicating and terminates the replication process.

## BIOCHEMISTRY PEARLS

▶ PCR is an in vitro method for the exponential amplification of a specific DNA region.

▶ PCR involves (1) denaturation, which separates the 2 DNA chains by heating the reaction mixture to 194 to 203°F (90-95°C), (2) annealing or cooling to 113 to 140°F (45-60°C) so that the oligonucleotide primers can bind or anneal to the separated strands of the target DNA, and (3) elongation with DNA polymerase (at 162°F [72°C] when *Taq* DNA polymerase used) adding nucleotides to the 3′ ends of the primers to a complete copy of the target DNA template.

▶ GC pairs have 3 hydrogen bonds, whereas AT pairs have only 2 hydrogen bonds and are therefore weaker.

▶ A heat-stable DNA polymerase obtained from the thermophilic bacterium *T. aquaticus* is used to synthesize the new strands in most PCR reactions.

▶ Endonucleases usually act at sites of palindromes.

## REFERENCES

Granner DK, Weil PA. Molecular genetics, recombinant DNA, & genomic technology. In: Murray RK, Granner DK, Mayes PA, et al, eds. *Harper's Illustrated Biochemistry.* 26th ed. New York: Lange Medical Books/McGraw-Hill; 2003.

Johnson G, Nelson S, Petric M, et al. Comprehensive PCR-based assay for detection and species identification of human herpesviruses. *J Clin Microbiol.* 2000;38(9):3274-3279.

# CASE 7

A 39-year-old woman presents to the clinic for a routine health maintenance examination. The patient reports she is feeling nervous and anxious all the time with frequent palpitations. Upon further questioning, she reports having diarrhea and has been losing weight. She has also noticed a change in hair and fingernail growth and frequently feels warm while others are cold or comfortable. She denies any history of depression or anxiety disorder and is not taking any medications. On examination, her heart rate is 110 beats/minute. She has a slight tremor and has increased reflexes in all extremities. A nontender thyroid enlargement is appreciated in the thyroid region. Her thyroid-stimulating hormone (TSH) level is low at 0.1 mIU/mL. The patient is told that she has an autoimmune antibody process.

▶ What is the most likely diagnosis?
▶ What is the biochemical mechanism for this disorder?

# ANSWERS TO CASE 7:

## Hyperthyroidism/Steroid Messenger Regulation of Translation

*Summary:* A 39-year-old woman has symptoms of nervousness, weight loss, gastrointestinal and skin alterations, heart palpitations, heat intolerance, and physical signs of hyperreflexia and a goiter.

- **Likely diagnosis:** Hyperthyroidism, likely Graves disease.

- **Biochemical mechanism:** The most frequent cause of hyperthyroidism, Graves disease, is an autoimmune process in which thyroid hypersecretion is caused by circulating immunoglobulins that bind to the TSH receptor on the thyroid follicular cells and stimulate thyroid hormone production. The diagnosis is confirmed by increased thyroid stimulating immunoglobulin (Ig) G antibodies and is frequently seen in other family members.

## CLINICAL CORRELATION

This 39-year-old woman has symptoms of hyperthyroidism, which is an excess of thyroid. This causes a tachycardia, tremor, nervousness, thin skin, weight loss through the hypermetabolic state, and hyperreflexia. If it is unchecked, then the high levels of thyroid hormone can sometimes even cause adrenergic crisis (so-called thyroid storm), which has a high rate of mortality. Normally, the thyroid hormone (thyroxine) is under tight control. The pituitary release of THS is stimulated by insufficient thyroxine, and suppressed by excess thyroxine. In cases of Graves disease, the most common cause of hyperthyroidism in the United States, an autoimmune immunoglobulin is produced that stimulates the TSH receptor of the pituitary. This is confirmed by either assaying for the thyroid-stimulating immunoglobulin, or a radionuclide scan revealing diffuse increased uptake throughout the thyroid gland. Treatment acutely includes β-adrenergic antagonists and agents that inhibit the catabolism of thyroid hormone, such as propylthiouracil (PTU).

# APPROACH TO:

## Steroid Messenger Regulation of Translation

### OBJECTIVES

1. Understand the general mechanisms of hormone action.

2. Know about some of the specific mechanisms by which hormones activate receptors.
   a. Know about hormones that bind to cell membrane receptors.
   b. Know about hormones that act through cyclic nucleotides.
   c. Know about hormones that act through calcium and the $PIP_2$ system.
   d. Know about hormones that bind intracellular receptors and activate genes.

3. Be familiar with how immunoglobulins of Graves disease cause hyperthyroidism.

4. Be aware of the mechanism of action of PTU and methimazole.

5. Understand the regulation of hormone levels.

## DEFINITIONS

**EFFECTOR:** The protein in a signal transduction pathway (eg, a hormonal response) that produces the cellular response.

**G PROTEIN:** A guanosine triphosphate (GTP)–binding protein that serves as a transducer in a signal transduction pathway. Upon binding GTP and releasing guanosine diphosphate (GDP), a G protein is able to activate the effector enzyme (eg, adenylate cyclase).

**GRAVES DISEASE:** An autoimmune disease in which the B lymphocytes synthesize an immunoglobulin (thyroid-stimulating immunoglobulin [TSIg]) that binds to and activates the TSH receptor in such a way that the thyroid hormones do not feedback inhibit the receptor–effector interaction, leading to a hyperthyroid condition.

**HORMONE:** A chemical signal that is produced in 1 set of cells and directs the activity in another set of cells that can be endocrine, paracrine, or autocrine.

**RECEPTOR:** A protein that will perceive the signal of a hormone or other chemical signal (eg, a neurotransmitter) by binding it and transmitting that signal further down the signal transduction pathway.

**SECOND MESSENGER:** A molecule that is synthesized within a cell in response to a receptor binding a hormone.

**TRANSDUCER PROTEIN:** A protein (such as the $\alpha$-subunit of a G protein) that transmits the signal from a hormone-bound receptor to the effector protein.

## DISCUSSION

Cellular biochemistry is a complex system of reactions and processes that must be efficiently regulated and integrated with processes underway in other cells and tissues. One method by which regulation is achieved is through the interaction of **hormones and their associated receptors** located either within or on the surface of the cell. A hormone is any substance in an organism that carries a signal to change metabolic processes within a cell.

The **hormonal-signaling process** is summarized in Figure 7-1. Hormones are released from secretory tissues in response to metabolic signals as well as electrical or chemical signals from the nervous system. The **released hormone binds to a receptor,** which can either be on the **cell surface** or, as in the case of **steroid and similar hormones, within the cell.** The hormone–receptor complex starts a series of events in which the signal is converted to other chemical forms that bring about **changes in the biochemical reactions within the cell.**

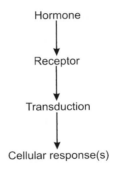

Figure 7-1. The hormonal-signaling process.

Hormones can be grouped into 3 main classifications based on their chemical structure and how they are synthesized. **Peptide hormones** include the **polypeptide hormones insulin and glucagon,** as well as the smaller peptides such as thyrotropin-releasing hormone (TRH) and the enkephalins. Some peptide hormones, like **thyrotropin** (TSH), are **glycoproteins. Amino acid-derived hormones** are synthesized from amino acid precursors. The catecholamines and serotonin are included in this grouping, as are the thyroid hormones, $T_3$ and $T_4$. The third classification is the steroid and steroid-like hormones, which includes the **progestogens, corticosteroids, androgens, estrogens, and calcitriol (the active form of vitamin D).**

The **cell-associated receptors** are the molecular entities primarily responsible for **recognizing the hormonal signal.** When the hormone binds to the receptor, the hormone–receptor complex initiates the events that culminate in the cellular response. These cell-associated hormone receptors can be classified into 2 main categories, nuclear receptors and cell-surface receptors. **Nuclear receptors** are intracellular **proteins present in either the cytosol or the nucleus** that bind hormones, which cross the cell membrane by simple diffusion. When **nuclear receptors** bind their cognate hormone, they undergo a **conformational change that enables them to bind to DNA at specific sites** called *cis*-**response elements.** When the hormone-nuclear receptor binds specifically to these response elements, they **influence transcription of the DNA genome into messenger RNA, either by activating or repressing it.**

**Cell-surface receptors,** as their name implies, **bind hormones on the extracellular side of the cell membrane.** When the hormone binds to its receptor on the cell surface, the **hormone-bound receptor either activates or forms a complex with a transducer protein in the membrane** that will cause the activation of some **enzymatic activity** in the cytoplasm of the cell. The enzymatic activity, sometimes called the **effector,** catalyzes the production of a second messenger that **mediates the intracellular response.**

Most transducer proteins that interact with cell-surface receptors are **GTP-binding proteins, commonly called G proteins.** G proteins typically are composed of **3 subunits:** $\alpha$, $\beta$, and $\gamma$. When the receptor is in the unbound state, all 3 subunits are bound together to form a heterotrimer that is in close association with the membrane-bound receptor.

**Figure 7-2.** Transduction by heterotrimeric G proteins.

In this state, GDP is bound to the α-subunit (Figure 7-2). Binding of the hormone by the receptor causes a conformational change such that the α-subunit is able to exchange the bound GDP for a molecule of GTP. The GTP-bound α-subunit separates from the βγ-dimer and can interact with the effector enzyme in either a stimulatory or inhibitory manner, depending on the nature of the α-subunit. Some different G protein families are presented in Table 7-1. **Common effector enzymes are adenylate cyclase, which converts ATP into 3′, 5′-cyclic AMP (cAMP) and phospholipase C (PLC),** which hydrolyzes the membrane lipid phosphatidylinositol-4,5-bisphosphate ($PIP_2$) to diacylglycerol and inositol-1,4,5-triphosphate ($IP_3$). While GTP is bound to the α-subunit, the interaction with the effector enzyme continues. However, the α-subunit also contains an intrinsic **GTPase activity** that will hydrolyze GTP to GDP and inorganic phosphate ($P_i$). This provides a mechanism by which the hormonal

| Table 7-1 • G-PROTEIN FAMILIES AND THEIR FUNCTIONS | | |
|---|---|---|
| **G Class** | **Initiating Signal** | **Downstream Signal** |
| $G_s$ | β-Adrenergic amines, glucagon, parathyroid hormone, thyrotropin (TSH), corticotrophin, many others | Stimulates adenylate cyclase |
| $G_i$ | Acetylcholine, α-adrenergic amines, many neurotransmitters, chemokines | Inhibits adenylate cyclase |
| $G_q$ | Acetylcholine, α-adrenergic amines, thyroid hormone receptor, many neurotransmitters | Increases $IP_3$ and intracellular calcium ion |
| $G_t$ (Transducin) | Photons | Stimulates cyclic guanosine monophosphate (cGMP) phosphodiesterase |

signal can be switched off, because GTP hydrolysis to GDP causes the α-subunit to release the effector enzyme and reassociate with the βγ subunits.

The hormonal cascade known as the **hypothalamic-pituitary-thyroid axis** employs **G-protein transducers that activate both adenylate cyclase and phospholipase C.** After receiving an electrochemical signal from the central nervous system (CNS), thyrotropin-releasing hormone (TRH) is released from the arcuate nucleus and median eminence of the **hypothalamus.** TRH is carried to the anterior pituitary via long portal vessels. In the anterior pituitary, **TRH binds to G protein–coupled TRH receptors on the cell surface of thyrotrophs.** This activates phospholipase C, releasing both DAG and $IP_3$. **DAG activates protein kinase C (PKC), which phosphorylates target proteins.** The release of $IP_3$ opens $Ca^{2+}$ channels in the endoplasmic reticulum, thus releasing $Ca^{2+}$ from storage and increasing cytoplasmic $[Ca^{2+}]$. Both of these events result in the increase in synthesis and release of thyrotropin, also known as TSH, which is stored in secretory granules within the thyrotroph. Circulating TSH binds to TSH receptors on the basolateral membranes of the thyroid follicular cell. The **TSH receptor is a G protein–coupled receptor that activates adenylate cyclase** to produce **cAMP** when hormone is bound. The **increase in cAMP triggers** a series of events within the follicular cell that result in the **secretion of the thyroid hormones thyroxine ($T_4$; 3,5,3′,5′-tetraiodo-L-thyronine) and 3,5, 3′α-triiodo-L-thyronine ($T_3$).** These events include increases in:

1. The transport of iodide ions across the basolateral membrane into the thyroid follicular cell via the Na/I cotransporter (NIS)

2. Iodination of tyrosine residues on colloidal thyroglobulin in the lumen of the follicle

3. Conjugation of iodinated tyrosines to form $T_3$ and $T_4$ on thyroglobulin

4. The endocytosis of thyroglobulin into the follicular cell from the lumen

5. The hydrolysis of thyroglobulin in the lysosome to release $T_3$ and $T_4$

6. The secretion of $T_3$ and $T_4$ into the bloodstream

Although the **thyroid hormones** are derived from amino acids, they **act in a fashion similar to that of the steroid hormones.** In the circulation, almost all of the thyroid hormones (99.98% of $T_4$ and 99.5% of $T_3$) are tightly bound to the proteins thyroxine-binding globulin (TBG), albumin, and transthyretin. However, the free, or "unbound," $T_3$ and $T_4$ **are responsible for the biologic effects** of the thyroid hormones. The **thyroid hormones enter the cell either by simple or carrier-mediated diffusion across the cell membrane.** Within the cytoplasm, approximately 50% of $T_4$ is deiodinated to form $T_3$. The **hormones enter the nucleus where they bind to the thyroid hormone receptor (THR).** The affinity of the THR is approximately 10 times greater for $T_3$ than it is for $T_4$, which is one reason why $T_3$ is more biologically active than $T_4$. When $T_3$ or $T_4$ bind to THR, the complex can bind to the thyroid response element of specific genes. The net effect of increased thyroid hormones is an increase in basal metabolic rate. This is accomplished by increasing the expression of genes that code for enzymes in both the **catabolic and anabolic pathways of** fats, carbohydrates, and proteins, as well as the expression of the Na-K pump. The careful regulation of thyroid hormone secretion is therefore important in the overall regulation of metabolism. Thus, $T_3$ and $T_4$ exert a negative feedback inhibition on the synthesis of TRH by the hypothalamus and the secretion of TSH by the anterior pituitary, so that the levels of $T_3$ and $T_4$ are tightly controlled.

Graves disease is an autoimmune disease in which the B lymphocytes synthesize Ig that binds to and activates the TSH receptor on the thyroid follicular cell membrane. This TSIg binds to and activates the TSH receptor in such a way that $T_3$ and $T_4$ do not feedback inhibit the receptor–effector interaction. Thus, all of the processes enumerated above that are sequelae of the TSH receptor–binding hormone are increased, resulting in a hyperthyroid condition.

Nonsurgical treatments for Graves disease include administration of thionamide antithyroid drugs, which include propylthiouracil (PTU) and methimazole, and/or treatment with radioactive iodine. The thionamides act by inhibiting the enzyme thyroid peroxidase, an enzyme on the apical membrane of the thyroid follicular cell that faces the lumen. This enzyme catalyzes the oxidation of iodide ion ($I^-$) to atomic iodine ($I^\circ$), which is required for the iodination of tyrosyl residues on thyroglobulin; these drugs decrease the amounts of $T_3$ and $T_4$ synthesized. They also decrease the amount of TSIg that is synthesized by mechanisms that are not understood. Radioactive iodine treatments cause the progressive destruction of thyroid cells, thus reducing thyroid function over a period of several weeks to months.

## COMPREHENSION QUESTIONS

7.1 The thyroid hormones $T_3$ and $T_4$ are synthesized in the follicular cells of the thyroid gland. From which of the following essential amino acids are the thyroid hormones synthesized?

A. Isoleucine
B. Lysine
C. Methionine
D. Phenylalanine
E. Valine

7.2 The thyroid hormones $T_3$ and $T_4$ bind to the THR in the target cells. Which of the following mechanisms best describes the role of the THR?

A. It activates adenylyl cyclase to produce cAMP.
B. It activates the phosphoinositide cascade.
C. It is a soluble guanylyl cyclase.
D. It is a tyrosine kinase.
E. It is a transcription factor.

7.3  A 26-year-old man presents complaining of heat intolerance, heavy sweating, tremulousness, and feeling "jittery inside." Physical examination reveals reddened conjunctiva and warm and moist palms, but the thyroid gland was not visibly enlarged. Which of the following tests would be most helpful to obtain an accurate diagnosis?

   A.  Electrocardiography
   B.  Free thyroxine level
   C.  Serum cortisol levels
   D.  Serum electrolytes
   E.  Serum glucose level

## ANSWERS

7.1  **D.** Thyroid hormones are synthesized from tyrosyl residues on thyroglobulin in the colloidal space of the thyroid follicular cells. Although tyrosine can be obtained from the diet, it can also be synthesized from the essential amino acid phenylalanine by the action of phenylalanine hydroxylase.

7.2  **E.** Thyroid hormones are similar to steroid hormones in that they bind to receptors in the nucleus of the cell. On binding to the receptor, the receptor–hormone complex binds to DNA affecting the transcription of messenger RNA.

7.3  **B.** This patient appears to have a hyperthyroid condition, even though the thyroid does not appear to be enlarged. Thyroid function tests would be most helpful to determine if this is the case. The free thyroxine level is a direct measure of the amount of free $T_4$, the biologically active $T_4$, in the serum. Elevation of the free $T_4$ indicates a hyperthyroid condition.

## BIOCHEMISTRY PEARLS

▶ Hormones bind to receptors, which can either be on the cell surface or, as in the case of steroid and similar hormones, within the cell.

▶ The hormone–receptor complex starts a series of events in which the signal is converted to other chemical forms that bring about changes in the biochemical reactions within the cell.

▶ Hormones that bind to cell–surface receptors activate or form a complex with a transducer protein in the membrane that will cause the activation of some enzymatic activity in the cytoplasm of the cell, producing a second messenger.

▶ Nuclear receptors are intracellular proteins present in either the cytosol or the nucleus that bind hormones (steroids), which cross the cell membrane by simple diffusion. The nuclear receptors undergo conformational changes that enable them to bind to DNA at specific sites.

# REFERENCES

Barrett EJ. The thyroid gland. In: Boron WF, Boulpaep EL, eds. *Medical Physiology: A Cellular and Molecular Approach.* 2nd ed. Philadelphia, PA: W.B. Saunders; 2011.

Farfel Z, Bourne HR, Iiri T. Mechanisms of disease: the expanding spectrum of G protein diseases. *N Engl J Med.* 1999;340(13):1012-1020.

Litwack G, Schmidt TJ. Biochemistry of hormones I: polypeptide hormones. In: Devlin TM, ed. *Textbook of Biochemistry with Clinical Correlations.* 7th ed. New York: Wiley-Liss; 2010.

A 3-year-old Caucasian boy is brought to the clinic for a chronic productive cough not responding to antibiotics given recently. He has no fever or sick contacts. His medical history is significant for abdominal distention, failure to pass stool, and emesis as an infant. He continues to have bulky, foul-smelling stools. No diarrhea is present. He has several relatives with chronic lung and "stomach" problems, and some have even died at a young age. The examination reveals an ill appearing, slender boy in moderate distress. Lung examination reveals poor air movement in the base of lungs bilateral and coarse rhonchi throughout both lung fields. A chloride sweat test was performed and was positive. What is the most likely diagnosis?

▶ What is the mechanism of the disease?
▶ How might gel electrophoresis assist in making the diagnosis?

# ANSWERS TO CASE 8:
## Cystic Fibrosis

*Summary:* A 3-year-old Caucasian boy has a history of chronic pulmonary and gastrointestinal problems and has a positive chloride sweat test. A family history of similar symptoms is also present.

- **Likely diagnosis:** Cystic fibrosis

- **Mechanism of disease:** Autosomal recessive disorder resulting in defective chloride ion channels of exocrine glands and epithelial tissues of the pancreas, sweat glands, and mucous glands in the respiratory, digestive, and reproductive tracts.

- **Gel electrophoresis:** Separates DNA chains of varying length and can allow identification of a specific gene sequences.

## CLINICAL CORRELATION

Cystic fibrosis is an inherited condition affecting approximately 1 in 2500 Caucasian individuals. Affected patients usually have abnormal mucous secretion and eccrine sweat glands leading to respiratory infections, gastrointestinal obstruction, pancreatic enzyme dysfunction, which in turn leads to malabsorption of nutrients, and excessive electrolyte secretion. The protein cystic fibrosis transmembrane conductance regulator (CFTR) is defective, leading to abnormal chloride transport. Approximately 70% of mutations are accounted for by deletion of 3 specific base pairs at the F 508 position of the CFTR. Oligonucleotide probes can be used to assay for this mutation, but other tests are required for the less common mutations.

# APPROACH TO:
## Gel Electrophoresis and Cloning

### OBJECTIVES

1. Understand the process of gel electrophoresis.

2. Know the difference between various types of blots.

3. Be familiar with DNA sequencing using the Sanger dideoxynucleotide method.

4. Understand the process and uses of cloning DNA.

### DEFINITIONS

**BLOTTING:** The transfer of proteins or nucleic acids from an electrophoresis gel to a membrane support (such as nitrocellulose or nylon). The membrane blot is then incubated with probes that bind the molecules of interest.

**COMPLEMENTARY DNA (CDNA):** A sequence of DNA copied from messenger RNA (mRNA), which does not contain introns present in native DNA.

**CFTR:** Cystic fibrosis transmembrane conductance regulator; a ligand-gated chloride channel regulated by phosphorylation. It is a member of the adenine nucleotide binding cassette (ABC) family of transport proteins.

**ELECTROPHORESIS:** The technique by which charged molecules in solution are separated in an electric field according to their different mobilities in the supporting medium.

**GEL ELECTROPHORESIS:** Electrophoresis using a gel as the supporting medium. Common gels are polyacrylamide and agarose.

**NORTHERN BLOT:** The technique by which molecules of RNA are separated by gel electrophoresis, transferred to a membrane support, and incubated with labeled oligonucleotide probes. Specificity is obtained by using oligonucleotide probes that have sequences complementary to the target RNA.

**SOUTHERN BLOT:** The technique by which molecules of DNA are separated by gel electrophoresis, transferred to a membrane support, and incubated with labeled oligonucleotide probes. Specificity is obtained by using oligonucleotide probes that have sequences complementary to the target DNA.

**WESTERN BLOT:** The technique by which protein molecules are separated by gel electrophoresis, transferred to a membrane support, and incubated with labeled antibodies. Specificity is obtained using antibodies that will bind the protein molecule of interest.

## DISCUSSION

Cystic fibrosis is the most common lethal autosomal recessive disease affecting the Caucasian population. It has a frequency of approximately 1 in 2500 and a carrier frequency of approximately 1 in 25. The protein affected is the CFTR, which is a chloride ion channel. There are more than 1000 mutations that have been discovered in the *CFTR* gene and more than 80% of these mutations lead to disease. The mutations lead to (1) defective or decreased protein production, (2) defective processing of the protein, (3) protein defective in the regulation of the chloride channel, or (4) defect in the transport of chloride ions. The most common mutation, a deletion of a phenylalanine residue at amino acid position 508 ($\Delta;F_{508}$), results in misfolding of the protein; it consequently does not traffic to the membrane.

Defects in the CFTR decrease the ability of cells to transport $Cl^-$ in a number of tissues, particularly the pancreas, airway epithelia, and sweat glands. When $Cl^-$ transport is defective in the pancreas, it leads to decreased $HCO_3^-$ secretion and decreased hydration that leads to thick secretions that block the pancreatic ducts and destruction of the organ. In the lungs, the decreased absorption of $Cl^-$ ions is thought to increase the absorption of the airway surface liquid thus increasing the viscosity of mucous, decreasing mucociliary clearance and increasing the incidence of airway infections. In sweat glands, defects in CFTR prevent the reabsorption of

Cl⁻ in the sweat gland duct, thus increasing the concentration of NaCl in sweat. The presence of salty sweat in children with cystic fibrosis gives rise to the northern Europe adage: "Woe to that child which when kissed on the forehead tastes salty. He is bewitched and soon must die."

**Gel electrophoresis** is a method routinely used in biochemistry and molecular biology to **separate, identify, and purify peptides, proteins, and DNA fragments based on their size. Electrophoresis** is a method by which **charged molecules in a solution are separated in an electric field because of their different mobilities.** The **mobility of an ion** in the electric field is dependent on the **charge of the ionized molecule, the voltage gradient of the electric field, and the frictional resistance** of the supporting **medium.** The supporting medium of choice for most protein and peptide analyses, as well as small DNA fragments, is **polyacrylamide gel.** For large DNA fragments, **agarose gel** gives the best results.

In general, **DNA molecules have a high negative charge-to-mass ratio** owing to their **sugar-phosphate backbone.** Therefore, when an electric field is applied, **DNA** will **migrate** through the agarose (or polyacrylamide) gel **toward the positive pole** in the electrophoresis apparatus. Because of the high charge-to-mass ratio, the relative electrophoretic mobility of DNA depends primarily on the size of the DNA molecule and porosity of the gel matrix, which can be varied by the concentration of agarose or polyacrylamide in the gel. **Small DNA strands will move fast, whereas large fragments will lag behind smaller fragments** as the DNA migrates through the gel. To estimate the size of DNA in the samples, molecular weight markers (a mixture of DNA fragments of known molecular size) are applied to one of the lanes in the gel. Gel electrophoresis separates DNA molecules based on their frictional coefficient, which is dependent on the length and conformation of the fragment. For most linear double-stranded DNA molecules, separation will be according to their molecular weight. However, **circular DNA molecules** (eg, from bacteria or plasmids) can adopt a super **coiled structure and therefore will pass through the gel with less resistance than the rod shape of linear DNA.**

Gel electrophoresis can be applied as a method for detection of genetic diseases such as cystic fibrosis. Larger deletions in the *CFTR* **gene** will cause it to move differently than the full-length wild type gene. In most cases, the DNA sample of the patient is amplified by a polymerase chain reaction (PCR) using specific primers. After the electrophoresis of the PCR samples, the bands are **visualized under ultraviolet (UV) light using ethidium bromide staining.**

Bands of molecules separated by electrophoresis can be detected in the gel by various staining and destaining methods, such as the above mentioned ethidium bromide. However, more specific information can be obtained by application of **blotting** techniques. There are 3 different blotting techniques based on whether DNA, RNA, or protein is being analyzed. However, **all blotting techniques have major steps in common.** These include (1) the **isolation of the biomolecules of interest** (DNA, RNA, or protein), (2) **separation of the mixture using gel electrophoresis**, and (3) subsequent transfer **of the sample molecules from the gel to a nitrocellulose or nylon membrane.** The final identification step involves **incubation of the membrane blot with probes** that bind specifically to the molecule of interest. DNA is analyzed using **Southern blotting,** named after E.M. Southern, who first described this procedure in 1975. Based on this initial terminology, **Northern and Western** blotting were given as names referring to RNA and protein-blotting transfer, respectively. The major difference between the procedures involves the probes used for detection and identification of the molecules of interest. **Southern and Northern blots take advantage of the ability of complementary nucleic acid strands to hybridize.**

In a Southern blot, after the DNA fragments have been transferred from the electrophoretic gel to the membrane, they are allowed to interact with a single-stranded DNA oligonucleotide that contains the sequence of nucleic acids in the gene of interest. The **oligonucleotide probe is usually radioactively labeled,** which allows the DNA band to be identified following exposure to x-ray film. **Northern blots are used to monitor the expression of a gene of interest by determining the amount of mRNA present.** Then the mRNA is isolated, separated by electrophoresis, and, after transfer to a membrane, is allowed to interact with a **radioactive DNA polynucleotide** that has a sequence of the gene of interest. **Visualization is by exposure to x-ray film.** In the case of a **Western blot** of a protein mixture, after the proteins have been transferred to the membrane, the membrane is **probed with an antibody that binds specifically to the target protein/antigen.** The antibody may be radioactive or coupled to a fluorescent chromophore to allow easy detection.

The ability to sequence DNA and analyze genes at the nucleotide level has become a powerful tool in many areas of analysis and research. The **Sanger dideoxynucleotide method of DNA sequencing** was first developed in 1975 by Frederick Sanger, after whom the technique was named. The strategy used in this method is to create **4 sets of labeled fragments, corresponding to the 4 deoxyribonucleotides.** It involves the enzymatic duplication of a DNA strand that is complementary to the strand of interest. In the Sanger method, **2′,3′-dideoxyribonucleotide triphosphates (ddNTPs) are used** in addition to deoxyribonucleotide triphosphates (dNTPs). Because the **ddNTPs lack the 3′-OH group, they will terminate DNA chain elongation** because they cannot form a phosphodiester bond with the next dNTP. Each of the 4 sequencing reaction tubes (A, C, G, and T) would then contain a single-stranded DNA template; a primer sequence; DNA polymerase to initiate synthesis where primer is hybridized to the template; mixture of the 4 deoxyribonucleotide triphosphates (dATP, dTTP, dCTP, and dGTP) to extend the DNA strand; one labeled dNTP (using a radioactive element or dye); and one ddNTP, which terminates the growing chain wherever it is incorporated. **Tube A would have ddATP, tube C ddCTP, and so forth.** Because the concentration of the ddNTP is low (approximately 1% of dNTP), the **chain will terminate randomly at various positions throughout the chain,** thus yielding an array of different length DNA fragments each terminated with the particular dideoxyribonucleotide. The **fragments of varying length are then separated by electrophoresis in parallel lanes** (each corresponding to the 4 deoxyribonucleotides) and the positions of the fragments analyzed to determine the sequence. The fragments are separated on the basis of size, with the shorter fragments moving faster and appearing at the bottom of the gel. The **sequence is then read from bottom to the top, yielding the 5′ to 3′ sequence.**

The ability to rapidly sequence DNA has become an important tool for molecular biology. For example, the PCR method needs the information of the sequence flanking the region of interest to be able to design **specific oligonucleotides (primers) to amplify the specific DNA region.** Another important use is identifying restriction sites in plasmids, which is useful in cloning a foreign gene into the plasmid. Before DNA sequencing, molecular biologists had to sequence proteins directly, which was a challenging and laborious process. Now amino acid sequences can be determined more easily by **sequencing a piece of cDNA and finding an open reading frame.** In eukaryotic gene expression, sequencing made it possible to identify conserved sequence motifs and determine important sites in the promoter regions. Furthermore, sequencing can be used to identify the site of a point mutation or other changes in the genome.

Recombinant DNA technology allows for a **transfer of a DNA fragment of interest into a self-replicating genetic element such as a bacterial plasmid or virus.** This technology has allowed many human genes to be cloned in *Escherichia coli*, yeast, or even mammalian cells, leading to easy production of human recombinant proteins in vitro. These include insulin for patients with diabetes, factor VIII for males with hemophilia A, human growth hormone (GH), erythropoietin (EPO) for treating anemia, 3 types of interferons, several interleukins, adenosine deaminase (ADA) for treating some forms of severe combined immunodeficiency (SCID), angiostatin and endostatin for trials as anticancer drugs, and parathyroid hormone with many more in development.

Efforts toward gene therapy make use of recombinant DNA technology. In the case of cystic fibrosis, which is the result of a defect in a single gene, direct insertion of the normal gene should theoretically restore the function of CFTR in the treated cells of the patient with cystic fibrosis. Because **respiratory failure is the major cause of deaths (95%) in cystic fibrosis,** lung cells have become the primary target for efforts at treating cystic fibrosis with gene therapy. Another advantage is the ability of delivering vectors containing the functional *CFTR* gene directly into the patient's airways by aerosol, without causing trauma to any other part of the body. To date, **trials of cystic fibrosis rely on adenovirus, adeno-associated virus (AAV), and cationic liposomes to mediate gene transfer** to nasal epithelial cells and respiratory epithelial cells. Adenoviruses do not integrate into the host chromosome; therefore, the vectors derived from these viruses have the advantage of negligible oncogenic potential. The disadvantages are the development of inflammation and the transient expression of the recombinant genes. Adeno-associated viruses are unique among animal viruses, because they require coinfection with an unrelated helper virus (either adenovirus or herpesvirus) for productive infection in cell culture. However, AAV has the ability to integrate into the host genome in the absence of a helper virus, but because it integrates at a specific location, the risk of virus-induced mutagenesis and oncogenesis is reduced. However, **liposomes** are synthetic lipid bilayers forming spherical vesicles, with size ranging from 25 nm to 1 mm in diameter depending on how they are made. Liposomes can transfect a variety of cell types, are biodegradable and hypoimmunogenic, and can be manufactured to a drug standard. Theoretically, there is no restriction on the size of the DNA to be delivered by liposome. The disadvantages are short-term expression of the transferred gene, no specific targeting ability, and a low transfection rate in vivo.

## COMPREHENSION QUESTIONS

8.1  A 30-month-old child whose growth rate has been in the lower tenth percentile over the last year presents with chronic, nonproductive cough and diarrhea with foul-smelling stools. She is diagnosed as having cystic fibrosis. For which of the following vitamins is this child most likely to be at risk of deficiency?

A.  Ascorbic acid (vitamin C)

B.  Biotin

C.  Folic acid

D.  Retinol (vitamin A)

E.  Riboflavin (vitamin $B_2$)

8.2  Some forms of genetic diseases such as cystic fibrosis and sickle cell anemia can be diagnosed by detecting restriction fragment length polymorphisms (RFLPs). Which of the following is most likely to be used in RFLP analysis?

A.  Dideoxynucleotides

B.  Mass spectrometry

C.  Northern blot

D.  Southern blot

E.  Western blot

8.3  Your patient has been diagnosed with cystic fibrosis and has been determined to have the most common mutation, the $\Delta;F_{508}$ gene. Which of the following is the most cost- and time-effective method for testing family members to see who are carriers of the mutation?

A.  Allele-specific oligonucleotide probe analysis

B.  DNA fingerprinting analysis

C.  DNA sequencing

D.  Restriction length fragment polymorphism analysis

## ANSWERS

8.1  **D.** Because cystic fibrosis leads to pancreatic damage and diminution of the ability to secrete $HCO_3^-$ and pancreatic digestive enzymes with the result that fat and protein are properly absorbed. Retinol is a fat-soluble vitamin that must be absorbed along with lipid micelles; other fat-soluble vitamins are E, D, and K. The other vitamins listed are water-soluble and their absorption is not significantly affected.

8.2  **D.** Restriction length fragment polymorphism analysis detects mutations in the DNA that either introduce or eliminate a recognition site for a restriction enzyme. This is detected by performing a Southern blot analysis on patient DNA after incubation with a specific restriction enzyme and comparing it to one performed on DNA obtained from a normal gene.

8.3 **A.** If the mutation is known, then radioactive or fluorescent probes can be produced for alleles that contain the mutation and for those that have a normal DNA sequence. The samples of DNA are spotted onto nitrocellulose paper in narrow bands. The paper is then incubated with the probe either for the normal or the mutant sequence. Because it does not involve an electrophoresis step, this type of analysis is less time consuming (and less expensive).

## BIOCHEMISTRY PEARLS

▶ Northern blot uses oligonucleotide probes to identify RNA, Southern blot identifies DNA, and Western blot identifies protein molecules.

▶ Recombinant DNA technology allows for a transfer of a DNA fragment of interest into a self-replicating genetic element such as a bacterial plasmid or virus.

▶ Restriction length fragment polymorphism analysis detects mutations in the DNA that either introduce or eliminate a recognition site for a restriction enzyme.

▶ Oligonucleotide probes can be directed against precise DNA sequences and yields a quick and accurate result.

## REFERENCES

Schwiebert LM. Cystic fibrosis, gene therapy, and lung inflammation: for better or worse? *Am J Physiol Lung Cell Mol Physiol*. 2004;286(4):L715-L716.

Welsh MJ, Ramsey BW, Accurso F, et al. Cystic fibrosis. In: Sriver CR, Beaudet AL, Sly WS, et al, eds. *The Metabolic & Molecular Bases of Inherited Disease*. 8th ed. New York: McGraw-Hill; 2001.

A 40-year-old man returned from a deer-hunting trip approximately 6 weeks ago and presents to clinic with multiple complaints. He states that recently he has had worsening joint pain and "arthritis" in multiple joints that seems to move to different spots. Patient also complains of some numbness in his feet bilaterally. The patient denies any medical problems and he had a normal annual physical examination prior to hunting trip. Upon further questioning, he remembered having a rash on his body and the lesions were circular and appeared to be resolving in the center. He noted that he felt really bad once he got home with muscle ache (myalgias), joint ache (arthralgias), stiff neck, and severe headache. He also remembered that many of his hunting friends had experienced flea and tick bites and is quite sure he was bitten as well. The physical examination is essentially normal except some joint tenderness of left knee and right shoulder. After making your diagnosis you gave him a prescription for erythromycin.

▶ What is the most likely diagnosis?
▶ What is the biochemical mechanism of action of erythromycin?

# ANSWERS TO CASE 9:

## Erythromycin and Lyme Disease

*Summary:* A 40-year-old man who presents with migrating arthralgias and neuro-logic changes, which were preceded by a centrally clearing circular rash, myalgias, and headache after a hunting trip where he was exposed to fleas and ticks.

- **Diagnosis:** Lyme disease
- **Biochemical site of action of erythromycin:** Inhibits bacterial protein biosynthe-sis at the translocation step of translation.

## CLINICAL CORRELATION

Lyme disease is a multisystem disease caused by the spirochete (spiral-shaped bacte-ria), *Borrelia burgdorferi*, nearly always transmitted by tick bite. Lyme disease is much more common in the New England area, usually during the late spring and early summer months. The deer tick is the main vector of transmission. The first stage is an acute infection with a red papule developing at the site of the bite, sometimes with lymphadenopathy and fever. The second stage includes disseminated infection and can lead to involvement of the heart, brain, joints, and skin. The typical target-shaped skin lesions may be seen. The third stage is a chronic infection and may last for years. Antibiotics are the treatment of choice, usually tetracyclines or penicillins.

# APPROACH TO:

## Protein Biosynthesis

## OBJECTIVES

1. Understand protein biosynthesis (initiation, elongation, translocation, termi-nation).

2. Know key differences between prokaryotic and eukaryotic protein synthesis.

3. Know the role of ribosomal RNA (rRNA).

4. Know the mechanism of action of different antibiotics with protein biosyn-thesis.

## DEFINITIONS

**A-SITE:** The acceptor site on the ribosome into which an aminoacyl-charged trans-fer RNA (tRNA) is brought that has an anticodon that is complementary to the messenger RNA (mRNA) codon. The ribosome will then catalyze the formation of a peptide bond with the aminoacyl group on this tRNA and the growing peptide chain.

**ANTICODON:** The 3-base sequence on a tRNA that will base pair with the 3-base sequence on the mRNA. The anticodon is specific for an amino acid; it translates the DNA sequence into an amino acid sequence in the protein produced.

**CODON:** The 3-base sequence of an mRNA that code for a particular amino acid.

**ELONGATION FACTORS:** Proteins required for bringing the aminoacyl-tRNA to the A-site, codon recognition, and translocation of the newly elongated peptidyl-tRNA from the A-site to the P-site.

**INITIATION FACTORS:** Proteins required for assembly of the ribosomal complex with mRNA and Met-tRNA so that protein synthesis can proceed.

**NUCLEOLAR ORGANIZING REGION (NOR):** Area of the nucleolus where a great deal of rRNA transcription and synthesis occurs.

**P-SITE:** The peptidyl site on the ribosome to which Met-tRNA is brought to base pair with the mRNA sequence AUG. It is also the site to which the peptidyl RNA is moved in a process known as translocation following the formation of a new peptide bond.

**POST-TRANSCRIPTION MODIFICATION OF tRNA:** The synthesis of tRNA involves modification of some uridine nucleotides to unusual nucleotides, such as pseudouridine, ribothymidine, and dihydrouridine.

**RIBOSOMES:** Complexes of proteins and rRNA on which protein synthesis occurs. There are 2 major subunits to all ribosomes, a larger subunit (50S for prokaryotes, 60S for eukaryotes) and a smaller subunit (30S for prokaryotes, 40S for eukaryotes).

## DISCUSSION

The **synthesis of proteins** involves **converting the nucleotide sequence of specific regions of DNA into mRNA (*transcription*)** followed by the **formation of peptide bonds** in a complex set of reactions that occur on **ribosomes (*translation*).** The amino acids incorporated into the protein are first **activated by being attached to a family of tRNA molecules,** each of which recognizes, by **complementary base-pairing interactions,** particular sets of **3 nucleotides (codons) in the mRNA.** Proteins are synthesized on ribosomes by linking amino acids together in the specific linear order stipulated by the sequence of codons in an mRNA. **Ribosomes are compact ribonucleoprotein particles found in the cytosol of all cells. All ribosomes are composed of a small and a large subunit.** The 2 subunits contain rRNAs of different lengths, as well as a different set of proteins. **All ribosomes consist of 2 major rRNA molecules** (23S and 16S rRNA in bacteria, 28S and 18S rRNA in eukaryotes) and 1 **or 2 small RNAs.** Small and large subunits are brought together by an mRNA molecule and protein synthesis starts immediately. After the protein is synthesized, the ribosomal subunits separate and are reused.

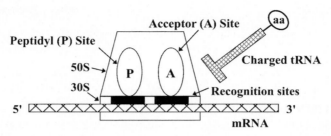

**Figure 9-1.** Various sites of antibiotic action in protein synthesis.

Protein synthesis is divided into 3 stages: initiation, elongation, and termination.

*Chain initiation:* Initiation requires the smaller ribosomal subunit, an initiation tRNA (with a 5'-CAU-3' anticodon), mRNA with its initiator codon (5'-AUG-3'), and several initiation factors, all of which form the ribosomal initiation complex. The initiation complex is near completion when a **tRNA carrying the amino acid methionine hydrogen bonds to the AUG codon on the mRNA.** When these components are in place, the larger ribosomal subunit joins the complex in such a way that the initiator met-tRNA$_{met}$ is localized in the P- or peptidyl site (Figure 9-1). The chain initiation phase ends and a second amino acid can be inserted.

*Chain elongation:* **Elongation** occurs by bringing an **aminoacyl-charged tRNA to the A- or acceptor site,** followed by **formation of the peptide bond and the translocation of a tRNA from the A- to the P-site.** Proteins called elongation factors are the workhorses in the process of elongating the nascent polypeptide chain by 1 amino acid at a time. Translation elongation factors are involved in the following 3-step cycle:

1. **Codon recognition:** A hydrogen bond forms between the mRNA codon and the anticodon of the next aminoacyl tRNA at the empty A-site of the ribosome.

2. **Peptide bond formation:** An enzyme called peptidyl transferase embedded in the large ribosomal subunit catalyzes the formation of a peptide bond between the polypeptide of the peptidyl-tRNA in the P-site and the newly arrived aminoacyl tRNA in the A-site.

3. **Translocation:** The tRNA in the P-site is ejected so that the newly formed peptidyl-tRNA located in the A-site can shift over to the P-site freeing up the A-site for the next aminoacyl-charged tRNA.

*Chain termination:* **Elongation comes to an end** when 1 (or more) of 3 **stop codons (UAA, UAG, UGA) is encountered.** A protein called a release factor binds directly to the termination codon in the A-site. The newly synthesized protein is hydrolyzed from the tRNA and both the tRNA and the protein are released from the ribosome.

A list of key differences between prokaryotes and eukaryotes with respect to protein synthesis is shown in Table 9-1. These include the existence of multiple eukaryotic initiation factors that facilitate the assembly of the ribosomal protein synthetic machinery, whereas there are **only 3 for prokaryotes.** An **initiation site**

| Table 9-1 • DIFFERENCES IN PROKARYOTIC AND EUKARYOTIC PROTEIN SYNTHESIS | | |
|---|---|---|
| ORGANISM | PROKARYOTE | EUKARYOTE |
| Start | fMet-tRNA$_f^{Met}$ | Met-tRNA$_i^{Met}$ |
| Recognition sequence | Shine-Dalgarno sequence | 5′ caps direct e-Ifs |
| Initiation factors (IFs) | IF-1, IF-2, IF-3 | Multiple e-IFs (>10) |
| Elongation factors (EFs) | EF-Tu, EF-G, EF-Ts | Multisubunit eEF-1, eEF-2, eEF-3 |

on bacterial mRNA consists of the AUG initiation codon preceded with a gap of approximately 10 bases by the Shine-Dalgarno polypurine hexamer, whereas the 5′ Cap (a 7-methylguanylate residue in a 5′→5′ triphosphate linkage) acts as an initiation signal in eukaryotes. In prokaryotes, the first or N-terminal amino acid is a formyl-methionine (fMet), but in eukaryotes it is usually a simple methionine. In addition, the size and nature of the prokaryotic ribosomes are quite different from the eukaryotic ribosomes.

rRNA is a component of the ribosomes, the protein synthesis factories in the cell. rRNA molecules are extremely abundant, making up at least 80% of the RNA molecules found in a typical eukaryotic cell. Virtually all ribosomal proteins are in contact with rRNA. Most of the contacts between ribosomal subunits are made between the 16S and 23S rRNAs such that the interactions involving rRNA are a key part of ribosome function. The environment of the tRNA-binding sites is largely determined by rRNA. The rRNA molecules have several roles in protein synthesis. 16S rRNA plays an active role in the functions of the 30S subunit. It interacts directly with mRNA, with the 50S subunit, and with the anticodons of tRNAs in the P- and A-sites. Peptidyl transferase activity resides exclusively in the 23S rRNA. Finally, the rRNA molecules have a structural role. They fold into 3-dimensional shapes that form the scaffold on which the ribosomal proteins assemble.

Many antibiotics act to inhibit protein synthesis in prokaryotes without affecting eukaryotic cells much. Several important targets in protein synthesis have been identified that are blocked by these agents to curb microorganism growth (see Figure 9-1). Aminoglycosides interfere with binding of fMet-tRNA to the ribosome, thereby preventing correct initiation of protein synthesis and partially freezing the complex. By contrast, Puromycin causes premature termination of protein synthesis because it resembles tyrosyl-tRNA. It can bind to the A-site on the ribosome, and the peptidyl transferase will form a peptide bond between the growing peptide and puromycin. However, since there is no anticodon to bind to the mRNA, the peptidyl-puromycin is released from the ribosome following formation of the peptide bond, thus stopping the synthesis. Tetracyclines inhibit protein synthesis in bacteria by blocking the A-site on the ribosome and inhibiting binding of aminoacyl tRNAs. Macrolides (see below) bind to the 50S subunit near the P-site to cause conformational changes and inhibit translocation of the peptidyl tRNA from the A-site to the P-site. Lincosamides bind near the P-site and interfere with binding of the aminoacyl end of the AA-tRNA. They occupy the site or change the ribosomal conformation such that it destabilizes the ribosomes and the growing chains fall off the mRNA. *Chloramphenicol* inhibits protein synthesis by bacterial ribosomes by blocking peptidyl transfer. It inhibits peptide bond formation between AA-tRNA and the growing chain on the *P*-site by inhibiting peptidyl transferase. *Neomycin, kanamycin,* and *gentamicin* interfere with the decoding site in the vicinity of nucleotide 1400 in 16S rRNA of 30S subunit. This region interacts with the wobble base in the anticodon of tRNA and blocks self-splicing of group I introns. *Streptomycin*, a basic trisaccharide, causes misreading of the genetic code in bacteria at relatively low concentrations but can inhibit initiation at higher concentrations.

Macrolide antibiotics constitute a group of 12- to 16-membered lactone rings substituted with 1 or more sugar residues, some of which may be amino sugars. Macrolides such as erythromycin (Figure 9-2) are generally bacteriostatic, although some of these drugs are bactericidal only at very high concentrations. Gram-positive bacteria accumulate approximately 100 times more erythromycin than do gram-negative microorganisms. Cells are considerably more permeable to the nonionized form of the drug, which explains increased antimicrobial activity observed at alkaline pH. The newer macrolides have structural modifications, such as methylation of the nitrogen atom in the lactone ring, that improve acid stability and tissue penetration of these agents. Macrolides act by binding reversibly to the ribosomal subunits of sensitive microorganisms and thereby inhibiting protein synthesis. Resistance to macrolides in clinical isolates is most frequently a result of posttranscriptional methylation of an adenine residue of 23S ribosomal RNA, which leads to coresistance to macrolides. Other mechanisms of resistance involving cell impermeability or drug inactivation have also been detected. It is believed that erythromycin does not inhibit peptide bond formation directly but rather inhibits the translocation step wherein a newly synthesized peptidyl tRNA molecule moves from the acceptor site on the ribosome to the peptidyl or donor site. Erythromycin, which does not reach the peptidyl transferase center, induces dissociation of peptidyl tRNAs containing 6, 7, or 8 amino acid residues.

Figure 9-2. Chemical structure of erythromycin.

## COMPREHENSION QUESTIONS

In questions 9.1 to 9.3, for each of the following steps in prokaryotic protein synthesis, indicate the most appropriate antibiotic (A-J) to inhibit the process.

    A.  Aminoglycosides

    B.  Chloramphenicol

    C.  Erythromycin

    D.  Gentamicin

    E.  Kanamycin

    F.  Lincosamides

    G.  Neomycin

    H.  Puromycin

    I.  Streptomycin

    J.  Tetracycline

9.1  Transfer of the peptide from the peptidyl tRNA to the aminoacyl-tRNA and formation of a peptide bond.

9.2  Binding of aminoacyl-tRNA in the A-site of the ribosomal complex.

9.3  Translocation of the peptidyl tRNA from the A-site to the P-site.

9.4  The 6-year-old son of a migrant worker is brought to a clinic with chills, headache, nausea, vomiting, and sore throat. The examining physician notes a persistent grayish colored membrane near the tonsils. History reveals that the patient has not been immunized against diphtheria. Diphtheria toxin is potentially lethal in this unimmunized patient because it causes which of the following?

    A.  Inactivates an elongation factor required for translocation in protein synthesis

    B.  Binds to the ribosome and prevents peptide bond formation

    C.  Prevents binding of mRNA to the 60S ribosomal subunit

    D.  Inactivates an initiation factor

    E.  Inhibits the synthesis of aminoacyl-charged tRNA

9.5  Replication of a particular DNA sequence is noted to be under inhibitory control usually. However, when substance "A" is added, it binds to a repressor, rendering the repressor inactive and allowing transcription to occur. Which of the following terms describes agent "A"?

    A.  Histone

    B.  Operon

    C.  Polymerase

    D.  Transcriber

    E.  Inducer

# ANSWERS

9.1 **B.** Chloramphenicol inhibits protein synthesis by inhibiting peptidyl transferase. This peptidyl group cannot be transferred to the aminoacyl-tRNA in the A-site.

9.2 **J.** Tetracyclines bind to the A-site of the prokaryotic ribosome and prevent aminoacyl-tRNAs from binding. Thus, protein synthesis is halted because new amino acids cannot be added to the growing protein.

9.3 **C.** Erythromycin and other macrolide antibiotics bind the 50S subunit near the P-site and cause conformational changes that inhibit the translocation of peptidyl tRNA from the A-site to the P-site.

9.4 **A.** Diphtheria toxin has 2 subunits. The B subunit binds to a cell surface receptor and facilitates the entry of the A subunit into the cell. The A subunit then catalyzes the ADP-ribosylation of elongation factor 2 (EF2). Thus, EF2 is inhibited from participating in the translocation process of protein synthesis; hence, protein synthesis stops.

9.5 **E.** An inducer is a small molecule that binds to and inactivates a repressor, which allows the sequence of DNA to be transcribed. An operon is a set of prokaryotic genes in close proximity that are coordinated as "all off" or "all on." An inducer may act to "turn on" the operon. One classic example is the *lac operon*. When allolactose is present, it serves as an inducer, and the operon is turned on, allowing proteins to be formed that metabolize lactose.

## BIOCHEMISTRY PEARLS

▶ The synthesis of proteins involves converting the nucleotide sequence of specific regions of DNA into mRNA (*transcription*), followed by the formation of peptide bonds in a complex set of reactions that occur on ribosomes (*translation*).

▶ Protein synthesis is divided into 3 stages: initiation, elongation, and termination.

▶ rRNA is a component of the ribosomes, the protein synthesis factories in the cell.

▶ Many antibiotics take advantage of the differences of the rRNA between eukaryotic and prokaryotic cells.

# REFERENCES

Alberts B, Johnson A, Lewis J, et al. *Molecular Biology of the Cell.* 5th ed. New York and London: Garland; 2007.

Lodish H, Berk A, Kaiser CA, et al. *Molecular Cell Biology.* 7th ed. New York: Freeman; 2012.

Petri WA. Anti-microbial agents. In: Goodman AG, Gilman LS, eds. *The Pharmacological Basis of Therapeutics.* 10th ed. New York: McGraw-Hill; 2001.

Prescott LM, Harley JP, Klein DA. *Microbiology.* 3rd ed. Boston, MA: W.C. Brown; 1996.

Voet D, Voet JG, Pratt CW. *Fundamentals of Biochemistry.* Upgrade ed. New York: John Wiley; 2002.

A 4-day-old male infant presents to the emergency department with vomiting and increasing lethargy. The patient was healthy at birth and experienced no delivery complications. The infant's feeding patterns have deteriorated over the previous 2 days and the parents deny any trauma. Upon examination, the patient is afebrile and his urine has a sweet odor. Alternating muscular hypotonia and hypertonia is observed. Computed tomography of the head reveals cerebral edema. Lumbar puncture results show clear cerebrospinal fluid (CSF), containing 4 WBC per high power field, no RBC, 45 mg% of protein, 46 mg% of sugar, and no bacteria in Gram stain smears. The CSF culture is negative. Ketone bodies and keto acids are detected in the urine. Serum analysis reveals elevated levels of branched-chain amino acids.

► What is the most likely diagnosis?
► What is the molecular mechanism behind this disorder?
► What is the pathophysiologic mechanism of his symptoms?

# ANSWERS TO CASE 10:

## Maple Syrup Urine Disease

*Summary:* A 4-day-old male infant with a history of poor feeding, signs consistent with encephalopathy, and laboratory evidence of metabolic dysfunction.

- **Most likely diagnosis:** Maple syrup urine disease (MSUD)

- **Molecular mechanism of disease:** Mutation in one or more of the subunits of the branched-chain α-ketoacid dehydrogenase complex (BCKD), inherited in an autosomal recessive manner.

- **Pathophysiologic mechanism of symptoms:** The dysfunctional enzyme complex is unable to degrade branched-chain amino acids (BCAAs), resulting in an accumulation of, among others, leucine. This leads to acute hyperosmolarity and cerebral edema.

### CLINICAL CORRELATION

MSUD is an autosomal recessive disorder caused by a dysfunctional BCKD unable to degrade BCAAs such as leucine, isoleucine, and valine. Elevated levels of leucine in the plasma and organs effects regulation of cellular volume leading to cerebral edema and the other neurologic problems (hypotonia/hypertonia). The characteristic urine odor is the result of elevated isoleucine metabolite found in the urine.

MSUD classically appears newborns; however, there are some forms of the disease that may present later. The diagnosis is confirmed by elevated plasma BCAAs and their metabolites. Newborn screening is also available immediately after birth. Treatment involves diet modification (limiting intake of BCAAs) and early recognition of metabolic decompensation with appropriate intervention.

# APPROACH TO:

## Maple Syrup Urine Disease

### OBJECTIVES

1. Describe the normal structure and function of the BCKD complex.

2. Explain how structure and function of the BCKD complex are altered in MSUD.

3. Relate the function of amino acid ratio maintenance in the brain to pathologic changes in MSUD.

### DEFINITIONS

**AUTOSOMAL MUTATION:** A genetic mutation that equally affects males and females. The chromosome affected is not a sex chromosome.

**BRANCHED-CHAIN AMINO ACID (BCAA):** An amino acid having aliphatic side-chains with a branch (a carbon atom bound to more than two other carbon atoms). Among the proteinogenic amino acids, there are 3 BCAAs: leucine, isoleucine, and valine.

**BRANCHED-CHAIN α-KETO ACID DEHYDROGENASE COMPLEX (BCKD):** Branched-chain α-keto acid dehydrogenase is a multienzyme complex associated with the inner membrane of mitochondria, and functions in the catabolism of branched-chain amino acids. The complex consists of multiple copies of 3 components: branched-chain α-keto acid decarboxylase (E1), lipoamide acyltransferase (E2), and lipoamide dehydrogenase (E3).

**FOUNDER MUTATION:** In genetics, a founder mutation is a mutation that appears in the DNA of one or more individuals who are founders of a distinct population. Founder mutations originate with changes that occur in the DNA and are passed down to other generations.

**KINASE:** An enzyme that catalyzes the transfer of a phosphate group or another high-energy molecular group to an acceptor molecule. Each of these kinases is named for its receptor, such as acetate kinase, fructokinase, or hexokinase.

**PHOSPHATASE:** Any of a group of enzymes capable of catalyzing the hydrolysis of esterified phosphoric acid, with liberation of inorganic phosphate, found in practically all tissues, body fluids, and cells, including erythrocytes and leukocytes.

**TRANSAMINASE:** Any of a group of enzymes that catalyze the transfer of an amino group from an amino acid to an acceptor keto-acid, resulting in the formation of a new amino acid and the conversion of the original amino acid to a keto-acid; also termed aminotransferase.

## DISCUSSION

MSUD is caused by a defect in BCAA (leucine, isoleucine, and valine) metabolism. These amino acids are normally degraded, through a sequence of reactions, to acetyl-CoA, acetoacetate, and succinyl-CoA. The second step in this process is catalyzed by the mitochondrial BCKD, which converts an α-keto acid to an acyl-CoA via oxidative decarboxylation. BCKD is a multienzyme complex consisting of 6 subunits. The complex contains 4 enzymatic subunits (E1 [α and β], E2, and E3), BCKD kinase, and BCKD phosphatase. Phosphorylation of the complex inactivates it and, conversely, it is activated by dephosphorylation. The genes encoding the enzymatic components are the BCKA decarboxylase (E1) α subunit gene, BCKA decarboxylase (E1) β subunit gene, dihydrolipoyl transacylase (E2) subunit gene, and lipoamide dehydrogenase (E3) subunit gene. The complex utilizes the coenzymes thiamine pyrophosphate, lipoamide, FAD, and the terminal oxidizing agent id $NAD^+$ (Figure 10-1).

MSUD is caused by an inherited autosomal mutation in either E1α (MSUD type 1A), E1β (MSUD type 1B), or E2 (MSUD type 2). Mutations may also occur in the E3 subunit but cause a different phenotype. The incidence rate in the general population is estimated to be 1:185,000 live births though it can increase to 1:176 live

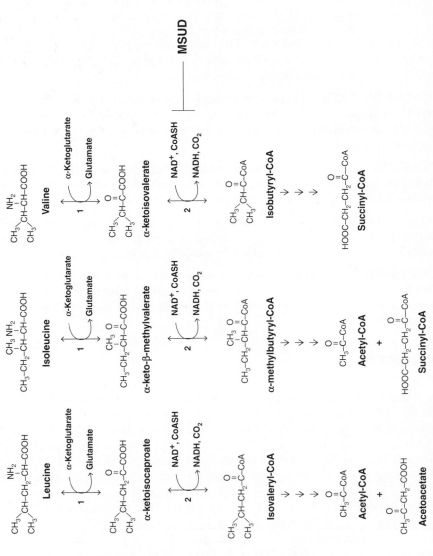

**Figure 10-1.** Abbreviated BCAA degradation pathway depicting the loss of function of the BCKD complex in the second step of the pathway observed in cases of MSUD. Steps 1 (BCAA transaminase) and 2 (BCKD complex) are common for leucine, valine and isoleucine. BCAA = branched-chain amino acid, BCKD = branched-chain α-ketoacid dehydrogenase complex, MSUD = maple syrup urine disease.

births when considering the Old World Mennonite population. A founder muta-tion in B *CKDHA* (E1 α) is believed to be prevalent in this group, with a classic MSUD carrier frequency of 1 in 10. This founder mutation results from a tyrosine to asparagine mutation in the E1 component that prevents the proper interaction of the α and β subunits. In the absence of this interaction, the normal tetrameric structure of the E1 subunit is disrupted, rendering an enzyme with decreased or no functional activity.

MSUD can be classified as classic, intermediate or intermittent and the criteria for classification depend largely on the level of enzyme activity. Classic cases of MSUD have little to no residual BCKDH activity (0%-2% of normal activity) and present with symptoms within a few days of birth. Intermediate and intermittent forms of the disease typically have some level of enzyme activity (3%-30% and 5%-20%, respectively). Patients with intermediate MSUD may appear normal in the neonatal period but present with the same phenotypic symptoms either in infancy or later (typically between the ages of 5 months and 7 years). Intermittent MSUD patients usually develop normally and only display symptoms during times of physiologic stress.

The lack of function of the BCKD complex results in accumulation of the BCAAs and their keto-acid derivatives. As these products build up, they become toxic to organs and, in particular, the brain. Elevated levels of leucine interfere with trans-port of other large neutral amino acids across the blood-brain barrier, reducing the availability of these required amino acids. This cerebral amino acid deficiency nega-tively affects brain growth and hinders the synthesis of neurotransmitters (dopamine, serotonin, norepinephrine, and histamine) required for cell-to-cell communication. Leucine is considered neurotoxic because it promotes a neurochemical syndrome that disturbs brain protein accretion, neurotransmitter synthesis, cell volume regula-tion, neuron growth, and myelin synthesis. Additionally, the cerebral accumulation of α-ketoisocaproic acid has been implicated in the inhibition of the mitochondrial electron transport chain, leading to the elevated cerebral lactate level observed in acute MSUD encephalopathy.

Treatment of MSUD involves limiting dietary intake of branched-chain amino acids, particularly leucine. Unlike leucine, elevated blood concentrations of valine and isoleucine seem to be more easily withstood. Restriction of dietary protein, which naturally contains less valine and isoleucine than leucine, can lead to defi-ciencies of valine and isoleucine even when leucine concentrations are elevated. Deficiencies of isoleucine and valine can be even more problematic for the brain, since all of the BCAAs use the same transporter to cross the blood–brain barrier. Thus, careful monitoring of BCAA levels in blood is imperative, and supplementa-tion of valine and isoleucine may be required.

## COMPREHENSION QUESTIONS

10.1 One hallmark of MSUD is the presence of ketones in the urine. A quick screen involves the addition of dinitrophenylhydrazine (2-DNP) to the patient's urine sample. A positive result is indicated by the formation of a yellow-white precipitate. The type of reaction responsible for this product can best be described as which of the following?

A.  Isomerization reaction

B.  Condensation reaction

C.  Combustion reaction

D.  Acid/base reaction

10.2 In addition to MSUD, there are a few additional inborn errors of metabolism that also present with neonatal encephalopathy. These include hyperketosis syndromes such as β-ketothiolase deficiency, urea cycle defects, glycine encephalopathy, and propionic or methylmalonic academia. Which of the following tests would allow the definitive diagnosis of MSUD?

A.  Urine protein analysis

B.  Cranial computed tomography

C.  CSF culture

D.  Plasma amino acid analysis

10.3 A healthy couple of Old World Mennonite descent is preparing to have a child. Given that the carrier incidence of the trait is 1 in 10, what is the probability that their child will have MSUD?

A.  1 in 10

B.  1 in 100

C.  1 in 400

D.  1 in 200

## ANSWERS

10.1 **B.** This reaction can be described as a condensation reaction, with 2 molecules joining together with a loss of water. In this case, the reaction is as follows:

$$RR'C = O + C_6H_3(NO_2)_2NHNH_2 \rightarrow C_6H_3(NO_2)_2NHNCRR' + H_2O$$

$$(\text{ketone} + \text{DNPH} \rightarrow \text{dinitrophenylhydrazone} + \text{water})$$

The other types of reactions do not apply. In an isomerization reaction, the structural arrangement of a compound is changed but its net atomic composition remains the same. A combustion reaction is a type of redox reaction in which a combustible material combines with an oxidizer to form oxidized products and generate heat. An acid-base reaction is type of double displacement reaction that occurs between an acid and a base. The $H^+$ ion in the acid reacts with the $OH^-$ ion in the base to form water and an ionic salt.

10.2  **D.** In cases of MSUD the levels of plasma BCAAs will be elevated. This will not be true for the other metabolic disorders described. Urine protein analysis and CSF culture would be negative for these disorders and would not allow for differentiation. Conversely, cranial computed tomography scans in each type of case could show signs of cerebral edema.

10.3  **C.** MSUD is inherited in an autosomal recessive manner, meaning that in order to be affected, the offspring would need to be homozygous for the trait. One in 4 offspring would have this genotype. Given the approximate incidence rate of the trait in the Mennonite population, each parent has a probability of 1/10 to be a carrier. Therefore, the probability that the child is affected is $(1/10) \times (1/10) \times (1/4) = 1/400$.

## BIOCHEMISTRY PEARLS

▶ The BCAAs are degraded, in part, by the multienzyme complex BCKD.

▶ MSUD results from a mutation in one of the enzymatic subunits of this enzyme.

▶ Symptoms of MSUD are caused by an accumulation of the BCAAs and branched-chain keto-acids.

## REFERENCES

Bodamer O, Hahn S, Tepas E. Overview of Maple Syrup Urine Disease. Up-to-date. August 8, 2012.

Chuang DT, Chuang JL, Wynn RM. Lessons from genetic disorders of branched-chain amino acid metabolism. *J Nutr.* 2006;136:243S-249S.

Chuang DT, Wynn RM, Shih VE. Maple syrup urine disease (branched-chain ketoacidosis). In: Valle D, et al, eds. *Scriver's The Online Metabolic & Molecular Bases of Inherited Disease.* McGraw-Hill; accessed June 12, 2012.

Strauss KA, Puffenberger EG, Morton DH. Maple syrup urine disease. In: Gene Reviews. [Internet.] Seattle (WA): University of Washington, Seattle; Initial Posting: January 30, 2006; Last Update: December 15, 2009.

Voet D, Voet JG. Amino acid metabolism. *Biochemistry.* 3rd ed. City, NJ: John Wiley & Sons, Inc; 2004.

A 32-year-old woman presents to your clinic with concerns over a recently detected right breast lump. Mammography revealed a right breast mass measuring 3 cm with numerous microcalcifications suggestive of breast cancer. During your discussion with the patient, she revealed that she had a sister who was diagnosed with breast cancer at the age of 39, a mother who passed away with ovarian cancer at the age of 40 years, and a maternal aunt who had both breast and colon cancers. Patient underwent an examination, which revealed a fixed and nontender breast mass on right side measuring 3 cm with mild right axillary lymphadenopathy. No skin involvement is noted. Biopsy was performed and revealed intraductal carcinoma.

▶ What cancer gene might be associated with this clinical scenario?
▶ What is the likely mechanism of the cancer gene in this case?

# ANSWERS TO CASE 11:

## Oncogenes and Cancer

*Summary:* A 32-year-old woman with strong family history of breast, colon, and ovarian cancers, who now presents with a fixed breast lesion that is proven via biopsy to be carcinoma.

- **Most likely cancer gene:** BRCA

- **Likely mechanism:** Inhibition of tumor-suppressor gene

## CLINICAL CORRELATION

This young woman has developed breast cancer at 32 years of age. Moreover, she has 2 first-degree relatives with breast, ovarian, or both cancers prior to menopause. This makes BRCA gene mutation likely. BRCA1 resides on chromosome 17. This gene encodes a protein that most likely is important in DNA repair. Thus, a mutation of the BRCA1 gene likely leads to abnormal cells propagating unchecked. A woman with a BRCA1 mutation has a 70% lifetime risk of developing breast cancer, and a 30%-40% risk of ovarian cancer. The vast majority of breast cancer is not genetically based, but occurs sporadically. However, familial-based breast cancers are most common because of BRCA1 mutation. BRCA2 is another mutation that is more commonly associated with male breast cancer. Other genetic mechanisms of cancer include oncogenes, which are abnormal genes that cause cancer usually by mutations. Proto-oncogenes are normal genes that are present in normal cells and involved in normal growth and development, but if mutations occur, they may become oncogenes.

# APPROACH TO:

## Oncogenes

### OBJECTIVES

1. Know the definitions of oncogenes and proto-oncogenes.

2. Understand the role of promoter and repressor functions of DNA synthesis.

3. Know the normal DNA replication.

4. Be familiar with DNA mutations (point mutations, insertions, deletions).

5. Know the process of DNA repair.

6. Understand the recombination and transposition of genes.

## DEFINITIONS

**OKAZAKI FRAGMENT:** Short segments of DNA (approximately 1000 nucleotides in prokaryotes, 100-200 nucleotides in eukaryotes) synthesized on the lagging strand during DNA replication. As the replication fork opens, the RNA polymerase primase synthesizes a short RNA primer, which is extended by DNA polymerase until it reaches the preceding Okazaki fragment. The RNA primer on the previous Okazaki fragment is removed, the gap filled in with DNA and the strands ligated.

**ONCOGENE:** Genes whose products are involved in the transformation of normal cells to tumor cells. Most oncogenes are mutant forms of normal genes (proto-oncogenes).

**PRIMASE:** An RNA polymerase that synthesizes a short RNA primer complementary to a DNA template strand that is being replicated. This RNA primer serves as the starting point for addition of nucleotides in the replication of the strand serving as a template.

**RECOMBINATION:** Any process in which DNA strands are cleaved and rejoined resulting in an exchange of material between molecules of DNA.

**TUMOR SUPPRESSOR GENES:** Genes that encode for proteins that normally inhibit the progress of a cell through the cell cycle. If these genes are mutated, a deficiency in the suppressor proteins creates unregulated cell growth, a condition permissive for tumorigenesis.

## DISCUSSION

**DNA replication** normally occurs during the **S phase of the cell cycle.** DNA replication occurs in a semiconservative fashion and this is because of the **intrinsic antiparallel nature of the double helix. All known DNA polymerases synthesize DNA in a 5′ to 3′ direction;** this means that 1 strand will be continuously synthesized and the other must be made through a **discontinuous mechanism and the production of Okazaki fragments.** After this process is finished, the cell will divide the newly replicated material in mitosis. In some aberrant cases, the cell will replicate its DNA over and over again without performing an intervening mitosis. This generates cells with abnormally high content of DNA, an abnormal form of DNA replication control.

**DNA replication begins by separating the parental DNA strands.** This is accomplished by enzymes called **helicases.** They **separate the strands** and move along the strands in a fixed direction at the expense of ATP, **opening up the strands so that the DNA polymerases can bind to them.** To prevent reannealing of the 2 strands, single-stranded binding proteins bind the 2 complementary strands. The **next step in the replication process is the laying down of an RNA primer,** which is catalyzed by the enzyme **primase. DNA polymerases extend the chain by adding deoxyribonucleotides to the 5′ end of the RNA primer.** It does this in a continuous **fashion on the leading strand,** but for the **lagging strand, the 1 with its 5′ end toward the replication fork, a series of short segments termed Okazaki fragments must be synthesized.** The RNA primers of the Okazaki fragments are removed as the DNA polymerase reaches the previous Okazaki fragment and the DNA segments are then joined by DNA ligase.

**DNA mutations arise from a variety of intrinsic and extrinsic factors.** Our genome is constantly under the assault of various **genotoxic agents such as ionizing radiation, oxygen free radicals, and UV light.** These agents serve to introduce **DNA double-strand breaks (DSBs) as well as thymine–thymine dimers into the DNA.** DSBs may generate deletion or insertion mutations and could alter the reading frame of the genetic code, an event that can easily lead to the malfunction of a protein. Ultraviolet (UV)-induced dimers may generate point mutations that also alter the reading frame.

To respond to the various forms of DNA damage, cells have evolved a host of DNA **repair mechanisms** that serve to restore the genetic material. Depending on the nature of the DNA damage (eg, DSB vs UV-induced thymine dimers), the cell will invoke a different mechanism of repair. In addition, the stage of the cell cycle at which the lesion is detected and processed can activate independent DNA repair pathways. For example, if a daughter chromatid template is present in S or $G_2$ **phase of the cell cycle, the cell will use this unperturbed partner molecule to fix a DSB.** This process is referred to as **homologous recombination (HR)** and represents a major branch of the DNA repair process. However, if the damage occurs during the $G_1$ **phase of the cell cycle, a period devoid of an existing chromatid template** that can be used for repair, **a general end joining process** will be used. This process, referred to as **nonhomologous end joining (NHEJ),** ligates the broken ends together with little to no regard for the loss of intervening sequences. Therefore, **NHEJ is considered an error prone process,** but given the large size of the genome and the presence of many forms of "junk DNA," the NHEJ process may not necessarily disrupt DNA sequences that encode proteins. By contrast to NHEJ, **HR is a process that is error free** by virtue of the fact that the **daughter chromatid is used as a template for repair.**

**Recombination and transposition of genes** are 2 processes that **mutate the genetic material.** As discussed above, recombination is integral to the process of DNA repair. When DNA recombination is impaired through mutation of specific genes (like *BRCA1* or *Rad51*), aberrant recombination takes place, generating abnormal chromosomes that possess translocations from 2 or more chromosomes. **Translocations transpose genes** from one chromosomal environment to another and often this leads to a disruption in gene expression. Such events are known to cause **gene amplification,** a phenomenon often associated with cancer. They may also generate chromosomes that possess 2 centromeres (dicentrics), leading to a variety of cellular defects in mitosis.

DNA replication is tightly controlled by a variety of proteins that act to promote the process (ie, DNA polymerases and *cis*-acting elements that bind to DNA and recruit factors involved in the process) as well as ones that inhibit the synthesis of DNA, either directly or indirectly. One factor that indirectly inhibits DNA synthesis is the **p53 tumor suppressor. Tumor suppressors refer to a general class of proteins that function to slow and alter cell growth** and development through a variety of mechanisms. In the absence of these factors, cells will have a reduced capacity to perform a variety of functions essential to maintain genomic stability. The **p53 functions to control the $G_1$ S boundary of the cell cycle,** and if the cell is not prepared to enter S phase, then DNA synthesis will be negatively regulated.

A major cause of familial breast cancer results from mutation in the breast cancer susceptibility gene, **BRCA1.** Originally identified in 1994, it was not until 1997 when David Livingston and colleagues demonstrated that *BRCA1* **is a nuclear protein** that its function began to be understood. They found that after treatment of cells with agents known to generate DNA damage (ie, hydroxyurea, UV light, ionizing radiation), **BRCA1 was found to localize to discrete nuclear structures typically called** *foci.* Such foci are known to correlate with sites of DNA damage or the sites of stalled replication forks in S phase of the cell cycle. In addition to the striking nuclear localization of *BRCA1* in response to DNA damaging agents, it was also observed that the **BRCA1 protein was phosphorylated in response to these agents.** Given this and the wealth of data obtained from studying the cell cycle in yeast model systems, it was concluded that *BRCA1* functioned as a cell cycle regulator in response to DNA damage.

Further studies have implicated *BRCA1* in the cellular response to DNA DSBs, a potentially lethal form of DNA damage. **Cells defective in BRCA1** possess numerous cytological and biologic features that have been known for years to be correlated with perturbation in the maintenance of chromosome stability. This includes **aneuploidy, centrosome amplification, spontaneous chromosome breakage, aberrant recombination events, sensitivity to ionizing radiation, and impaired cell cycle checkpoints.** In addition, a variety of experiments have demonstrated roles for *BRCA1* in enforcing the $G_2/M$ cell cycle transition, homologous recombination between sister chromatids, as well as the restart of stalled replication in S phase.

The **BRCA1 tumor suppressor interacts with numerous cellular proteins in large complexes.** This includes a variety of proteins implicated in various DNA repair and cell cycle processes. In fact, *BRCA1* has been reported to interact with as many as **50 proteins.** Moreover, *BRCA1* has been shown to function in various transcriptional mechanisms, suggesting that the function of this important protein may go well beyond its well-documented role in DSB repair. How the inactivation of *BRCA1*, a gene that appears to operate in DNA repair pathways that appear generic to various cell types and predisposes women to inherited forms of breast cancer, remains a mystery and the subject of much debate. Given that *BRCA1* appears to have key roles in transcriptional regulation, it has been suggested that *BRCA1* could influence mammary tissue through pathways that impinge on the biology of estrogen and estrogen-related metabolites. In addition, it has been suggested that breast tissue differs from other tissues in the types of DNA repair processes that are used. Perhaps there are redundant DNA repair pathways in nonmammary tissue. In any event, the complex behavior of *BRCA1* promises to challenge future researchers as they search for the underlying mechanisms that initiate familial breast cancer.

## COMPREHENSION QUESTIONS

11.1 Hereditary retinoblastoma is a genetic disease that is inherited as an autosomal dominant trait. Patients with hereditary retinoblastoma develop tumors of the retina early in life, usually in both eyes. The affected gene (*RB1*) was the first tumor suppressor gene to be identified. Which of the following best describes the function of the protein encoded by *RB1*?

A. It binds transcription factors required for expression of DNA replication enzymes.

B. It allosterically inhibits DNA polymerase.

C. It binds to the promoter region of DNA and prevents transcription.

D. It phosphorylates signal-transduction proteins.

11.2 Mutations in the tumor suppressor gene *BRCA1* are transmitted in an autosomal dominant fashion. When a cell is transformed to a tumor cell in individuals who have inherited 1 mutant allele of this tumor suppressor gene, which of the following most likely occurs?

A. Overexpression of a transcription factor

B. Deletion or mutation of the normal gene on the other chromosome

C. Chromosomal translocation

D. Gene duplication of the mutant gene

11.3 Women who inherit 1 mutant *BRCA1* gene have a 60% chance of developing breast cancer by the age of 50 years. The protein produced by *BRCA1* has been found to be involved in the repair of DNA DSBs. Which of the following processes is most likely to be adversely affected by a deficiency in the *BRCA1* protein?

A. Removal of thymine dimers

B. Removal of RNA primers

C. Removal of carcinogen adducts

D. Homologous recombination

E. Correction of mismatch errors

## ANSWERS

11.1 **A.** The RB1 protein binds to E2F transcription factors, preventing them from activating transcription of the genes encoding enzymes required for DNA replication, such as DNA polymerase. The RB1–E2F complex acts as a transcription repressor. Midway through $G_1$ phase, RB1 is phosphorylated by cyclin-dependent kinases, releasing E2F to activate transcription. A deficiency of RB1 leads to unregulated transcription of DNA replicatory enzymes and DNA synthesis.

11.2 **B.** Because *BRCA1* is inherited in an autosomal dominant fashion, then 1 allele is sufficient to produce the BRCA1 protein. However, if the normal allele is somatically mutated or deleted, then the affected cell cannot produce the BRCA1 protein and can be transformed into a tumor cell.

11.3 **D.** BRCA1 plays a significant role in the repair of DSBs; therefore, since homologous recombination requires a cleavage of both strands of a DNA molecule, this event is most likely to be affected by a deficiency in this protein. Thymine dimers, mismatches, and adducts of DNA with carcinogens are effectively removed by a process of excision repair, in which a section of 1 strand of DNA is removed.

## BIOCHEMISTRY PEARLS

▶ DNA replication normally occurs during the S phase of the cell cycle.

▶ DNA replication occurs in a semiconservative fashion and this is because of the intrinsic antiparallel nature of the double helix.

▶ All known DNA polymerases synthesize DNA in a 5′ to 3′ direction.

▶ To respond to the various forms of DNA damage, cells have evolved a host of DNA repair mechanisms that serve to restore the genetic code.

▶ Tumor suppressors refer to a general class of proteins that function to slow and alter cell growth and development through a variety of mechanisms. *BRCA* tumor suppressor gene, when mutated, increases the risk of breast cancer.

▶ Inactivation of *BRCA1*, a gene that appears to operate in DNA repair pathways that appear generic to various cell types, predisposes women to inherited forms of breast cancer, but the exact mechanism has been elusive.

## REFERENCES

Couch FJ, Weber BL. Breast cancer. In: Scriver CR, Beaudet AL, Sly WS, et al, eds. *The Metabolic and Molecular Basis of Inherited Disease.* 8th ed. New York: McGraw-Hill; 2001:999-1031.

Edenberg HJ. DNA replication, recombination, and repair. In: Devlin TM, ed. *Textbook of Biochemistry with Clinical Correlations.* 7th ed. New York: Wiley-Liss; 2010.

Scully R, Chen J, Ochs RL. Dynamic changes of BRCA1 subnuclear location and phosphorylation state are initiated by DNA damage. *Cell.* 1997;90(3):425-435.

Scully R, Livingston DM. In search of the tumor-suppressor functions of BRCA1 and BRCA2. *Nature.* 2000;408(6811):429-432.

# CASE 12

A 25-year-old Mediterranean woman presents to her obstetrician at 12-weeks gestation for her first prenatal visit. This is her first pregnancy, and she is concerned about her baby and the risk of inheriting a "blood" disease like others in her family. The patient reports a personal history of mild anemia but nothing as severe as her brother who required frequent transfusions and died at the age of 10 years. The patient was told by her physician that she did not need to take iron supplementation for her anemia. Patient denies having any anemic symptoms. Her physical examination is consistent with a 12-week pregnancy and ultrasonography confirmed an intrauterine pregnancy at 12-weeks gestation. The patient's hemoglobin (Hb) level shows a hypochromic, microcytic (small-sized red cell) anemia (Hb, 9 g/dL) and Hb electrophoresis demonstrated increased Hb A2 level (4.0%) and increased fetal Hb level, a pattern consistent with β-thalassemia minor. The patient underwent chorionic villus sampling to assess whether the fetus was affected, and the diagnosis returned in several hours.

▶ What is the molecular genetics behind this disorder?
▶ What was the likely test and what is the biochemical basis?

# ANSWERS TO CASE 12:

## Thalassemia/Oligonucleotide Probe

*Summary:* A 25-year-old Mediterranean pregnant woman has a history of asymptomatic mild hypochromic, microcytic anemia, elevated Hb A2 and F on electrophoresis. Her brother had severe hemolytic disease that required transfusions and ultimately caused his premature death at the age of 10 years. She is diagnosed with β-thalassemia minor.

- **Molecular genetics:** Impaired production of β-globin peptide chain. Numerous mutations have been identified in the production of RNA, including in the promoter region and splice junctions.

- **Likely test:** Oligonucleotide probe. After chorionic villus sampling is performed, a radioactive probe can be used and hybridized with specific genetic mutations in fetus DNA, allowing for prompt detection and prenatal diagnosis.

## CLINICAL CORRELATION

Anemia is the abnormally low level of Hb or red blood cell mass, which has the potential of limiting the delivery of oxygen to tissue. By far, the most common cause of anemia is iron deficiency, leading to small volume of red blood cells (microcytic). Another common cause of microcytic anemia is thalassemia. Certain ethnicities have higher incidences of thalassemia (eg, Mediterranean, East Asian descent).

This patient is of Mediterranean descent, making thalassemia more likely. Furthermore, the microcytic (small red blood cell size) anemia in the face of elevated Hb A2 and F is consistent with β-thalassemia minor. Patients with β-thalassemia major (Cooley anemia) typically have severe anemia requiring frequent transfusions and shortened life expectancy. Infants will appear healthy after birth, but as the HbF levels fall, the infant becomes severely anemic. Females with β-thalassemia major who survive beyond childhood are usually sterile.

# APPROACH TO:

## Oligonucleotide Probes

### OBJECTIVES

1. Know about the use of oligonucleotide probes for detection of mutations.

2. Know how oligonucleotide segments are synthesized.

3. Be familiar with common mutations that cause thalassemias (substitutions in TATA box, mutations in splice junction, and changes in stop codon).

## DEFINITIONS

**ERYTHROPOIESIS:** Erythropoiesis is the development of mature red blood cells containing Hb (erythrocytes) from pluripotential stem cells via a linear cascade.

**FRAMESHIFT MUTATION:** Insertion or deletion of a number of nucleotides that are not divisible by 3 into a coding sequence, thereby causing an alteration in the reading frame of the entire sequence downstream of the mutation.

**LOCUS CONTROL REGION:** Regulatory region which is believed to regulate transcription by opening and remodeling chromatin structure. It may also have enhancer activity.

**PROMOTER SEQUENCE:** A regulatory region present at a short distance upstream from the 5′ end of a transcription start site that acts as the binding site for RNA polymerase to initiate transcription. The TATA box and CAAT box are DNA consensus sequences in the promoter region.

**THALASSEMIA:** A group of genetic disorders that is characterized by the absence of or reduced synthesis of 1 or more of the 4 globin chains in Hb. The sequelae can range from benign to fatal, depending on the severity of the decrease in the globin chain.

**TRANSPOSONS:** These are segments of DNA that can move around to different positions in the genome of a single cell. In the process, they may cause mutations and increase (or decrease) the amount of DNA in the genome. These mobile segments of DNA are sometimes called "**jumping genes.**"

## DISCUSSION

Thalassemia is a common condition in the Mediterranean region, and its clinical features were described as early as 1925. The term *thalassemia* is coined from the Greek word, which means "the sea." Mendelian transmission of thalassemia was discovered in 1938. Later, it became apparent that thalassemia is not a single disease but a **group of genetic disorders,** all of which arise from **abnormalities in Hb synthesis.** The thalassemias are characterized by the **absence or reduced synthesis of 1 or more of the 4 globin chains of Hb.** There are 4 different genetic loci that control the formation of $\alpha$-, $\beta$-, $\gamma$-, and $\delta$-chains of Hb. **Fetal Hb (HbF)** is formed from **2 $\alpha$- and 2 $\gamma$-chains.** In adults, the $\gamma$-chain is replaced by the $\beta$- and $\delta$-chains, which combine with 2 $\alpha$-chains to form **HbA** ($\alpha_2\beta_2$, approximately 97%) and HbA$_2$ ($\alpha_2\gamma_2$, approximately 3%; Figure 12-1). In the late 1970s, the $\alpha$-gene was found to be localized to chromosome 16, whereas the $\beta$-, $\gamma$-, and $\delta$-genes were clustered on chromosome 11. Thus, although thalassemia does not occur in the fetus since the *$\beta$-globin* genes are activated only after birth, prenatal diagnosis is possible.

**Thalassemias are named according to the affected globin chain:** Thus, a disorder of the $\alpha$-chain would be an $\alpha$-**thalassemia,** and a disorder of the $\beta$-chain would be a $\beta$-**thalassemia.** There are 2 major forms of thalassemia, one in which the $\beta$-globin chain is not produced ($\beta^0$) and another in which there is significantly reduced level of $\beta$-globin chain ($\beta^+$). The positive category includes variants with unusually high levels of HbF or HbA$_2$, variants with normal levels of HbA$_2$, silent

**Figure 12-1.** Maturation of hemoglobin from the fetal form to the adult form. In β-thalassemias, because of a defect in the β-globin gene, the γ-chain cannot be effectively replaced with the β-chain.

or benign variants, those that are inherited in a dominant fashion, and variants that are not linked to the *β-gene* cluster.

A severe decrease in β-globin levels leads to the precipitation of the α-chain, which, in turn, causes a defect in the maturation of the erythroid precursor, and erythropoiesis, thus reducing red cell survival. The profound anemia in the affected individual stimulates the production of erythropoietin leading to the expansion of bone marrow and subsequent skeletal deformities. The hyperplasia of the bone marrow induces increased iron absorption leading to the deposition of iron in tissues. If the concentration of iron in the tissues becomes too high, then this can lead to organ failure and death if appropriate therapeutic steps are not taken.

There are at least **200 β-thalassemia alleles** that have been characterized to date. β-Thalassemias are caused primarily by **point mutations** within the *β-globin* gene and the neighboring flanking region. There are 2 exceptions that are attributed to larger deletions ranging from 290 base pairs (bp) to more than 60 kbp. One is a family of upstream deletions, which down regulates the locus control region, and the other affects the promoter region of *β-globin* gene. The **promoter region deletions** typically include the messenger RNA (mRNA) cap site, TATA box, and CAAT elements. Apart from deletions, there are insertions of 6 to 7 kbp retrotransposons in the *β-globin* gene that decrease the transcript level to 15% in comparison with the control. In addition, there are also a few thalassemia mutations that segregate independently of the *β-globin* gene, such as those involving the trans-acting regulatory factors that affect the expression of *the β-globin* gene. One can thus broadly classify the different classes of mutations which result in β-thalassemia as follows:

1. **Transcription** (eg, deletion, insertion)

2. **mRNA processing** (eg, cryptic splice sites, consensus sequence, poly A addition site)

3. **Translation** (initiation, nonsense, frameshift mutations)

4. **Post-translation stability** (highly unstable β-chain)

5. Determinants unlinked to the *β-globin* gene cluster

The **most common point mutations** occur in the **CAAT or TATA box** in the **promoter** sequence. The single base substitution A to G at position –29 in individuals of African descent leads to a mild form of the disease, whereas the substitution A to C in those of Chinese descent leads to thalassemia major. In addition, a single nucleotide substitution in the GT/AG splice junction can lead to a misspliced mRNA that does not allow the translation of a functional β-globin chain. The C to T mutation at position –101 causes an extremely mild deficit in *β-globin* gene. The effect is so mild that it is a "silent" or benign mutation in heterozygotes. All the point mutations that prevent the translation of the β-globin mRNA (eg, changing the start codon ATG to GTG, or TGT to the stop codon TGA) or a single nucleotide frame shift lead to the $β^0$-phenotype.

There are several biochemical techniques that can be used to accurately determine the genetic defect that results in a particular thalassemia. Many of these techniques make use of the **polymerase chain reaction (PCR)**, which amplifies the DNA and allows detection of multiple mutations at once.

The **amplification refractory mutation system** (ARMS) is a technique in which the target DNA is amplified using a common primer and either mutation specific primer for β-thalassemia or the correct sequence primer to the target. This method provides quick screening of the DNA to detect if the patient carries the mutant gene or not. When both the primers are used in the same PCR reaction, they compete to amplify the target, and the technique is termed competitive oligonucleotide priming, and the primers are labeled with different fluorescent dyes to allow detection.

**A PCR restriction enzyme analysis** takes advantage of the occurrence of approximately 40 thalassemia mutations that either introduce or remove a restriction endonuclease site. The PCR amplified target sequence is digested using restriction enzymes (enzymes that cleave DNA at particular nucleotide sequences) and the pattern of fragmentation on an agarose gel defines the presence or absence of a particular mutation.

Radiolabeled single stranded DNA oligonucleotide probes are allowed to anneal with the target strand in an **oligonucleotide hybridization analyses.** Typically, the target DNA is fixed onto nitrocellulose or nylon membrane. The probe forms stable duplexes with target sequences from the heterogenous mixture of many sequences in genomic DNA and is detected by autoradiography using x-ray film. In populations that have predominantly one common mutation, a very successful and efficient hybridization analysis is the **PCR allele-specific oligonucleotide assay.** This requires that the sequence of the common mutation is known. The amplified genomic DNA is transferred onto a nylon membrane and probed using an allele-specific oligonucleotide, that is, one that is complementary to the sequence of the DNA that contains the mutation. The membrane is probed both with oligonucleotides having the mutant and the correct DNA sequence of the β-globin gene. The genotype of the DNA is determined by the presence or the absence of the hybridization signal. Recently, **microchips,** which are an array of oligonucleotides immobilized on a glass plate, have been used to detect thalassemias. Fluorescent-labeled DNA from an individual is hybridized onto this microchip and the reaction is monitored with a fluorescent microscope. This technique allows the study of a specific mutation using several hundred oligonucleotides simultaneously. It is highly sensitive with a low background; however, the resolving power is low.

Using 1 or a more of the DNA analysis tools described above, effective prenatal detection of various mutations in the β-*globin* gene cluster has been successfully achieved. Although gene therapy for genetic diseases is in its infancy, hopefully the future will bring effective treatment options for patients affected with thalassemia.

## COMPREHENSION QUESTIONS

12.1 Micawley Talltwin is a 7-year-old child star brought to his pediatrician by his parents after they noticed that he felt very fatigued. They also noted that his abdomen seemed to be enlarged. Examination reveals an enlarged spleen. Further history reveals that he has been taking vitamins and iron supplements over the last few months. Laboratory tests show a microcytic anemia and elevated iron levels in tissues. Which of the following conditions is most consistent with the findings in this patient?

    A.  Aplastic anemia

    B.  Cooley anemia

    C.  Pernicious anemia

    D.  Thalassemia major

    E.  Thalassemia minor

12.2 After diagnosing the patient in question 12.1 and ascertaining that he is not agranulocytic, his physician prescribes subcutaneous infusion of deferoxamine, an iron chelator, and monitors him for several weeks. What is his condition most likely to be on reexamination?

    A.  Iron levels decrease, but he remains anemic.

    B.  Iron levels decrease, and anemia recovers.

    C.  He develops irreversible and severe agranulocytosis.

    D.  Iron and vitamin C levels decrease.

12.3 An electrophoretic analysis of Hb level in the patient in questions 12.1 and 12.2 indicates that, although there is a decrease in the relative amount of the β-chain with respect to the α-chain, both the β- and the α-chains migrate at the same position as normal chains. His anemia is most likely caused by which of the following?

    A.  Defect in an enzyme involved in heme synthesis

    B.  Point mutation in the coding region of the gene coding for the β-chain

    C.  Frameshift mutation in the coding region of the gene coding for the β-chain

    D.  Mutation in the promoter of the *β-chain* gene

    E.  Mutation in the structural gene of the β-chain

12.4  As a medical geneticist, you analyze the DNA of the patient from question 12.1 and find that he is homozygous for thalassemia. Assuming the disease is autosomal recessive, what can you deduce about the genotype of Mr. and Mrs. Talltwin?

A.  Dad Talltwin is a carrier of the disease and Mom Talltwin is normal.

B.  Mom Talltwin is a carrier of the disease and Dad Talltwin is normal.

C.  Dad Talltwin is homozygous and Mom Talltwin is normal.

D.  Mom Talltwin is homozygous and Dad Talltwin is normal.

E.  Both Mom and Dad Talltwin are carriers of the disease.

## ANSWERS

12.1  **E.** The correct diagnosis is thalassemia minor because the patient had been asymptomatic until the age of 7 years. If he had thalassemia major or Cooley anemia, then he would have exhibited symptoms as early as his first birthday. Pernicious anemia leads to a macrocytic or megaloblastic anemia, whereas aplastic anemia is characterized by normal sized erythrocytes.

12.2  **A.** The iron chelator helps in excreting iron but has no role in increasing red blood cell production to counteract anemia.

12.3  **D.** Because the β-chain is decreased with respect to the α-chain, it is most likely that there is a mutation that decreases the expression of the *β-chain* gene, in which a mutation in the promoter region could result. A point mutation in the β-chain leading to an amino acid substitution could lead to changes in electrophoretic mobility but would not alter the levels of expression. A frameshift mutation in the β-chain would result in decreased β-chain on the electrophoregram.

12.4  **E.** Thalassemia is autosomal recessive; therefore, Micawley Talltwin can get the disease only if both the parents were to be heterozygotes (or a carrier) of that particular trait.

## BIOCHEMISTRY PEARLS

▶ The thalassemias are characterized by the absence or reduced synthesis of 1 or more of the 4 globin chains of Hb.

▶ Thalassemias are named according to the affected globin chain; thus, a disorder of the α-chain would be an α-thalassemia and a disorder of the β-chain would be a β-thalassemia.

▶ The **ARMS** is a technique in which the target DNA is amplified using a common primer and either mutation specific primer for β-thalassemia or the correct sequence primer to the target.

▶ **PCR restriction enzyme analysis** takes advantage of the occurrence of approximately 40 β-thalassemia mutations that either introduce or remove a restriction endonuclease site.

▶ Radio-labeled single stranded DNA oligonucleotide probes are allowed to anneal with the target strand in an **oligonucleotide hybridization analyses.**

▶ With 1 common mutation, a very successful and efficient hybridization analysis is the **PCR allele-specific oligonucleotide assay.** This requires that the sequence of the common mutation is known.

## REFERENCES

Kanavakis E, Traeger-Synodino J, Vrettou C, et al. Prenatal diagnosis of the thalassaemia syndromes by rapid DNA analytical methods. *Mol Hum Reprod.* 1997;3(6):523-528.

Weatherall DJ, Clegg, JB. *The Thalassaemia Syndromes.* 4th ed. London: Blackwell Science; 2001.

An 8-year-old boy is brought to his pediatrician by his mother because she was concerned that he was having language-speech problems, was hyperactive, and was told by teachers that he may have mental retardation. The mother reports a strong family history of mental retardation in males. On examination, the boy is found to have a large jaw, prominent ears, and enlarged testes (macroorchidism). The mother was told her family had a genetic problem causing the mental retardation. The patient underwent a series of blood tests and was scheduled to see a genetic counselor who expressed that the etiology of the genetic defect was likely transmitted from his mother. The genetic counselor states that his mother likely has a silent mutation.

► What is the most likely diagnosis?
► Which chromosome is likely to be affected?
► What are some types of biochemical mutations?
► What is the biochemical basis of the different types of mutations?

# ANSWERS TO CASE 13:
## Fragile X Syndrome

*Summary:* An 8-year-old boy has mental retardation, speech-language problems, hyperactivity, physical findings of large jaw, prominent ears, and macroorchidism and has a strong family history of mental retardation. The genetic counselor informs the mother that she is the carrier and that she has a silent mutation.

- **Most likely diagnosis:** Fragile X syndrome (most common form of familial mental retardation)

- **Affected chromosome:** Chromosome X

- **Types of mutations:** *Silent* means protein product not affected; *missense* means single amino acid substitution leading to significant alteration (such as sickle cell); and *nonsense* means that a stop codon is formed.

- **Molecular basis of disease:** Mutation resulting in an increased number of CGG repeats on the X chromosome. When the number of repeats reaches a critical size, it can be methylated and inactivated resulting in the disorder. Individuals who carry 50 to 199 repeats are phenotypically normal and carry a premutation. If repeats exceed 200, then the patient has a full mutation; and if methylation occurs, then he or she will be affected.

## CLINICAL CORRELATION

Fragile X is the most common inherited form of mental retardation, affecting primarily males. The clinical presentation can vary, but usually the affected male has moderate to severe mental retardation, hyperactivity, and typical facies such as large jaw and large ears. Pigmented skin lesions (café au lait) can also be seen. Because females have 2 copies of the X chromosome, they are "resistant" to mutations on one gene. Fragile X affects the long arm of the X chromosome, with multiple copies of triplicate repeats, usually CGG, leading to methylation of the DNA. The *FMR* gene product is affected and, through a little-understood mechanism, leads to mental retardation.

# APPROACH TO:
## Mutations

### OBJECTIVES

1. Know the definitions of point mutations (silent, missense, and nonsense), insertions, deletions, and frameshift mutations.

2. Be familiar with the defect in fragile X syndrome.

## DEFINITIONS

**POINT MUTATION:** The substitution of a single nucleotide in the genetic material of an organism. These include silent, missense, and nonsense mutations.

**SILENT MUTATION:** A single nucleotide is exchanged by another, but this alteration does not change the amino acid for which the codon codes. The final protein product remains unchanged.

**MISSENSE MUTATION:** A single nucleotide is exchanged by another, and this alteration does have an effect on the coding amino acid. The final protein product is also modified. The modification may or may not be deleterious to the final protein, depending on the function of the amino acid.

**NONSENSE MUTATION:** A single nucleotide is exchanged by another, which produces a new stop codon at this position. This premature stop codon generally results in a truncated form of the protein and most often leaves it as an inactive form.

**DELETION:** One or more nucleotides are removed from the genetic sequence. If the deletions are multiples of 1 or 2, a frameshift will be the result, which will likely damage the final protein product. A deletion of 3 or a multiple of 3 does not shift the reading frame; rather, it would merely remove a codon(s). The final protein product would lose amino acid(s), which may or may not leave it inoperative.

**INSERTION:** One or more nucleotides are added to the genetic sequence. These are the opposite of deletions.

**TRINUCLEOTIDE REPEAT EXPANSION:** Amplification from one generation to the next of 3 nucleotide repeats in the coding or noncoding regions of DNA. The mechanism may arise from DNA complimentary strand slippage. This is associated with fragile X syndrome and myotonic dystrophy.

**DNA METHYLATION:** Process by which methyl groups are added to DNA bases (most often cytosine). Methylation functions to regulate gene expression because heavily methylated genes are not expressed. In addition, bacteria use methylated DNA as a defense mechanism. Every organism has different patterns of methylated DNA, and bacteria take advantage of this by destroying foreign DNA via nucleases, enzymes that cut DNA at specific sites.

## DISCUSSION

**Replication** often produces **changes in the chemical makeup of DNA**. Many of these changes are easily repaired; however, those **alterations in the DNA base sequence that do not get repaired are referred to as mutations.** There are various types of mutations including **point mutations, deletions, and insertions.**

   **Point mutations** arise when **one base pair is substituted for another,** and they are the **most common types of mutations.** Point mutations can be further subdivided into 3 categories: **silent, missense, and nonsense. Silent mutations do not affect the**

| Table 13-1 • EXAMPLES OF MUTATIONAL EVENTS SILENT MUTATION | | | | | |
|---|---|---|---|---|---|
| **Genetic Code** | | **Silent Mutation Encountered** | | | |
| **CODON** | **AMINO ACID** | **CODON** | **AMINO ACID** | **MUTANT CODON** | **AMINO ACID** |
| GCC | Alanine | GCC | Alanine | GCT | Alanine |
| GCT | Alanine | | | | |
| GCA | Alanine | | | | |
| GCG | Alanine | | | | |

translated mRNA or final protein product–thus, the name *silent*. The genetic code is degenerate, which means that most amino acids are encoded by several different codons or triplets of DNA/RNA bases. Therefore, it is possible to switch a single base but not alter the resulting protein product (Table 13-1). The **sickle cell trait** is a result of a **missense mutation.** This type of point mutation actually **does alter the protein product.** In the case of sickle cell hemoglobin, adenine is replaced by thymine, causing a hydrophilic glutamic acid to be replaced with a hydrophobic valine in the resulting protein (Table 13-2). In a **nonsense mutation, the mutation brings about a premature stop in the gene of interest** because the altered codon now represents a stop codon (Table 13-3). These are commonly seen in muscular dystrophies and some cystic fibrosis cases. **Aminoglycosides are currently being used to treat premature stop codons** as they affect the translational accuracy of transfer RNA (tRNA), thereby allowing recognition of incorrect codons including the stop codon. Ultimately, the translation machinery reads through the premature stop codon because of altered amino acid insertion by tRNA and produces full-length protein instead of a truncated protein or degraded messenger RNA (mRNA).

| Table 13-2 • MISSENSE MUTATION | | | | | | | |
|---|---|---|---|---|---|---|---|
| **β-Chain of normal hemoglobin** | GTG | CAC | **CTG** | **ACT** | CCT | GAG | GAG |
| | Gly | His | Leu | Thr | Pro | **Glu** | Glu |
| A missense mutation found in β-chain of sickle cell hemoglobin | GTG | CAC | CTG | ACT | CCT | GTG | GAG |
| | Gly | His | Leu | Thr | Pro | **Val** | Glu |

| Table 13-3 • NONSENSE MUTATION | | | | | | | |
|---|---|---|---|---|---|---|---|
| **Normal** | **GGC** | **CTG** | **ACA** | **GGG** | **CAA** | **AAA** | **CTG** |
| | Gly | Leu | Thr | Gly | Gln | Lys | Leu |
| A nonsense mutation found in Duchenne muscular dystrophy | GGC | CTG | ACA | GGG | TAA | AAA | CTG |
| | Gly | Leu | Thr | Gly | **STOP** | | |

## Table 13-4 • FRAMESHIFT MUTATION

**Frameshift Resulting in Altered Protein**

| CCC | GCA | TAT | | | CAT | TTT | ACC |
|---|---|---|---|---|---|---|---|
| Pro | Ala | Tyr | | | His | Phe | Thr |

↓
Deletion of **TA**

| CCC | GCA | TCA | | | TTT | TAC | |
|---|---|---|---|---|---|---|---|
| Pro | Ala | **Ser** | | | **Phe** | **Tyr** | |

**Frameshift Causing Premature Stop**

| CCC | GCA | TAT | CAT | | TTT | ACC | |
|---|---|---|---|---|---|---|---|
| Pro | Ala | | | | His | Thr | |

↓
Deletion of **TC**

| CCC | GCA | TAA | | | | | |
|---|---|---|---|---|---|---|---|
| Pro | Ala | **STOP** | | | | | |

Another type of mutation is a **deletion in which 1 or more DNA bases have been removed.** However, an insertion is a mutation wherein 1 or more DNA bases have been added. These 2 types of mutations can cause a shift in the open reading frame, called **frameshift mutations,** of a gene if the **insertion or deletion is a multiple of 1 or 2 bases.** Typically, a frameshift mutation will result in **disease either as result of altering the protein product, leaving it nonfunctional, or generation of a premature stop codon,** which confers a truncated form of the altered protein (Table 13-4). Both cases present major problems because the altered protein will not likely be able to carry out the normal duties required of it. Because codons are read as multiples of 3, an insertion or deletion of 3 or a multiple of 3 may or may not be as deleterious to the gene as multiples of 1 or 2. In this situation, the resulting protein could include extra amino acids in the case of insertions or lose amino acids in the case of deletions. It is possible that this could hinder the protein from functioning normally.

**Many forms of fragile X syndrome** are examples of **insertions in multiples of 3** where the outcome is detrimental not because of altered amino acid sequence but rather a **loss of protein expression. Deletions and insertions** typically occur in highly **repetitive sequences, and this is exactly what is seen in fragile X. Fragile X syndrome is the most common form of inherited mental retardation.** It affects approximately 1 in 4000 males and 1 in 8000 females. Mutations of the X chromosome, including fragile X, may account for the higher number of male patients in mentally handicapped facilities. The **FMR1 gene is highly conserved. Normal individuals have 7 to 60 (CGG) repeats** in the 5′-untranslated region, and the repeats are often broken up by AGG. **Many fragile X individuals have an increase in the number of CGG repeats, which may expand to more than 230 repeats.** This is termed the *full mutation*. Repeats ranging from 60 to 230 are called a premutation. The premutation carrier has normal **fragile X mental retardation protein (FMRP)** levels, but the gene is unstable in its passage to offspring.

The fragile X phenotype is mainly caused by the **loss of FMRP resulting from CGG trinucleotide repeat expansion of FMR1.** However, some point mutations and deletions in the *FMR1* gene show the same phenotype as the repeat expansion. The alteration arising from the trinucleotide repeated expansion within the promoter region of *FMR1* leads to enhanced local methylation and, ultimately, transcriptional silencing. DNA methylation causes protrusions in the DNA helix where the methylated cytosines interfere with transcription factor binding. This is a common property used for gene regulation. However, in the case of fragile X, the methylation signals to halt all expression of FMRP. Loss of FMRP gives the phenotypical characteristics commonly seen in patients with fragile X.

## COMPREHENSION QUESTIONS

13.1 A 6-year-old boy visits his physician because his parents have noticed autistic behavior and speech problems. The mother's family does have a history of mental retardation. Therefore, the physician suggested a genetic screen of *FMR1* for fragile X syndrome. Polymerase chain reaction (PCR) revealed borderline fragile X syndrome. What situation most likely explains this result?

A. Complete loss of FMRP

B. *FMR1* gene CGG repeated expansion of 60 with partial DNA methylation

C. *FMR1* gene CGG repeated expansion of 230 with minor DNA methylation

D. *FMR1* gene CGG repeated expansion of 280 with complete DNA methylation

Using the genetic code below, predict the type of mutation that had to occur to show these alterations in the final protein product for questions 13.2 and 13.3:

|   | T | C | A | G | |
|---|---|---|---|---|---|
| **T** | Phe | Ser | Tyr | Cys | T |
| | Phe | Ser | Tyr | Cys | C |
| | Leu | Ser | STOP | STOP | A |
| | Leu | Ser | STOP | Trp | G |
| **C** | Leu | Pro | His | Arg | T |
| | Leu | Pro | His | Arg | C |
| | Leu | Pro | Gln | Arg | A |
| | Leu | Pro | Gln | Arg | G |
| **A** | Ile | Thr | Asn | Ser | T |
| | Ile | Thr | Asn | Ser | C |
| | Ile | Thr | Lys | Arg | A |
| | Met | Thr | Lys | Arg | G |
| **G** | Val | Ala | Asp | Gly | T |
| | Val | Ala | Asp | Gly | C |
| | Val | Ala | Glu | Gly | A |
| | Val | Ala | Glu | Gly | G |

13.2

| Phe | Thr | Val | Tyr | Leu | Gly | Met | → | Phe | Thr | Val | STOP |
|-----|-----|-----|-----|-----|-----|-----|---|-----|-----|-----|------|
| TTT | ACA | GTT | TAT | CTC | GGG | ATG |   |     |     |     |      |

A. Missense mutation
B. Nonsense mutation
C. Silent mutation
D. Repeat expansion

13.3

| Phe | Thr | Val | Tyr | Leu | Gly | Met | → | Phe | Thr | Phe | Ile | STOP |
|-----|-----|-----|-----|-----|-----|-----|---|-----|-----|-----|-----|------|
| TTT | ACC | GTT | TAT | CTA | GGG | ATG |   |     |     |     |     |      |

A. Deletion of G in third codon
B. Deletion of A in second codon
C. Insertion of T between second and third codons
D. Insertion of GT between AC and A of second codon

## ANSWERS

13.1 **C.** A CGG repeat expansion of 230 base pairs is just at the limit of the number of repeats required to have the full mutation. Expansions from 7 to 60 are seen in normal patients and those exceeding 230 are positive for fragile X syndrome. Because some of the DNA was methylated, this could help to silence the expression of *FMRP* and cause some of the phenotype seen in the patient. Therefore, this scenario would be considered borderline fragile X.

13.2 **B.** A nonsense mutation causes a premature stop codon on a single nucleotide substitution. The original sequence, TAT, coding for a tyrosine, must have been mutated to either TA**A** or TA**G**, leaving a stop codon in place of the tyrosine.

13.3 **A.** Deletion of G in the third codon gives the sequence:

TTT ACC GTT TAT CTA GGG ATG →
TTT ACC TTT ATC TAG GGA TG

This causes a frameshift and a premature stop codon to be generated. Therefore, the final protein product would look like the one in question.

| Phe | Thr | Val | Tyr | Leu | Gly | Met | → | Phe | Thr | Phe | Ile | STOP |
|-----|-----|-----|-----|-----|-----|-----|---|-----|-----|-----|-----|------|
| TTT | ACC | GTT | TAT | CTA | GGG | ATG |   | TTT | ACC | TTT | ATC | TAG  |

## BIOCHEMISTRY PEARLS

▶ Mutations are alterations in the DNA base sequence that do not get repaired.

▶ There are various types of mutations including point mutations, deletions, and insertions.

▶ Point mutations arise when one base pair is substituted by another, and they are the most common types of mutations.

▶ Point mutations can be further subdivided into 3 categories: silent, missense, and nonsense.

▶ Many individuals with fragile X have an increase in the number of CGG repeats, which may expand to more than 230 repeats.

## REFERENCES

Crawford DC, Acuna JM, Sherman SL. FMR1 and the fragile X syndrome: human genome epidemiology review. *Genet Med.* 2001;3(5):359-371.

Warren ST, Sherman SL. The fragile X syndrome. In: Scriver CR, Beaudet AL, Sly WS, et al, eds. *The Metabolic and Molecular Basis of Inherited Disease.* 8th ed. New York: McGraw-Hill; 2001.

A 40-year-old woman presents to the emergency department with complaints of lower back pain, fever, nausea, vomiting, malaise, chills, syncope, dizziness, and shortness of breath. Patient states that she has some burning with urination (dysuria). Her fever was as high as 103°F (39.4°C) at home earlier in the day. She has a history of non–insulin-dependent diabetes mellitus but denies any other medical problems. On examination, she is in moderate distress with a temperature of 102°F (38.9°C), pulse of 110 beats/minute, respiratory rate of 30 breaths/minute, and blood pressure of 70/30 mm Hg. Her extremities are cool to the touch with thready pulses. Her chest is clear to auscultation bilaterally, and heart is tachycardic but with regular rhythm. She has significant costovertebral tenderness on the right side. Her white blood cell (WBC) count was elevated at 20,000/mm$^3$. The hemoglobin and hematocrit were normal. Her glucose was moderately elevated at 200 mg/dL, and her serum bicarbonate level is low. Arterial blood gas demonstrated a pH of 7.28 and parameters consistent with a metabolic acidosis. Her urinalysis shows an abnormal number of gram-negative rods.

▶ What is the most likely diagnosis?
▶ What is the biochemical mechanism of the metabolic acidosis?

# ANSWERS TO CASE 14:
## Anaerobic Metabolism

*Summary:* 40-year-old woman with diabetes presents with fever 102°F (38.9°C), chills, nausea, vomiting, back pain (costovertebral tenderness), chills, increased WBC count, hypotension, and metabolic acidosis.

- **Most likely diagnosis:** Septic shock and pyelonephritis.

- **Likely cause of the metabolic acidosis:** Lactic acid produced from cells undergoing anaerobic metabolism as a result of tissue hypoperfusion from shock.

## CLINICAL CORRELATION

This patient developed septic shock, infection-related hypotension, and low blood pressure. The decreased blood pressure then led to insufficient red blood cells and oxygen to be delivered to the various tissues in the body. Thus, the tissue had to switch from aerobic metabolism to anaerobic metabolism. Lactate accumulates, leading to acidemia. The treatment of septic shock is initially intravenous fluids, since the body is relatively volume depleted as a result of the vasodilation response to the infection. Sometimes, the blood pressure remains low despite several liters of intravenous fluids; in these cases, so-called vasoactive drugs are used such as dopamine infusion to cause vasoconstriction and, therefore, elevate the blood pressure. Antibiotics are also important to treat the infection. Finally, control of the source of the sepsis is critical. This may include surgery to remove an abscess or necrotic bowel, or removal of a foreign body, or simply debridement. Thus, septic shock is treated by supporting the blood pressure, as well as providing antibiotics and source control. Worsening of the acidemia and accumulation of lactate is a poor prognostic sign in septic shock.

# APPROACH TO:
## Aerobic and Anaerobic Metabolism

### OBJECTIVES

1. Be very familiar with the tricarboxylic acid (TCA) cycle.

2. Know about the differences in energy production in aerobic and anaerobic conditions.

### DEFINITIONS

**ACCEPTOR CONTROL:** The regulation of the rate of an enzymatic reaction by the concentration of 1 or more of the substrates.

**ANAEROBIC GLYCOLYSIS:** The biochemical process by which glucose is converted to lactate with the production of 2 moles of adenosine triphosphate (ATP). This process is increased when the cellular demand for ATP is greater than the ability of the TCA cycle and oxidative phosphorylation to produce it because of decreased oxygen tension or heavy exercise.

**GLYCOLYSIS:** The biochemical process by which glucose is converted to pyruvate in the cytosol of the cell. It results in the production of 2 mol of ATP and 2 mol of the reduced cofactor nicotinamide adenine dinucleotide (NADH), which transfers its reducing equivalents to the mitochondrion for the production of ATP via oxidative phosphorylation.

**KREBS CYCLE:** Citric acid cycle, TCA cycle, the mitochondrial process by which acetyl groups from acetyl-CoA are oxidized to $CO_2$. The reducing equivalents are captured as NADH and $FADH_2$, which feed into the electron transport system of the mitochondrion to produce ATP via oxidative phosphorylation.

## DISCUSSION

**Most of the energy** that the body requires for maintenance, work, and growth is obtained by the **terminal oxidation of acetyl coenzyme A (acetyl-CoA) produced by the catabolism of carbohydrates, fatty acids, and amino acids.** The oxidation of acetyl-CoA is **achieved by mitochondrial enzymes that make up the tricarboxylic acid cycle (TCA cycle, also called the citric acid cycle or the Krebs cycle). All of the enzymes** in this metabolic pathway are **located in the matrix of the mitochondria except one, succinate dehydrogenase. Succinate dehydrogenase is a membrane-bound protein located on the inner mitochondrial membrane facing the matrix.** The 2 carbons that enter the TCA cycle as an **acetyl group** are effectively **oxidized to carbon dioxide. Oxygen** is not directly involved in this process; instead, reducing equivalents are captured by the electron carriers $NAD^+$ and flavin adenine dinucleotide (FAD) producing 3 (NADH + $H^+$) and 1 $FADH_2$. A high-energy phosphate bond is also produced in the form of GTP. The reduced cofactors NADH and $FADH_2$ are then reoxidized by passing their reducing equivalents to $O_2$ through the electron transport system (ETS) of the mitochondria with the production of water and ATP via oxidative phosphorylation.

The **TCA cycle** is shown in Figure 14-1. In the first step, **acetyl-CoA is condensed with oxaloacetate** to produce citrate with the release of free coenzyme A in a reaction catalyzed by **citrate synthase.** Citrate is then **isomerized to isocitrate by the enzyme aconitase.** The next step involves the **oxidative decarboxylation of isocitrate to produce α-ketoglutarate.** The enzyme catalyzing this reaction, **isocitrate dehydrogenase,** requires the oxidized **electron carrier $NAD^+$** to accept the electrons released in the oxidation and produce the first NADH + $H^+$. **α-Ketoglutarate is then converted to succinyl-CoA** in a second oxidative decarboxylation reaction catalyzed by **α-ketoglutarate dehydrogenase.** This reaction requires the participation of 2 cofactors, oxidized $NAD^+$ and CoA, and results in the production of a second NADH + $H^+$. **Succinyl-CoA** is then transformed to **succinate by succinate thiokinase with the release**

**Figure 14-1.** The tricarboxylic acid (TCA) cycle, also known as the citric acid cycle and the Krebs cycle.
The overall reaction is:

$$AcCOA + 3NAD^+ + FAD + GDP + P_i \rightarrow 2CO_2 + 3NADH + FADH_2 + GTP + CoA$$

1. Citrate synthase
2. Aconitase
3. Isocitrate
4. $\alpha$-Ketoglutarate dehydrogenase
5. Succinate thiokinase
6. Succinate dehydrogenase
7. Fumarase
8. Malate dehydrogenase

of free CoA. The high energy released in the hydrolysis of the thioester bond of succinyl-CoA drives the **phosphorylation of GDP to produce GTP. Succinate is then converted to oxaloacetate** in a series of reactions reminiscent of the β-oxidation of fatty acids. A double bond is introduced into succinate in an oxidation catalyzed by **succinate dehydrogenase, the only membrane-bound enzyme in the TCA cycle.** The reducing equivalents are captured as $FADH_2$. The resulting **fumarate is then hydrated to form malate by the enzyme fumarase.** Oxaloacetate is then **regenerated by the oxidation of malate by malate dehydrogenase** with the production of another NADH + H$^+$.

Although the TCA cycle does not directly involve the participation of molecular **oxygen** as a substrate, the reduced cofactors NADH and $FADH_2$ **must be reoxidized** by the mitochondrial ETS for continued operation of the cycle. Thus, the **rate of oxidation of acetyl-CoA by the TCA cycle** is to a large degree **regulated** by the availability of the **oxidized cofactors NAD$^+$ and FAD.** When tissues do not receive enough oxygen as a result of hypoperfusion, the ETS cannot regenerate these cofactors at a sufficient rate and the reactions that use them are inhibited because one of the required substrates is lacking (acceptor control). Thus, acetyl-CoA builds up in the mitochondria, depleting free CoA levels. Decreased levels of NAD$^+$ and CoA also inhibit the conversion of pyruvate to acetyl-CoA by pyruvate dehydrogenase.

When the ETS and oxidative phosphorylation are compromised by a **lack of oxygen, cytosolic levels of ATP drop while ADP and AMP levels increase.** The flow of glucose through the glycolytic pathway is increased because of **allosteric activation of phosphofructokinase and pyruvate kinase** by the drop in ATP and rise in AMP concentrations. This results in an **increased production of NADH and pyruvate by the glycolytic pathway.** However, since electron transport is inhibited by a lack of oxygen, **regeneration of NAD$^+$ by the glycerol 3-phosphate or malate-aspartate shuttles,** and the **ETS is also inhibited.** To continue the production of ATP by the glycolytic pathway, **NAD$^+$ must be regenerated** to accept more reducing equivalents when **glyceraldehyde 3-phosphate is oxidized to 1,3-bisphosphoglycerate. Lactate dehydrogenase** is activated by increased levels of pyruvate and NADH and converts pyruvate to lactate with the regeneration of NAD$^+$ (Figure 14-2). **Lactate** that cannot be reused by the cells that produce it is **transported out of the cell to the bloodstream.**

Lactate has 2 metabolic fates, either complete combustion to $CO_2$ and $H_2O$ or conversion back to glucose through gluconeogenesis. Both processes require

**Figure 14-2.** The conversion of pyruvate to lactate by the enzyme pyruvate dehydrogenase. The reaction, which is reversible, uses the reducing equivalents from NADH and regenerates NAD$^+$ for the continuation of the glycolytic pathway when oxygen is limiting.

an active ETS and oxidative phosphorylation. Reduced oxygenation of cells thus decreases the utilization of lactate and increases its production with a resulting **lactic acidosis.**

When tissues are hypoperfused, the resulting **anaerobic** conditions have energetic consequences. First, **all catabolic processes that require an active ETS and oxidative phosphorylation (eg, β-oxidation of fatty acids and amino acid breakdown) are inhibited.** Thus, certain energy stores cannot be used by the cell. Energy needs must be met by catabolism of carbohydrates through the glycolytic pathway. However, since under these anaerobic conditions, **pyruvate dehydrogenase, the TCA cycle and oxidative phosphorylation are compromised,** only a fraction of the chemical energy that is obtained from the oxidation of glucose under aerobic conditions is produced. Glucose completely oxidized to $CO_2$ and $H_2O$ under aerobic conditions will produce between **36 and 38 mol of ATP per mole of glucose** depending on the shuttle used to transport cytosolic reducing equivalents to the mitochondria. **Only 2 mol of ATP are produced per mole of glucose converted to lactate through anaerobic glycolysis.** The ATP needs of the cell are met by the increased rate of the glycolytic pathway.

## COMPREHENSION QUESTIONS

14.1 Phil Hardy has decided to train for an upcoming marathon. Nearing the age of 50 years, Phil figures that after he trains he should be able to maintain a 9 minute-per-mile pace, which would mean that he would finish the race in approximately 4 hours. Given that he would be adequately hydrating himself at the various water stations along the way, as he is about to finish the 26-mile and 385-yard course, what is the primary fuel that his leg muscles would be using?

A. Fatty acids from the blood

B. Glycerol from the blood

C. Glycogen stored in muscle

D. Glucose from the blood

E. Ketone bodies from the blood

14.2 A postoperative patient on intravenous fluids develops lesions in the mouth (angular stomatitis). Urinalysis indicates an excretion of 15 μg riboflavin/mg creatinine, which is abnormally low. Which of the following TCA cycle enzymes is most likely to be affected?

A. Citrate synthase

B. Isocitrate dehydrogenase

C. Fumarase

D. Malate dehydrogenase

E. Succinate dehydrogenase

14.3  After excessive drinking over an extended period of time while eating poorly, a middle-aged man is admitted to the hospital with "high output" heart failure. Which of the following enzymes is most likely inhibited?

A.  Aconitase

B.  Citrate synthase

C.  Isocitrate dehydrogenase

D.  α-Ketoglutarate dehydrogenase

E.  Succinate thiokinase

## ANSWERS

14.1  **A.** After 4 hours of heavy exercise, glycogen stored in muscle cells has been expended. Free glycerol cannot be used by the muscle cell because it does not have the enzyme (glycerol kinase) that will phosphorylate it so that it can enter the glycolytic pathway. Although glucose and ketone bodies can be taken up by the muscle cells and used for energy, fatty acid oxidation provides most of the ATP for the marathon runner at this point in the race.

14.2  **E.** The patient has demonstrated a deficiency in riboflavin (urinary excretion of less than 30 µg/mg creatinine is considered clinically deficient). Riboflavin is a component of the cofactor FAD, which is required for the conversion of succinate to fumarate by succinate dehydrogenase.

14.3  **D.** This patient has exhibited symptoms of beri-beri disease, which is a result of a nutritional deficiency in vitamin B$_1$ (thiamine). The active form of the vitamin, thiamine pyrophosphate, is a required cofactor for α-ketoglutarate dehydrogenase.

## BIOCHEMISTRY PEARLS

▶ Most of the energy that the body requires for maintenance, work, and growth is obtained by the terminal oxidation of acetyl-CoA, which is produced by the catabolism of carbohydrates, fatty acids, and amino acids.

▶ The oxidation of acetyl-CoA is achieved by mitochondrial enzymes that make up the TCA cycle (also called the citric acid cycle or the Krebs cycle).

▶ When the ETS and oxidative phosphorylation are compromised by a lack of oxygen, cytosolic levels of ATP drop, while ADP and AMP levels increase.

▶ The flow of glucose through the glycolytic pathway is increased because of allosteric activation of phosphofructokinase and pyruvate kinase by the drop in ATP and rise in AMP concentrations.

▶ The 4 carbon intermediates of the TCA cycle may be replenished or increased by metabolites of the glucogenic amino acids entering at α-ketoglutarate, succinyl-CoA, or oxaloacetate. In addition, the C$_4$ pool can also be increased by the carboxylation of pyruvate to oxaloacetate catalyzed by pyruvate carboxylase.

## REFERENCES

Beattie DS. Bioenergetics and oxidative metabolism. In: Devlin TM, ed. *Textbook of Biochemistry with Clinical Correlations*. 7th ed. New York: Wiley-Liss; 2010.

Harris RA. Carbohydrate metabolism I: major metabolic pathways and their control. In: Devlin TM, ed. *Textbook of Biochemistry with Clinical Correlations*. 7th ed. New York: Wiley-Liss; 2010.

A 59-year-old man is brought to the emergency department (ED) by the emergency medical services after a family member found him extremely confused and disoriented, with an unsteady gait and strange irregular eye movements. The patient has been known in the past to be a heavy drinker. He has no known medical problems and denies any other drug usage. On examination, he is afebrile with a pulse of 110 beats/minute and a normal blood pressure. He is extremely disoriented and agitated. Horizontal rapid eye movement on lateral gaze is noted bilaterally. His gait is very unsteady. The remainder of his examination is normal. The urine drug screen was negative and he had a positive blood alcohol level. The ED physician administers thiamine.

▶ What is the most likely diagnosis?
▶ What is importance of thiamine in biochemical reactions?

# ANSWERS TO CASE 15:
## Thiamine Deficiency

*Summary:* A 59-year-old man with a history of heavy alcohol use presents with mental confusion, ataxia, and ophthalmoplegia.

- **Most likely diagnosis:** Wernicke-Korsakoff syndrome (thiamine deficiency) often associated with chronic users of alcohol.

- **Importance of thiamine:** An important water-soluble vitamin used as a cofactor in enzymatic reactions involving the transfer of an aldehyde group. Without thiamine, individuals can develop dementia, macrocytic anemia (folate deficiency), gastritis, peptic ulcer disease, liver disease, depression, nutritional deficiencies, cardiomyopathy, and pancreatitis.

## CLINICAL CORRELATION

Thiamine, also known as vitamin $B_1$, is fairly ubiquitous. Thiamine deficiency is uncommon except in alcoholics as a result of nutritional deficiencies and malabsorption. The classic clinical triad of dementia, ataxia (difficulty with walking), and eye findings may be seen, but more commonly, only forgetfulness is noted. Sometimes, thiamine deficiency can lead to vague symptoms such as leg numbness or tingling. Because thiamine is water soluble, it can be added to intravenous fluids and administered in that way. Other manifestations include beri-beri disease, which is cardiac involvement leading to a high cardiac output, and vasodilation. Affected patients often feel warm and flushed, and they can have heart failure.

# APPROACH TO:
## Thiamine Pyrophosphate

### OBJECTIVES

1. Know about the role of thiamine pyrophosphate (TPP) in pyruvate dehydrogenase.

2. Understand the role of TPP in $\alpha$-ketoglutarate dehydrogenase and the role of TPP in transketolase in pentose phosphate pathway.

3. Be familiar with how thiamine deficiency results in decreased energy generation and how it results in decreased ribose and NADPH production.

### DEFINITIONS

**CARBANION:** A carbon within a molecule that has a negative charge because of the removal of a proton (hydrogen ion).

**DECARBOXYLATION:** The process of removing a carboxyl group (–COOH) from a molecule. Frequently this is achieved by oxidizing the compound in a process known as oxidative decarboxylation.

**DEHYDROGENASE:** An enzyme that oxidizes a molecule by the removal of a pair of electrons and 1 or 2 protons.

**NUCLEOPHILIC ADDITION:** The process of forming a bond between an electron-rich group (nucleophile) and an electron-deficient atom (electrophile).

**OXIDATION:** The removal of electrons from an atom or compound.

**THIAMINE:** Vitamin $B_1$; a water-soluble vitamin containing a thiazolium ring. The active form of the vitamin is thiamine pyrophosphate, which is an important coenzyme for many biochemical reactions.

## DISCUSSION

**Thiamine (vitamin $B_1$) is an important water-soluble vitamin** that, in its **active form of thiamine pyrophosphate,** is used as a **cofactor in enzymatic reactions that involve the transfer of an aldehyde group.** Thiamine can be synthesized by plants and some microorganisms, but not usually by animals. Hence, **humans must obtain thiamine from the diet,** though small amounts may be obtained from synthesis by intestinal bacteria. Because of its importance in metabolic reactions, it is present in large amounts in skeletal muscle, heart, liver, kidney, and brain. Thus, it has a widespread distribution in foods, but there can be a substantial loss of thiamine during cooking above 212°F (100°C).

Thiamine is absorbed in the intestine by both active transport mechanisms and passive diffusion. The active form of the cofactor, **TPP (thiamine pyrophosphate), is synthesized by an enzymatic transfer of a pyrophosphate group from ATP to thiamine** (Figure 15-1). The resulting TPP has a reactive carbon on the thiazole ring

**Figure 15-1.** Activation of thiamine (vitamin $B_1$) to the active cofactor, thiamine pyrophosphate (TPP) by the enzyme TPP synthetase.

**Figure 15-2.** The catalytic mechanism shared by the enzymes pyruvate dehydrogenase, α-ketoglutarate dehydrogenase, and branched-chain α-ketoacid dehydrogenase. $E_1$ is the dehydrogenase complex; $E_2$ is the dihydrolipoyl transacetylase subunit; and $E_3$ is the dihydrolipoyl dehydrogenase component. $E_1$ and $E_2$ are specific to each enzyme, and $E_3$ is common to all 3 enzymes.

that is easily ionized to form a carbanion, which can undergo nucleophilic addition reactions.

**Thiamine pyrophosphate is an essential cofactor** for enzymes that catalyze the **oxidative decarboxylation of α-keto acids to form an acylated coenzyme A (acyl CoA).** These include **pyruvate dehydrogenase (pyruvate → acetyl-CoA), α-ketoglutarate dehydrogenase (α-KG → succinyl-CoA) and branched-chain α-keto acid dehydrogenase.** These 3 enzymes operate by a similar catalytic mechanism (Figure 15-2). Each of these enzymes is a multi-subunit complex with 3 enzymatic activities that require the participation of several cofactors. The first activity ($E_1$) is the **dehydrogenase complex**, which has TPP as the enzyme-bound cofactor. The carbanion form of TPP attacks the carbonyl carbon of the α-keto acid, releasing $CO_2$ and leaving a hydroxyalkyl-TPP intermediate. The hydroxyalkyl group reacts with the oxidized form of lipoamide, the prosthetic group of dihydrolipoyl transacetylase ($E_2$), which is the second component of the complex. The resulting acyllipoamide reacts with coenzyme A (HSCoA) to form the product, acyl CoA, and leaving lipoamide in the fully reduced form. To regenerate the fully oxidized form of lipoamide for further rounds of the reaction, it interacts with the **third component of the complex, dihydrolipoyl dehydrogenase ($E_3$)**, which has covalently bound FAD. The FAD accepts the reducing equivalents from the reduced lipoamide to form $FADH_2$ **and oxidized lipoamide.** The reducing equivalents are then transferred to **NAD⁺ to form NADH, which is regenerated via the electron transport system with the production of ATP.**

The $E_1$ and $E_2$ components are specific for each of the pyruvate dehydrogenase, α-ketoglutarate dehydrogenase, and branched-chain α-keto acid dehydrogenase complexes. However, the $E_3$ component is identical for all of the enzymes.

**Figure 15-3.** The reaction catalyzed by the enzyme transketolase, which transfers a glycoaldehyde group from a ketose to an aldose.

Thiamine pyrophosphate is also an important cofactor for the **transketolase** reactions in the **pentose phosphate pathway of carbohydrate metabolism** (Figure 15-3). These reactions are important in the **reversible transformation of pentoses into the glycolytic intermediates fructose 6-phosphate and glyceraldehyde 3-phosphate.** Again, it is the reactive carbon on the thiazole ring of TPP that reacts with a ketose phosphate (xylulose 5-phosphate) to cause the release of an aldose phosphate with 2 fewer carbons (glyceraldehyde 3-phosphate). The TPP-bound glycoaldehyde unit is then transferred to a different aldose phosphate (ribose 5-phosphate or erythrose 4-phosphate) to produce a ketose phosphate that has 2 carbons more (sedoheptulose 7-phosphate or fructose 6-phosphate).

A **deficiency in thiamine will decrease the efficiency of the enzymes for which TPP is required as a cofactor.** Thus, the rate of conversion of pyruvate to acetyl-CoA and the flow of acetyl-CoA through the tricarboxylic acid cycle will be depressed as a result of the inefficiency of the TPP-requiring enzymes pyruvate dehydrogenase and α-ketoglutarate dehydrogenase. The production of the reduced electron carrier, NADH, and the ATP produced from it via oxidative phosphorylation will be decreased as a consequence. Because **nervous tissue and heart use at high rates ATP** synthesized from the **oxidation of NADH produced from pyruvate conversion to acetyl-CoA** and from the tricarboxylic acid (TCA) cycle, **these tissues are most affected by a deficiency in thiamine.** When deficient in thiamine, the brain can no longer efficiently metabolize pyruvate through the TCA cycle to produce ATP and thus must convert it to lactate to produce ATP. This increased conversion of pyruvate to lactate decreases the pH in areas of the brain that have rapid ATP turnover rates and leads to cellular destruction.

A **deficiency in thiamine also adversely affects the flux of glucose metabolized by the pentose phosphate pathway. Transketolase activity requires the cofactor TPP to transfer the glycoaldehyde unit from a ketose to an aldose** in the remodeling reactions of the pathway. When these reactions cannot proceed, precursor metabolites build up, and the flow through the pathway is decreased.

This results in a **decreased production of NADPH and decreased conversion of glucose to pentose, including ribose.** This can lead to decreased regeneration of reduced glutathione and **susceptibility to oxidative stress.**

Thiamine turnover is rapid because of the ubiquitous presence of **thiaminase enzymes** that **hydrolyze thiamine into its pyrimidine and thiazole components.** Thus, **symptoms of thiamine deficiency can appear within 2 weeks of a diet depleted in thiamine.** In Western societies, severe thiamine deficiency is most frequently found in **alcoholics.** Patients who chronically misuse alcohol are prone to thiamine deficiency arising from a number of factors including poor nutrition and poor absorption and storage, as well as an increased breakdown of TPP. Alcohol is known to inhibit the active absorption of thiamine.

Thiamine deficiency is most frequently assessed by assaying erythrocyte transketolase activity in the presence as well as the absence of added TPP. If the red blood cells have sufficient thiamine, then the transketolase will be fully saturated with TPP, and no increase in activity will be observed when TPP is added to the assay system. An increase in transketolase activity indicates that the patient is thiamine deficient.

## COMPREHENSION QUESTIONS

15.1 A full-term female infant failed to gain weight and showed metabolic acidosis in the neonatal period. A physical examination at 6 months showed failure to thrive, hypotonia, small muscle mass, severe head lag, and a persistent acidosis (pH 7.0–7.2). Blood lactate, pyruvate, and alanine were greatly elevated. Treatment with thiamine did not alleviate the lactic acidosis.

Which of the following enzymes is most likely deficient in this patient?

A. Alanine aminotransferase

B. Phosphoenolpyruvate carboxykinase

C. Pyruvate carboxylase

D. Pyruvate dehydrogenase

E. Pyruvate kinase

15.2 A 3-month-old male infant developed seizures and progressively worsened, showing hypotonia, psychomotor retardation, and poor head control. He had lactic acidosis and an elevated plasma pyruvate level, both of which were more than 7 times the normal amount. Pyruvate carboxylase activity was measured using extracts of fibroblasts and was found to be less than 1% of the normal level. Oral administration of which of the following amino acids would you recommend as the best therapy for this patient?

A. Alanine

B. Glutamine

C. Leucine

D. Lysine

E. Serine

15.3   A deficiency in thiamine (vitamin B₁) would most likely lead to which of the
following clinical manifestations?

A. Decrease in carboxylase enzyme activity

B. Decrease in serum lactate concentrations

C. Decrease in red blood cell transketolase activity

D. Increase in urinary methylmalonate

E. Increase in prothrombin time

## ANSWERS

15.1   **D.** The increased concentrations of pyruvate, lactate, and alanine indicate
that there is a block in the pathway leading from pyruvate toward the TCA
cycle. A deficiency in pyruvate dehydrogenase would lead to a buildup of pyruvate. Pyruvate has 3 fates other than conversion to acetyl-CoA by pyruvate
dehydrogenase: conversion to oxaloacetate by pyruvate carboxylase, reduction to lactate by lactate dehydrogenase, and transamination to the amino
acid alanine. Thus, because pyruvate builds up, an increase in lactate and alanine would be expected if pyruvate dehydrogenase was deficient.

15.2   **B.** A deficiency in pyruvate carboxylase results in a diminution of oxaloacetate, the $C_4$ acid that acts as the acceptor for an acetyl group from acetyl-
CoA. In order for the TCA cycle to continue efficiently, $C_4$ acids must be
replenished. Amino acids whose carbon skeletons feed into the TCA cycle
and increase the $C_4$ pool will accomplish this. Glutamine, which is converted
to α-ketoglutarate, will lead to an increase in all of the $C_4$ acids (succinate,
fumarate, malate, and oxaloacetate). Alanine and serine are converted to
pyruvate, which as a result of the deficiency in pyruvate carboxylase will not
increase the $C_4$ pool. Lysine and leucine are ketogenic amino acids and thus
also do not increase the $C_4$ pool.

15.3   **C.** In addition to being an important cofactor for the enzymes involved in
the oxidative decarboxylation of pyruvate, α-ketoglutarate, and branched-
chain α-ketoacids, thiamine is also a cofactor for the enzyme transketolase,
the enzyme that transfers a glycoaldehyde group from a ketose sugar to an
aldose sugar in the pentose phosphate pathway. One of the diagnostic tools
in determining thiamine deficiency is determination of the activity of red
blood cell transketolase in the presence and absence of added thiamine.
Thiamine deficiency would be expected to increase blood lactate concentrations. Biotin deficiency would lead to decreased carboxylase activity,
whereas an increased methylmalonate concentration would be observed
with vitamin B₁₂ deficiency. Vitamin K deficiency would lead to an increase
in prothrombin time.

## BIOCHEMISTRY PEARLS

▶ Thiamine (vitamin $B_1$) is an important water-soluble vitamin that, in its active form of TPP, is used as a cofactor in enzymatic reactions that involve the transfer of an aldehyde group.

▶ Thiamine deficiency is uncommon except in people who abuse alcohol who, as a consequence of nutritional deficiencies and malabsorption, may become deficient.

▶ The classic clinical triad of dementia, ataxia (difficulty with walking), and eye findings may be seen, but more commonly, forgetfulness alone is noted.

▶ Thiamine pyrophosphate is also an important cofactor for many dehydrogenase reactions as well as the transketolase reactions in the pentose phosphate pathway of carbohydrate metabolism.

## REFERENCES

Murray RK, Bender DA, Botham KM, et al, eds. *Harper's Illustrated Biochemistry*. 29th ed. New York: Lange Medical Books/McGraw-Hill; 2012.

Wilson JD. Vitamin deficiency and excess. In: Longo D, Fauci AS, Kaspar D, et al, eds. *Harrison's Principles of Internal Medicine*. 18th ed. New York: McGraw-Hill; 2011.

A 68-year-old woman in a hypertensive crisis is being treated in the intensive care unit with intravenous nitroprusside for 48 hours. The patient's blood pressure was brought back down to normal levels; however, she was complaining of a burning sensation in her throat and mouth followed by nausea and vomiting, diaphoresis, agitation, and dyspnea. The nurse noticed a sweet almond smell in her breath. An arterial blood gas revealed a significant metabolic acidosis. A serum test suggests a metabolite of nitroprusside, thiocyanate, is at toxic levels.

► What is the likely cause of her symptoms?
► What is the biochemical mechanism of this problem?
► What is the treatment for this condition?

# ANSWERS TO CASE 16:
## Cyanide Poisoning

*Summary:* A 69-year-old woman with new onset burning sensation in mouth and throat, nausea and vomiting, agitation, and diaphoresis after a medication error was noted. Metabolic acidosis is seen on the arterial blood gas. A thiocyanate level is in the toxic range.

- **Diagnosis:** Cyanide poisoning from toxic dose of nitroprusside.

- **Biochemical mechanism:** Cyanide inhibits mitochondrial cytochrome oxidase, blocking electron transport, and preventing oxygen utilization. Lactic acidosis results secondary to anaerobic metabolism.

- **Treatment:** Supportive therapy, gastrointestinal decontamination, oxygen, and antidotal therapy with amyl nitrite, sodium nitrite, and sodium thiosulfate.

## CLINICAL CORRELATION

Hypertensive emergencies are defined as episodes of severely elevated blood pressure, such as systolic levels of 220 mm Hg and/or diastolic blood pressures exceeding 120 mm Hg *with* patient symptoms of end-organ dysfunction. These symptoms may include severe headache, neurologic deficits, chest pain, or heart failure symptoms. Hypertensive emergencies require immediate lowering of the blood pressure to lower (but not necessarily to normal) levels. In contrast, hypertensive urgencies are circumstances of markedly elevated blood pressures in the absence of patient symptoms; lowering the blood pressure over 24 to 48 hours is reasonable in these cases.

One hazard of abruptly lowering the blood pressure is causing hypotension and subsequent ischemia to the brain or heart. In other words, the very treatment designed to prevent end-organ disease may cause the problem. To avoid precipitous hypotension, agents that induce a smooth fall in blood pressure are preferable, such as sodium nitroprusside, a titratable intravenous agent used for malignant hypertension. Its desirable properties include the ability to precisely increase or decrease the infusion to affect the blood pressure. One side effect of sodium nitroprusside is that its metabolite is thiocyanate, and with prolonged use, cyanide poisoning may result, which inhibits the electron transport chain. Thus, in clinical practice, short-term nitroprusside is used, or serum thiocyanate levels are drawn.

# APPROACH TO:
## Electron Transport System and Cyanide

## OBJECTIVES

1. Know about the function of the electron transport chain (ETC).

2. Understand what factors may inhibit the ETC.

3. Be familiar with the biochemical process by which the therapy for cyanide poisoning works.

4. Recognize other ETC sites and agents of inhibition.

## DEFINITIONS

**OXIDATIVE PHOSPHORYLATION:** The mitochondrial process whereby electrons from NADH or reduced flavin bound in enzymes are transferred down the electron transport chain to oxygen forming water and providing energy through the formation of an hydrogen ion gradient across the inner mitochondrial membrane. The hydrogen ion gradient is used to drive the formation of ATP from ADP and inorganic phosphate ($P_i$). This process is also called *coupled oxidative phosphorylation* to emphasize that ATP formation from ADP and $P_i$ is coupled to and linked with electron transport such that inhibition of one also inhibits the other.

**HYDROGEN ION GRADIENT:** A situation developed across the inner mitochondrial membrane wherein the concentration of hydrogen ions outside the mitochondrion is higher than the concentration inside. Hydrogen ions are extruded from the mitochondrion by the transfer of electrons from complex I to coenzyme Q, from coenzyme Q to complex III, and from complex III to complex IV. The gradient is discharged by ATP synthase, which admits hydrogen ions into the mitochondrion thereby driving the phosphorylation of ADP by $P_i$.

**ELECTRON TRANSPORT CHAIN:** Present in the mitochondrial membrane, this linear array of redox active electron carriers consists of NADH dehydrogenase, coenzyme Q, cytochrome c reductase, cytochrome c, and cytochrome oxidase as well as ancillary iron sulfur proteins. The electron carriers are arrayed in order of decreasing reduction potential such that the last carrier has the most positive reduction potential and transfers electrons to oxygen.

**REDUCTION POTENTIAL:** The tendency of an electron carrier to give up electrons, stated in electron volts, is called reduction potential. In any reduction–oxidation reaction electrons flow from the species with the more negative reduction potential to the more positive reduction potential.

**CYTOCHROME:** A heme (protoporphyrin IX) containing electron transfer protein. Some heme moieties are covalently attached to the protein components (cytochrome c), whereas others have isoprenoid side chains (cytochromes a and $a_3$).

**IRON SULFUR PROTEINS:** These carry 1 electron and contain centers that chelate iron with organic and inorganic sulfur. Some centers contain a single iron atom chelated by 4 cysteine sulfurs; others contain 2 iron atoms chelated through 4 cysteine sulfurs and 2 inorganic sulfurs; yet others contain 4 iron atoms chelated by 4 cysteine sulfurs and 4 inorganic sulfurs.

**COENZYME Q (UBIQUINONE):** A 2 electron accepting quinone that can accept and transfer 1 electron at a time allowing it to exist in a semiquinone state as well as the fully oxidized quinone or fully reduced dihydroxy state. It is bound to multiple isoprenoid units (ubiquinone has ten units), allowing it to bind to the membrane.

**FLAVIN MONONUCLEOTIDE (FMN):** An isoalloxazine ring bound to ribosyl monophosphate in an N-glycosidic bond. FMN can accept 2 electrons or donate 1 at a time to another electron acceptor.

**FLAVIN ADENINE DINUCLEOTIDE (FAD):** An isoalloxazine ring bound to ribosyl monophosphate in an N-glycosidic bond, which is attached to adenosine monophosphate. Like FMN, FAD can accept or donate 2 electrons 1 at a time to another electron acceptor.

## DISCUSSION

The **ETC or electron transport system (ETS)** is located on the **inner membrane of the mitochondrion** and is responsible for the **harnessing of free energy** released as **electrons travel from more reduced (more negative reduction potential, $E_0'$) to more oxidized (more positive $E_0'$) carriers** to drive the phosphorylation of ADP to ATP (Figure 16-1). Complex I accepts a pair of electrons from NADH ($E_0' = -0.32$ V) and passes the electron pair through the intervening carriers to **complex IV**, which passes the electrons to 1 atom of molecular oxygen ($E_0' = +0.82$ V) to form water with hydrogen ions ($H^+$) from the medium.

The transport of electrons through the carriers is **highly coupled to the formation of ATP from ADP and $P_i$** through the formation and relaxation of the **proton gradient formed across the inner mitochondrial membrane by electron transport**. Each time **electrons are transported between complexes I and III**, between **complexes III and IV**, or **between complex IV** and **oxygen, protons are extruded from the mitochondrial matrix** across the inner membrane to the intermembrane space/cytosol. (The outer membrane poses no barrier to proton passage.) In other words, the energy gained from these electron transfers is used to pump protons from the mitochondrial matrix side to the cytosol side. Because the mitochondrial membrane is impermeable to protons, there is a gradient that develops with a higher concentration of protons outside the matrix. The protons then come through the ATP synthase complex through proton pores, and, as they come back into the mitochondrial matrix, ADP is phosphorylated to ATP. Thus, because the process of electron transport is tightly coupled to ADP phosphorylation, ADP must be present for electron transport to proceed, and therefore the ADP/ATP translocase must be able to exchange a molecule of ADP in the cytosol for a molecule of ATP (newly made) in the matrix of the mitochondria. When these **various processes operate in concert the mitochondria** are said to exhibit **coupled respiration**.

The components of the electron transport chain have various **cofactors**. **Complex I, NADH dehydrogenase**, contains a **flavin cofactor and iron sulfur centers**, whereas **complex III, cytochrome reductase**, contains cytochromes b and $c_1$. **Complex IV, cytochrome oxidase**, which transfers electrons to **oxygen**, contains **copper ions** as well as **cytochromes a and $a_3$**. The general structure of the cytochrome cofactors is shown in Figure 16-2. Each of the cytochromes has a heme cofactor, but they vary slightly. The b-type cytochromes have

**Figure 16-1.** Schematic diagram of electron transport chain ATP synthase and ATP/ADP translocase.

**Figure 16-2.** Heme active center of cytochromes a, b, and c components of electron transport chain.

protoporphyrin IX, which is identical to the heme in hemoglobin. The c-type cytochromes are covalently bound to cysteine residue 10 in the protein. The a-type cytochromes have a long isoprenoid $[(CH_2-CH = C(CH_3)-CH_2)_n]$ tail bound at one side-chain position.

Inhibition of the electron transport chain in coupled mitochondria can occur at any of the 3 constituent functional processes; electron transport per se, formation of ATP, or antiport translocation of ADP/ATP (Table 16-1). **The best known inhibitor of the ADP/ATP translocase is atractyloside** in the presence of which **no ADP for phosphorylation is transported across the inner membrane to the ATP synthase** and **no ATP is transported out.** In the absence of ADP phosphorylation the proton gradient is not reduced allowing other protons to be extruded into the intermembrane space because of the elevated [H⁺], and, thus, electron transfer is halted. Likewise the antibiotic oligomycin directly inhibits the ATP synthase, causing a cessation of ATP formation, buildup of protons in the intermembrane space, and a halt in electron transfer. Similarly, a blockade of complex I, III, or IV that inhibits electron flow down the chain to $O_2$ would also stop both ATP formation and ADP/ATP translocation across the inner mitochondrial membrane.

**Cyanide ion (CN⁻)** is a potent inhibitor of complex IV, the cytochrome c oxidase component of the electron transport system in the oxidized state of the heme ($Fe^{3+}$). It can be delivered to tissue electron transport systems as a dissolved gas

| Table 16-1 • RESPIRATORY CHAIN SITES AND INHIBITORS | |
|---|---|
| **Respiratory Chain Sites** | **Inhibitor** |
| Complex I: NADH: CoQ reductase | Piericidin<br>Amytal<br>Rotenone |
| Complex III: Cytochrome c reductase | Antimycin A |
| Complex IV: Cytochrome oxidase | Cyanide ion<br>Carbon monoxide |
| ATP synthase | Oligomycin |
| ADP/ATP translocase | Atractyloside, Bongkrekate |

$$Hb(Fe^{+2})O_2 + NO_2^- \longrightarrow MetHb(Fe^{+3})OH + NO_3^-$$

$$MetHb(Fe^{+3})OH + cyt\ a/a_3(Fe^{+3})\text{-}CN^- \longrightarrow cyt\ a/a_3(Fe^{+3}) + MetHb(Fe^{+3})\text{-}CN^-$$

$$MetHb(Fe^{+3})\text{-}CN^- + S_2O_3^{-2} \xrightarrow{Rhodanese} SCN^- + SO_3^{-2} + MetHb(Fe^{+3})OH$$

**Figure 16-3.** Strategy for reversal of cyanide binding to cytochrome oxidase (cyt a/a$_3$Fe$^{3+}$).

after breathing HCN or ingested as a salt such as KCN or as a medication leading to the formation of CN⁻ such as nitroprusside. **CN⁻ competes effectively with oxygen for binding to cytochrome c oxidase at the oxygen-binding site.** Cyanide binding—and therefore, cyanide poisoning—is reversible if treated properly and early. The treatment strategy depends on dissociation of cyanide from cytochrome a/a$_3$ (Fe$^{3+}$). **Increasing the percentage of oxygen breathed will increase the competition of oxygen over cyanide for the cytochrome a/a$_3$ (Fe$^{3+}$).** Two other medications foster this competition. Nitrite ion (NO$_2^-$) is administered to convert some oxyhemoglobin [HbO$_2$(Fe$^{2+}$)] to methemoglobin [met-HbOH(Fe$^{3+}$)], another competitor for cyanide binding (Figure 16-3). The cyanide adduct of methemoglobin is formed releasing cytochrome oxidase in the Fe$^{3+}$ form ready to bind oxygen and disinhibit the electron transport chain. To remove the cyanide adduct in a nontoxic fashion, thiosulfate ion is administered. The mitochondrial enzyme rhodanese catalyzes the conversion of cyanide and thiosulfate to thiocyanate and sulfite. Thiocyanate is incapable of inhibiting cytochrome oxidase and is excreted. The methemoglobin can be reconverted to oxyhemoglobin by NADH and methemoglobin reductase.

Other sites of the electron transport chain can be targets of inhibitors based on similarity in structure to enzyme components or to substrates of the various components. For instance, the fish poison rotenone resembles the isoalloxazine ring of the FMN cofactor of complex I, the NADH CoQ reductase. Rotenone binds the enzyme quite avidly and prevents transfer of electrons from NADH to coenzyme Q through the iron sulfur centers and thus inhibits oxidation of NADH and subsequent reduction of oxygen to water. By contrast, carbon monoxide resembles molecular oxygen and binds with a higher affinity than oxygen to complex IV, the cytochrome oxidase component, inhibiting transfer of electrons to oxygen.

## COMPREHENSION QUESTIONS

16.1  A 16-month-old girl was found to have ingested approximately 30 mL of an acetonitrile-based cosmetic nail remover when she vomited 15 minutes postingestion. The poison control center was contacted, but no treatment was recommended because it was confused with an acetone-based nail polish remover. The child was put to bed at her normal time, which was 2 hours following ingestion. Respiratory distress developed sometime after the child was put to bed, and she was found dead the next morning. Inhibition of which of the following enzymes was the most likely cause of this child's death?

A.  Cytochrome c reductase

B.  Cytochrome oxidase

C.  Coenzyme Q reductase

D.  NADH dehydrogenase

E.  Succinate dehydrogenase

16.2  Which of the following best describes the reason for the latency of acetonitrile toxicity and why prompt treatment would have prevented this child's respiratory distress and death?

A.  Acetonitrile crosses the mitochondrial membrane slowly.

B.  Acetonitrile induces hemolysis by inhibiting glucose 6-phosphate dehydrogenase.

C.  Acetonitrile is only poorly absorbed by the intestinal system.

D.  Complex IV of the electron transport system binds acetonitrile weakly.

E.  Cytochrome P450 enzymes oxidize acetonitrile and slowly release cyanide.

16.3  Inhibition of oxidative phosphorylation by cyanide ion leads to increases in which of the following?

A.  Gluconeogenesis to provide more glucose for metabolism

B.  Transport of ADP into the mitochondria

C.  Utilization of fatty acids substrates to augment glucose utilization

D.  Utilization of ketone bodies for energy generation

E.  Lactic acid in the blood causing acidosis

16.4  Which of the following procedures best describes the emergency intervention for cyanide poisoning?

A.  Decrease the partial pressure of oxygen

B.  Treatment with nitrites to convert hemoglobin to methemoglobin.

C.  Treatment with thiosulfate to form thiocyanate

D.  Use of N-acetylcysteine taken orally

16.5  An unskilled worker in a water garden/plant nursery was sent to sweep up a spill of a white powder in the storage shed. Later he was found with labored breathing and convulsions. On further examination, the white powder was identified as rotenone. Respiratory distress is induced on rotenone exposure because it inhibits the complex that catalyzes which of the following?

  A.  Electron transfer from NADH to coenzyme Q
  B.  Oxidation of coenzyme Q
  C.  Reduction of cytochrome c
  D.  Electron transfer from cytochrome c to cytochrome $a_1/a_3$
  E.  Electron transfer from cytochrome $a_1/a_3$ to oxygen

16.6  The major metabolic consequence of perturbation of the electron transfer in mitochondria is which of the following?

  A.  Increased production of NADPH
  B.  Increased oxidation of NADH
  C.  Increased reduction of $O_2$ to $H_2O$
  D.  Decreased regeneration of $NAD^+$
  E.  Decreased reduction of FAD

## ANSWERS

16.1  **B.** The culprit here is cyanide produced from acetonitrile. Cyanide inhibits the electron transport chain of cytochrome oxidase.

16.2  **E.** Acetonitrile itself is not the toxicant but undergoes metabolism and produces cyanide, which is the toxic agent here.

16.3  **E.** Gluconeogenesis requires ATP, which is in short supply, turning up the catabolism of glucose to lactate in the absence of an intact electron transport chain. ADP cannot be transported into the mitochondrion because ATP, its antiporter partner, is not made by oxidative phosphorylation as a result of cyanide inhibition of cytochrome oxidase. Metabolism of fatty acids and ketone bodies requires a functional electron transport chain for their metabolism, and these possibilities are also ruled out.

16.4  **B.** Increased oxygen competes with cyanide bound to cytochrome oxidase displacing it. Nitrites bind to hemoglobin, converting it to methemoglobin, which binds cyanide more tightly than cyanhemoglobin and pulls cyanide from cyanhemoglobin to form cyanomethemoglobin. Thiosulfate is used to displace cyanide from cyanomethemoglobin to form thiocyanate, which can be excreted, a happy ending for cyanide poisoning. N-acetylcysteine is used for acetaminophen toxicity, not cyanide toxicity.

16.5  **A.** Rotenone binds avidly to the flavoprotein NADH CoQ reductase, complex I (also called NADH dehydrogenase). The central portion of the rotenone structure resembles the isoalloxazine ring of the FMN molecule, and when it binds to complex I, rotenone prevents the transfer of electrons from NADH to coenzyme Q.

16.6  **D.** Inhibition of the electron transport chain shuts down the major pathway of regenerating $NAD^+$ from the NADH produced in intermediary metabolism. This forces the cytosolic conversion of pyruvate to lactate to regenerate $NAD^+$ so that glycolysis can continue in the absence of a functioning electron transport system.

## BIOCHEMISTRY PEARLS

▶ The ETC or ETS is located on the inner membrane of the mitochondrion and is responsible for the harnessing of free energy. The chain consists of a series of carriers arranged along the inner membrane of mitochondria that transport electrons from NADH and reduced flavin carriers to molecular oxygen.

▶ Energy is released as electrons travel from more reduced (more negative reduction potential, $E'_0$) to more oxidized (more positive $E'_0$) carriers to drive the phosphorylation of ADP to ATP.

▶ The components of the electron transport chain have various cofactors, which form vital complexes.

▶ The disruption of various complexes may interfere with the ETC, leading to inability to manufacture ATP.

▶ The energy gained from electron transfer is used to drive protons out of the inner mitochondrial matrix to the cytosol, establishing a gradient of protons. Because the protons come back into the matrix via the ATP synthase complex, ADP is phosphorylated to ATP.

▶ The normal mitochondria produce ATP as they transport electrons to oxygen; any interference with ATP synthesis or translocation across the mitochondrial membrane will inhibit electron transfer.

▶ Rotenone binds avidly to the flavoprotein NADH CoQ reductase, complex I (also called NADH dehydrogenase).

## REFERENCES

Brunton L, Chabner B, Bjorn Knollman, eds. *Goodman and Gilman's The Pharmacological Basis of Therapeutics.* 12th ed. New York: McGraw-Hill; 2010.

Davidson VL, Sittman DB. *National Medical Series–Biochemistry.* Philadelphia, PA: Harwol; 1994:381-383.

Devlin TM, ed. *Textbook of Biochemistry with Clinical Correlations.* 7th ed. New York: Wiley-Liss; 2010.

McGilvery RW. *Biochemistry: A Functional Approach.* Philadelphia, PA: W.B. Saunders; 1979:397-400.

A 42-year-old man presents to the emergency department (ED) with complaints of severe epigastric pain and intractable nausea and vomiting for the past 3 days. He reports drinking heavily for the past week but quit drinking and eating a couple of days before his N/V begun. He is currently homeless and is known to be an alcoholic with frequent visits to the ED. He denies any other medical conditions. On examination, he is malnourished, lethargic, and obtunded. He is afebrile but is noted to be slightly hypotensive and tachypneic. His abdominal examination reveals epigastric tenderness but no signs of an acute surgical abdomen. A fruity odor is noticed from his breath. Laboratory values reveal a high anion gap metabolic acidosis with high serum ketone levels. His serum glucose level is noted to be low.

▶ What is the most likely diagnosis?
▶ What is the initial treatment?

# ANSWERS TO CASE 17:
## Alcoholic Ketoacidosis

*Summary:* A 42-year-old man who abuses alcohols presents to the ED after a binge-drinking episode and a period of fasting with lethargy/epigastric pain, an elevated anion gap metabolic acidosis, and an elevated serum ketone level.

- **Diagnosis:** Alcoholic ketoacidosis (AKA) results from decreased carbohydrate intake (malnourishment) and alcohol-induced inhibition of gluconeogenesis. The 2 combine to increase free fatty acid delivery to the liver and formation of ketoacids seen in the blood and urine.

- **Best treatment:** Administration of intravenous (IV) fluids containing dextrose. Thiamine should be given prior to glucose to prevent Wernicke encephalopathy or Korsakoff syndrome. Complications of alcoholic ketoacidosis include seizures, arrhythmias, cardiac arrest, pulmonary edema, and delirium tremens.

## CLINICAL CORRELATION

Although ketoacidosis is primarily seen as a complication of uncontrolled diabetes mellitus, there are other causes of this condition. Patients with poor nutrition and alcoholism are also at risk of developing this metabolic derangement. When the body is faced with poor nutrition and decreased carbohydrate intake, the body decreases its insulin secretion and increases its glucagon secretion. The main symptoms are nausea, vomiting, and abdominal pain. Physical examination findings include tachycardia, tachypnea, hypotension, and abdominal distention and tenderness. The arterial blood gas will reveal an anion gap metabolic acidosis, and the glucose level may be normal or decreased. Alcohol inhibits gluconeogenesis and increases lipolysis. The effects from both the malnutrition and alcoholism lead to the formation of ketoacids. Treatment of AKA is based on reversing the 3 key underlying causes: (1) fluid depletion, (2) glycogen depletion, and (3) an elevated ratio of NADH to $NAD^+$. Thus, treatment is with IV fluids containing dextrose increases insulin secretion and decreases glucagon secretion, reversing the underlying biochemical derangement.

# APPROACH TO:
## Alcoholic Ketoacidosis

## OBJECTIVES

1. Describe how ethanol is metabolized by the liver.
2. Explain the mechanism by which consumption of large quantities of alcohol followed by fasting results in a ketoacidotic state.
3. Compare the metabolic profiles of AKA with diabetic ketoacidosis (DKA).

## DEFINITIONS

**ALCOHOL DEHYDROGENASE:** A family of cytosolic isozymes that oxidize alcohols to the corresponding aldehydes using $NAD^+$ as the electron acceptor, converting it to $NADH + H^+$. With ethanol as the substrate, the product is acetaldehyde.

**ACETALDEHYDE DEHYDROGENASE:** An enzyme that oxidizes acetaldehyde to acetate while converting $NAD^+$ to $NADH + H^+$. The majority of acetaldehyde is metabolized in liver mitochondria (~ 80%) by ALDH2, but there is a cytosolic isozyme (ALDH1) that metabolizes the remainder.

**KETOSIS:** The metabolic state in which the production of ketone bodies is elevated leading to hyperketonemia, or elevated ketones in the blood.

**KETOACIDOSIS:** A pathologic metabolic state characterized by uncontrolled ketosis that leads to a lowering of the pH of the blood due to the increased presence of ketoacids. Acetone, a breakdown product of acetoacetate, can usually be detected on the breath.

**KETONE BODIES:** The metabolites acetoacetate, β-hydroxybutyrate and acetone, which are produced by the catabolism of fatty acids and ketogenic amino acids.

**MICROSOMAL ETHANOL OXIDIZING SYSTEM (MEOS):** A cytochrome P450 enzyme system located in the endoplasmic reticulum of the liver that oxidizes ethanol to acetaldehyde. The enzyme system consists of cytochrome P450 reductase and CYP2E1, the cytochrome P450 that has the greatest specificity for ethanol. While ethanol is oxidized to acetaldehyde, NADPH is oxidized to $NADP^+$ and $O_2$ is reduced to $H_2O$.

## DISCUSSION

Ethanol is a small, amphipathic molecule that is readily absorbed in the intestinal tract by simple passive diffusion and enters the blood stream. The majority of ingested ethanol is metabolized in the liver, although a small percentage (< 10%) is excreted via the breath or urine. As the liver filters ethanol from the bloodstream, hepatocytes oxidize it to acetaldehyde using the cytosolic enzyme alcohol dehydrogenase using $NAD^+$ as the electron accepter to produce NADH as a product (Figure 17-1). Acetaldehyde is a toxic product and is further metabolized to acetic acid. The acetaldehyde must first enter the mitochondrion where an enzyme called acetaldehyde dehydrogenase oxidizes it to acetic acid while reducing $NAD^+$ to NADH (Figure 17-2). Thus, both steps in the conversion of ethanol to acetic acid result in the production of NADH at the expense of $NAD^+$, thereby increasing the [NADH]/[$NAD^+$] ratio in the liver. Although the acetate produced can be activated to acetyl-CoA in the liver and used for energy generation, most of it is secreted into the blood stream, which delivers it to muscle tissue, where it can be activated to acetyl-CoA and completely oxidized to $CO_2$ via the tricarboxylic acid (TCA) cycle and generate ATP via oxidative phosphorylation.

NAD$^+$    NADH + H$^+$

CH$_3$CH$_2$OH   —Alcohol Dehydrogenase→   CH$_3$C$\overset{O}{\underset{H}{}}$

Ethanol       Acetaldehyde

**Figure 17-1.** Conversion of ethanol to acetaldehyde by alcohol dehydrogenase.

NAD$^+$    NADH + H$^+$

CH$_3$C$\overset{O}{\underset{H}{}}$   —Acetaldehyde Dehydrogenase→   CH$_3$C$\overset{O}{\underset{OH}{}}$

Acetaldehyde       Acetate

**Figure 17-2.** Conversion of acetaldehyde to acetate by acetaldehyde dehydrogenase.

The liver also has an alternate system that accounts for 10%-20% of the metabolism of ethanol. The MEOS is located in the endoplasmic reticulum and utilizes a cytochrome P450 enzyme system to convert ethanol to acetaldehyde. The MEOS is a mixed function oxidase enzyme complex that is bound to the endoplasmic reticulum membrane (Figure 17-3). The complex consists of cytochrome P450 reductase and cytochrome P450 2E1 (CYP2E1), and together they oxidize ethanol to acetaldehyde and reduce molecular oxygen to water. The additional reducing equivalents needed for the reaction are obtained by cytochrome P450 reductase converting NADPH to NADP$^+$ and passing those electrons to CYP2E1.

AKA is a sequela of the increased [NADH]/[NAD$^+$] from metabolism of ethanol and low blood glucose levels from decreased food intake. Most patients with AKA have just had a period of binge drinking. Because of repeated vomiting and epigastric pain, they have refrained from eating, resulting in a low blood glucose concentration and the depletion of stored liver glycogen. The increased [NADH]/[NAD$^+$] from alcohol metabolism impairs gluconeogenesis by inhibiting the conversion of lactate to pyruvate and glycerol to dihydroxyacetone phosphate (DHAP), processes that both require NAD$^+$. Pyruvate and DHAP are both major sources of carbon for the synthesis of glucose via gluconeogenesis.

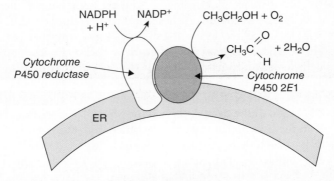

**Figure 17-3.** The microsomal ethanol oxidizing system.

Low blood glucose from decreased food intake promotes the secretion of glucagon and lipolytic hormones, which stimulate the release of free fatty acids from stored triglyceride in adipose into the bloodstream. After being taken up by the liver, the free fatty acids are activated to fatty acetyl-CoA. Although the rate of β-oxidation is decreased due to the high $[NADH]/[NAD^+]$, the acetyl-CoA produced from the fatty acids that do undergo β-oxidation is directed to the production of the ketone bodies acetoacetate and β-hydroxybutyrate. This is because the high $[NADH]/[NAD^+]$ in the mitochondrion favors the reduction of oxaloacetate to malate, making it less available for condensation with acetyl-CoA to form citrate. To liberate free CoA for further reactions, 2 molecules of acetyl-CoA recombine to form acetoacetyl-CoA, which is then converted to acetoacetate and β-hydroxybutyrate (Figure 17-4). The excess production of these ketone bodies leads to the ketoacidosis. While in the bloodstream, acetoacetate can undergo a spontaneous, nonenzymatic decarboxylation to yield acetone, which is exhaled and can often be smelled on the breath.

While patients that present with DKA or AKA have similarities in their biochemical profiles, there are some important differences. In addition to elevated ketone bodies and decreased blood pH, patients that present usually exhibit a severe depression of insulin levels along with increases in glucagon, cortisol and catecholamines.

**Figure 17-4.** Metabolic pathway for the formation of ketone bodies.

For patients with DKA, this altered hormonal profile usually results in hypergly-cemia due to increased glucose production from gluconeogenesis and decreased uptake of glucose by peripheral tissues. However, with AKA, blood glucose levels are usually low due to decreased nutrient intake because of nausea and vomiting. The increased [NADH]/[NAD⁺] that results from metabolizing large quantities of ethanol depresses gluconeogenesis. The elevated [NADH]/[NAD⁺] also leads to a higher lactate/pyruvate ratio and an increased ratio of β-hydroxybutyrate/acetoacetate than is observed with DKA. Because patients with AKA have a higher β-hydroxybutyrate/acetoacetate ratio, the amount of ketone bodies in urine can be underestimated if only tested by ketone test strips, which only measure acetoacetate. Using these ketone test strips to monitor treatment can also give the false impres-sion that ketoacidosis is worsening, when in reality β-hydroxybutyrate is being oxidized back to acetoacetate as the ratio of NADH/NAD⁺ returns to normal.

## COMPREHENSION QUESTIONS

Questions 17.1 to 17.3 refer to the following clinical scenario:
A disoriented man with severe nausea and vomiting and reeking of alcohol is brought to the ED by two persons who found him collapsed on their front lawn. Laboratory samples were taken during his examination and revealed very low blood glucose levels and elevated serum ketone levels.

17.1  Which of the following is the most probable cause of the elevated ketone and low glucose readings?

A.  Increased flux of acetyl CoA through the TCA cycle

B.  Inadequate dietary intake

C.  Increased protein mobilization

D.  Increased pyruvate carboxylase activity

17.2  The disorientation observed in the patient is most likely caused by which of the following?

A.  Alcohol damage to the kidney

B.  Decreased lung surfactant efficacy caused by excessive alcohol intake

C.  Increased ketone bodies stimulate diuresis

D.  Mentation is suppressed by elevated ketone bodies

E.  Neuronal and glial metabolism is reduced

17.3  The patient is treated by IV thiamine and glucose solutions. Although the patient appears to be improving, ketone test strip analysis indicates an increase in urinary ketones. This is best explained by which of the following?

A.  Conversion of β-hydroxybutyrate to acetoacetate

B.  Decreased activity of the TCA cycle

C.  Increased catabolism of ketogenic amino acids

D.  Inhibition of pyruvate dehydrogenase

E.  Conversion of lactate to pyruvate

17.4  Alcohol metabolism is accomplished in various cellular compartments including the cytosol, mitochondria, and endoplasmic reticulum. Which reaction is least likely to inhibit the synthesis of glucose?

A.  Ethanol → Acetaldehyde by cytosolic alcohol dehydrogenase

B.  Ethanol → Acetaldehyde by the microsomal ethanol oxidizing system

C.  Acetaldehyde → Acetic acid by mitochondrial acetaldehyde dehydrogenase

D.  β-Hydroxybutyrate → Acetoacetate

## ANSWERS

17.1  **B.** Increased pyruvate carboxylase would favor increased gluconeogenesis. Increased protein mobilization would also favor an increase in glucose synthesis. Increasing the flux of acetyl CoA through the TCA cycle would decrease the production of ketone bodies. A lack of adequate nutrition due to nausea and vomiting as a result of excessively consuming alcohol would lead to low blood glucose. Gluconeogenesis is slowed due a high NADH/NAD$^+$, but fatty acids continue to be oxidized to elevate ketone body production.

17.2  **E.** None of the first 4 alternatives affects brain function. Neurons and glia require glucose as the sole source for energy production. With low blood glucose as a result of repressed gluconeogenesis, neurons and glia lack the energy that is required for function.

17.3  **A.** The increase in ketone bodies detected by ketone test strips is most likely due to conversion of β-hydroxybutyrate to acetoacetate as the NADH/NAD$^+$ returns to normal levels. Treatment with IV glucose solutions will resolve the low concentration of blood glucose, which will decrease the need for β-oxidation of fatty acids and the production acetyl CoA, ketone bodies, and NADH. As the NADH/NAD$^+$ decreases, the equilibrium between acetoacetate and β-hydroxybutyrate shifts toward acetoacetate.

17.4  **B.** The conversion of ethanol to acetaldehyde by alcohol dehydrogenase, acetaldehyde to acetic acid, and β-hydroxybutyrate to acetoacetate all produce NADH + H$^+$ as products. Increased NADH/NAD+ inhibits those reactions that require NAD+ as an electron acceptor. Several reactions in gluconeogenesis require NAD+; therefore, these reactions would be inhibited by low NAD+. The MEOS does not produce NADH; rather, it requires NADPH as a source of reducing equivalents. Thus, oxidation of ethanol to acetaldehyde by the MEOS would not inhibit gluconeogenesis.

## BIOCHEMISTRY PEARLS

▶ Poor nutrition and decreased carbohydrate consumption leads to an increase in glucagon secretion and decreased insulin secretion.

▶ The increased [NADH]/[NAD$^+$] from alcohol metabolism impairs gluconeogenesis by inhibiting the conversion of lactate to pyruvate and glycerol to DHAP.

▶ Compared with DKA, glucose levels in AKA are low.

## REFERENCES

Umpierrez GE, DiGirolamo M, Tuvlin JA, et al. Differences in metabolic and hormonal milieu in diabetic- and alcohol-induced ketoacidosis. *J Crit Care*. 2000;15(2):52-59.

Ngatchu T, Sangwaiya A, Dabiri A, et al. Alcoholic ketoacidosis with multiple complications: a case report. *Emerg Med J*. 2007;24(11):776-777.

A 27-year-old man presented to the emergency department with the signs and symptoms of acute appendicitis. He was promptly sent to the operating room for emergency appendectomy. The patient was prepped and draped for the surgery, and halothane was given as an inhalation anesthetic. A total of 2 minutes after the anesthetic was given, the patient was noted to have an extremely elevated temperature, muscle rigidity, and tachypnea. Arterial blood gas test revealed metabolic acidosis, and a serum electrolytes study demonstrated hyperkalemia. A nurse quickly went to talk to the family about the events, and the family mentioned that the only other person to have surgery in their family had a similar reaction and died. The physician makes a diagnosis of malignant hyperthermia (MH).

▶ What is the biochemical basis of this disease?
▶ What is the best treatment for this condition?

# ANSWERS TO CASE 18:
## Malignant Hyperthermia

*Summary:* 27-year-old man with acute appendicitis undergoing a halothane inhaled anesthetic with acute onset of hyperthermia, tachypnea, respiratory acidosis, hyperkalemia, and family history of similar events. The tentative diagnosis is MH.

- **Biochemical mechanism:** Uncoupling of oxidative phosphorylation.

- **Treatment:** Supportive care with attempts to bring temperature down, correct blood gas and electrolyte abnormalities, and give dantrolene.

## CLINICAL CORRELATION

MH is an untoward response of susceptible individuals to preoperative anesthesia utilizing halothane and succinylcholine, although other inhalation anesthetics such as enflurane and isoflurane have been recognized as milder prompts for this complication of anesthesia. The frequency of occurrence is 1 in 15,000 children and 1 in 100,000 adults. The inheritance is dominant in 50% of cases and recessive in 20%, suggesting a more complex basis for this response. The clinical findings are muscle rigidity, hyperthermia, seizure, cardiac arrhythmias, and sometimes death. Prevention is the key, in that every patient should be queried about personal or family history of complications during surgery. Once a patient is found to have MH, the health care professional should alert other family members to the same possibility. The muscle relaxant, dantrolene, is the treatment of choice. Even with prompt recognition and therapy, the mortality rate is as high as 5%.

# APPROACH TO:
## Oxidative Phosphorylation (Uncoupling)

### OBJECTIVES

1. Understand how MH is caused by the uncoupling of oxidative phosphorylation.

2. Understand the biochemical mechanism for the heat production.

3. Be familiar with the mechanism of how dantrolene reverses the effects.

### DEFINITIONS

**MALIGNANT HYPERTHERMIA (MH):** An unusual adverse response to some inhalation anesthetics such as halothane in which there is an acute dramatic elevation in body temperature as well as tachypnea, muscle rigidity, and hyperkalemia.

$Ca^{2+}$ **SIGNALING:** Many enzymes in metabolism and signaling pathways are responsive to $Ca^{2+}$ concentrations. Calcium is sequestered within tissues (eg, within cisternae in the sarcoplasmic reticulum of muscle) and released on signal increasing the $Ca^{2+}$ concentration in the cytosolic compartment and eliciting $Ca^{2+}$-induced responses. Increased calcium concentration stimulates the activity of muscle phosphorylase kinase and activates pyruvate dehydrogenase phosphatase to increase the metabolic flow of glucose to $CO_2$ and $H_2O$.

$Ca^{2+}$ **CHANNEL:** A transport system allowing passage of the charged calcium ion through a hydrophobic membrane.

## DISCUSSION

**Hyperthermia is a rare complication of anesthesia** not completely understood. Most of the evidence points to the **ryanodine receptor (chromosome 19q13.1) as the defective gene product.** This receptor is the $Ca^{2+}$ **release channel of muscle sarcoplasmic reticulum.** Stimulation of this channel leads to **excessive $Ca^{2+}$ release from the cisternae of the sarcoplasmic reticulum, and that $Ca^{2+}$ prompts muscle contraction, an increase in body temperature, tachycardia, and subsequent metabolic acidosis.**

The scheme in Figure 18-1 summarizes the effects of $Ca^{2+}$ release on processes that bring about the complex of symptoms seen in malignant hyperthermia. **Increased $Ca^{2+}$ release triggers the binding of** adenosine triphosphate **(ATP)-charged myosin to actin to initiate muscle contraction.** This muscle contraction may be repeated to the point of **muscle rigidity with attendant muscle damage and release of myoglobin.** The sustained muscle contraction uses increased amounts of **ATP** increasing demands on **glycolysis,** tricarboxylic acid **(TCA) cycle, and oxidative phosphorylation.** $Ca^{2+}$ release serves to activate, at least partially, **phosphorylase kinase,** which speeds the mobilization of glycogen stores for ATP generation. Sympathetic outflow

**Figure 18-1.** Direct and indirect effects of $Ca^{2+}$ release in aberrant response to anesthetics halothane and succinylcholine.

**Figure 18-2.** Electron transport system showing development of proton gradient outside the mitochondrial membrane by the passage of electrons down the chain.

triggered by these changes leads to increased activation of glycogen breakdown and lipolysis. Fatty acids serve as a signal to increase the levels of **uncoupling proteins** in various tissues. **The uncoupling proteins form channels in mitochondria allowing proton reentry into the mitochondrial matrix.** Because the phosphorylation of adenosine diphosphate (ADP) to ATP depends on the proton gradient through the ATP synthase, these channels **collapse the proton gradient allowing electron transport to occur without the phosphorylation of ADP** (Figure 18-2). Because ATP is being consumed at an elevated rate and mitochondrial production of ATP is compromised, glycolysis increases to compensate for the shortfall in ATP production. **Pyruvate and lactate, the end products of glycolysis, increase in concentration, giving rise to the metabolic acidosis** observed.

The uncoupling proteins (UCPs; numbered 1-5) are a physiologic mechanism for maintaining body temperature through selective uncoupling of electron transport from ATP synthesis. The free energy release normally captured in the formation of the high-energy phosphate bond when phosphorylating ADP to ATP is lost as heat and changes body temperature. Physiologically, sympathetic outflow and catecholamine hormone release prompt new synthesis of the uncoupling proteins in response to the hypothalamus sensing lowered body temperature. In the case of malignant hyperthermia, this mechanism is triggered by anesthetic challenge to the calcium release channel, and the subsequent metabolic and signaling changes assembled above unfold.

Treatment of MH depends on cessation of anesthesia, mechanical means to reduce the temperature, and the correction of blood electrolyte and gas parameters to normal. In addition, dantrolene is infused initially intravenously and then may be given orally (Figure 18-3). **Dantrolene brings about the reduction in contraction of skeletal muscles by decreasing the amount of $Ca^{2+}$ released from the sarcoplasmic reticulum.** A serious adverse event of dantrolene use is its potential hepatotoxicity.

**Figure 18-3.** Structure of dantrolene (1-{[5-(4-nitrophenyl)-2-furyl]methylideneamino}imidazolidine-2, 4-dione).

The hepatotoxicity is fatal to 0.1% to 0.2% of patients treated for 60 days or longer. Thus, use of dantrolene for longer than 45 days requires monitoring of hepatic markers.

## COMPREHENSION QUESTIONS

18.1 A young and otherwise healthy student undergoing preparation for a simple surgical procedure was noticed to have an elevating temperature and respiratory rate with muscle rigidity following the onset of anesthesia using halothane and succinylcholine. Laboratory findings revealed elevated levels of calcium, hydrogen ion, pyruvate, and lactate. The diagnosis was MH. The muscle rigidity observed in this patient is most likely prompted by which of the following?

A. Patient's fear of surgery

B. Increased levels of hydrogen ion, causing the muscles to become immobile

C. Increased $Ca^{2+}$ levels in muscle tissue, triggering muscle contraction

D. Increased pyruvate and lactate, causing precipitation of muscle protein

E. Increased body temperature

18.2 Rapidly elevating body temperature was observed in the patient in question 18.1. The underlying cause for this pyretic episode is which of the following?

A. Hypothalamic upward adjustment of body temperature set point in response to cold operating room temperature

B. Muscles producing heat from exertion of contraction

C. Uncoupling proteins allowing dissipation of the mitochondrial hydrogen ion gradient releasing energy as heat

D. Metabolism of fatty acids from lipid storage depots releasing heat

E. Elevated consumption of ATP to support muscle contraction releasing heat

18.3 Which of the following best describes the mechanism of action of dantrolene in the treatment of MH?

A. Decrease of $Ca^{2+}$ release

B. Reduction of body temperature with hypothalamic set temperature

C. Effect on mitochondrial ATP production

D. Nuclear transcription attenuation

E. Recoupling of the sodium and ATP channels

## ANSWERS

18.1 **C.** Release of $Ca^{2+}$ triggers actin–myosin reaction, prompting muscle contraction. Neither fear of surgery nor hydrogen ion levels causes concerted muscle contraction. Increased pyruvate/lactate or temperature tends to counteract contraction.

18.2 **C.** MH does not involve central brain control of temperature but is caused by metabolic alterations. Regardless of the source of energy—whether fatty acids or the utilization of ATP to support muscle contraction—the electron transport chain is involved. Uncoupling of oxidation from ADP phosphorylation is caused by uncoupling proteins that dissipate energy as heat. This causes the elevation of body temperature seen in this patient.

18.3 **A.** Dantrolene brings about reduction in contraction of skeletal muscles by decreasing the amount of $Ca^{2+}$ released from the sarcoplasmic reticulum. In addition, supportive care is aimed at decreasing body temperature and correcting the metabolic acidosis and electrolyte balance.

## BIOCHEMISTRY PEARLS

▶ MH is most likely, given that anesthetic agents stimulate a calcium release channel, leading to excessive $Ca^{2+}$ release from the cisternae of the sarcoplasmic reticulum, in turn causing muscle contraction, increased body temperature, tachycardia, and subsequent metabolic acidosis—"most likely" at beginning makes this a pearl about this case, not about MH in general.

▶ Although the UCPs 1 to 5 are a physiologic mechanism for maintaining body temperature through selective uncoupling of electron transport from ATP synthesis, MH is a pathologic exaggeration of this process.

▶ The treatment of MH includes stopping the anesthesia, cooling the patient, and administration of dantrolene, which reduces muscle contractions by decreasing the amount of $Ca^{2+}$ released from the sarcoplasmic reticulum.

## REFERENCE

Brunton L, Chabner B, Bjorn Knollman, eds. *Goodman and Gilman's The Pharmacological Basis of Therapeutics*. 12th ed. New York: McGraw-Hill; 2010.

A 40-year-old obese woman presents to the emergency department with complaints of worsening nausea, vomiting, and abdominal pain. Her pain is located in the midepigastric area and right upper quadrant. She reports a subjective fever and denies diarrhea. Her pain is presently constant and sharp in nature but previously was intermittent and cramping only after eating "greasy" foods. On examination she has a temperature of 100°F (37.8°C) with otherwise normal vital signs. She appears ill and in moderate distress. She has significant midepigastric and right upper-quadrant tenderness. Some guarding is present but no rebound. Her abdomen is otherwise soft with no distention and active bowel sounds. Laboratory values were normal except for increased liver function tests, white blood cell count, and serum amylase. Ultrasonography of the gallbladder revealed numerous gallstones and a thickening of the gallbladder wall. A surgery consult was immediately sought.

▶ What is the most likely diagnosis?
▶ What is the role of amylase in digestion?

# ANSWERS TO CASE 19:
## Pancreatitis

*Summary:* 40-year-old woman with history of intermittent right upper-quadrant pain worsening after "greasy" meals and now with constant midepigastric pain, nausea, and vomiting with elevated liver function tests and amylase.

- **Diagnosis:** Gallstone pancreatitis.

- **Role of amylase:** Enzyme for carbohydrate metabolism, used to digest glycogen and starch.

## CLINICAL CORRELATION

**Acute pancreatitis** is an inflammatory process in which pancreatic enzymes are activated and cause autodigestion of the gland. In the United States, **alcohol use is the most common cause,** and episodes are often precipitated by binge drinking. The next most common cause is biliary tract disease, usually passage of a gallstone into the common bile duct. Hypertriglyceridemia is also a common cause, and that occurs when serum triglyceride levels are above 1000 mg/dL, as is seen in patients with familial dyslipidemias or diabetes. When patients appear to have "idiopathic" pancreatitis, that is, no gallstones are seen on ultrasound, and no other predisposing factor can be found, biliary tract disease is still the most likely cause: either biliary sludge (microlithiasis), or sphincter of Oddi dysfunction. **Abdominal pain is the cardinal symptom of pancreatitis,** and it is often severe, typically in the **upper abdomen with radiation to the back.** The pain is often relieved by sitting up and bending forward and is exacerbated by food. Patients also **commonly have nausea and vomiting,** also precipitated by oral intake. The treatment includes nothing by mouth, intravenous hydration, pain control, and monitoring for complications.

# APPROACH TO:
## Amylase and Carbohydrate Metabolism

### OBJECTIVES

1. Be aware of the role of amylase in carbohydrate metabolism.

2. Understand the cause for increased amylase in pancreatitis.

3. Understand why conservative treatment (intravenous [IV] fluids, nothing by mouth (NPO), pain medication, and possibly a nasogastric tube) is effective in treatment of this condition.

## DEFINITIONS

**α-AMYLASE:** An endosaccharidase that catalyzes the hydrolysis of $\alpha(1\rightarrow4)$ glycosidic bonds present in glycogen and starch. It is present in both saliva and pancreatic digestive juice. (Refer to Figure 25-1b in Case 25 for a diagram showing the $\alpha[1\rightarrow4]$ glycosidic bonds in starch.)

**ENDOSACCHARIDASE:** An enzyme that randomly hydrolyzes glycosidic bonds within polysaccharides.

**LIPASE:** An enzyme that hydrolyzes the ester linkage between a fatty acid and glycerol in a triglyceride.

**PANCREAS:** A major endocrine and exocrine organ located behind the stomach. It secretes pancreatic juice into the duodenum to neutralize the effluent from the stomach and supply digestive enzymes. It also synthesizes and secretes the hormones insulin, glucagon, and somatostatin into the bloodstream from cells within the islets of Langerhans.

**ZYMOGEN:** A proenzyme; an inactive precursor of an enzyme stored in secretory granules. After secretion, the zymogen is activated by cleavage of certain peptide bonds either by low pH or by other enzymes.

## DISCUSSION

The **pancreas** is a **major exocrine organ** that **synthesizes and secretes digestive enzymes.** It also produces and secretes $NaHCO_3$ to neutralize the acidic effluent from the stomach. The pancreas also has an important endocrine role because it synthesizes and secretes the hormones **insulin, glucagon, and somatostatin** into the bloodstream from cells within its islets of Langerhans.

The exocrine gland is divided into small globules that are drained by an intralobular duct. The intralobular ducts feed into the interlobular duct, which is joined to the main pancreatic duct. The pancreatic duct joins with the common bile duct (usually) in the hepatopancreatic ampulla, which exits into the duodenum. The secretory unit of the pancreas consists of the acinus and the intercalated duct. The epithelial cells of the intercalated duct have high concentrations of the enzyme carbonic anhydrase, which generates $HCO_3^-$ from $CO_2$ and $H_2O$ for neutralization of stomach acid entering the duodenum. The acinus is a cluster of acinar cells that are grouped around the intercalated duct. The acinar cells are specialized epithelial cells that synthesize and secrete the 20 or so enzymes that will be used to digest the macromolecules in the lumen of the intestine. Most of the digestive enzymes, particularly those used to degrade proteins, are synthesized as zymogens or proenzymes that must be activated. These proenzymes are synthesized on ribosomes on the rough endoplasmic reticulum. They are then transported to the Golgi apparatus and are sequestered in zymogen granules until they are secreted. Storing these inactive enzymes in zymogen granules protects the acinar cell from digesting itself. Secretion of these zymogens is regulated by cholecystokinin receptors and muscarinic acetylcholine receptors. The proenzymes are activated in the intestine, usually by the action of trypsin. There are some enzymes that are synthesized and stored as the active enzymes in the zymogen granules. These include **α-amylase, carboxyl ester lipase, lipase, colipase,** RNase, and DNase.

**Acute pancreatitis** is a result of anatomical changes that arise from 2 events. The first is the autodigestion of the acinar cells by inappropriate activation of the pancreatic enzymes (especially trypsinogen) within the cell. The second is the cellular injury response that is mediated by proinflammatory cytokines. The mechanisms by which the digestive enzymes become activated within the acinar cell are unclear. However, such inappropriate activation of pancreatic enzymes leads to destruction of the acinar cell and surrounding fat deposits, and it weakens the elastic fibers of the blood vessels, resulting in leakage.

**Obstruction of the main pancreatic duct** as a result of a **gallstone** lodged in or near to the hepatopancreatic ampulla can result in acute pancreatitis. One theory is that obstruction increases the pressure in the main pancreatic duct. The increase in pressure causes interstitial edema, which impairs the blood flow to the acinus. The lack of blood flow leads to ischemic injury of the acinar cell, resulting in release of the digestive enzymes into the interstitial space. How this leads to premature activation of the proenzymes stored in the acinar cell is unclear.

**α-Amylase and lipase are 2 digestive enzymes** that are synthesized and stored in the acinar cell as the active enzymes. Amylase is an endosaccharidase that catalyzes the hydrolysis of the $\alpha(1 \rightarrow 4)$ glycosidic bonds that form the main polymeric backbone of the polysaccharides starch and glycogen. Present in both saliva and pancreatic juice, it is the pancreatic form of the enzyme that breaks down most of the dietary polysaccharides. α-Amylase hydrolyzes dietary starch and glycogen to glucose, maltose, maltotriose, and an oligosaccharide referred to as the α-limit dextrin.

**Pancreatic lipase is the primary digestive enzyme for the breakdown of triglycerides.** It acts on triglycerides to hydrolyze the fatty acyl ester bonds. Lipase is specific for the ester bonds in the 1′- and 3′-positions to produce free fatty acids and β-monoacylglycerols. Pancreatic lipase is strongly inhibited by bile acids and therefore requires the presence of colipase, a small protein that binds to the lipase and activates it.

Since both α-amylase and lipase are stored in the pancreas as the active enzymes, they are important blood markers to help diagnose acute pancreatitis. The serum level of α-amylase will increase in the first 12 hours following the onset of acute pancreatitis. During the next 48 to 72 hours, the levels will usually fall back to normal values. Serum lipase levels also rise, but they remain elevated after the α-amylase levels have returned to normal and may take 7 to 10 days to normalize.

**Most cases** (85%-90%) of **acute pancreatitis** that are caused by **gallstones** will resolve on their own, and therefore conservative treatment modalities are appropriate. These include pain management with analgesics, administration of intravenous fluids to maintain the intravascular volume and electrolyte balance, as well as removal of oral alimentation to decrease the secretion of pancreatic juice. Nasogastric suction has also been used to decrease gastrin release from the stomach and to eliminate gastric emptying into the duodenum. However, controlled trials have not demonstrated the efficacy of nasogastric suction in the treatment of mild to moderate acute pancreatitis.

## COMPREHENSION QUESTIONS

19.1 Prior to a race, many marathon runners will try to increase their glycogen concentrations by loading up with foods with high starch content, such as pasta. α-Amylase secreted by the pancreas will digest the starch into which of the following major products?

A. Amylose, amylopectin, and maltose

B. Glucose, galactose, and fructose

C. Glucose, sucrose, and maltotriose

D. Limit dextrins, maltose, and maltotriose

E. Limit dextrins, lactose, and sucrose

19.2 A 3-month-old infant presents with hepatosplenomegaly and failure to thrive. Liver biopsy reveals glycogen with an abnormal, amylopectin-like structure with long outer chains. Which of the following enzymes would most likely be deficient?

A. α-Amylase

B. Branching enzyme

C. Debranching enzyme

D. Glycogen phosphorylase

E. Glycogen synthase

19.3 A 3-year-old Caucasian girl presents with chronic diarrhea and a failure to thrive. Stools were oily. History reveals that she was breastfed and had no problems until she was weaned. Which of the enzymes would be expected to be deficient following stimulation with secretin?

A. Cholesteryl esterase

B. Gastric lipase

C. Hormone sensitive lipase

D. Lipoprotein lipase

E. Pancreatic lipase

For questions 19.4 to 19.6, match the following enzymes:

A. Sucrose and lactose

B. Glucose and fructose

C. Glucose and galactose

D. Glucose

19.4 Lactase

19.5 Sucrase

19.6 Maltase

## ANSWERS

19.1 **D.** α-Amylase hydrolyzes α(1→4) glycosidic bonds present in starch (amylose and amylopectin) in a random fashion leaving primarily the disaccharide maltose, the trisaccharide maltotriose, and an oligosaccharide known as the α-limit dextrin, which is composed of 6 to 8 glucose residues with 1 or more α(1→6) glycosidic bonds. Galactose and fructose are not present in starch.

19.2 **B.** Amylopectin is plant starch that has some α(1→6) branch points, but not as many as normal glycogen. Glycogen, which has an amylopectin-like structure, has fewer branch points than normal glycogen and would be less soluble within the cell. A deficiency in the branching enzyme will introduce fewer α(1→6) branch points.

19.3 **E.** Neither hormone sensitive lipase nor lipoprotein lipase is a digestive enzyme. The patient's symptoms are consistent with an inability to absorb triglycerides, which would eliminate cholesteryl esterase from consideration. Since the patient did not have any problems while being breast-fed, then the most likely enzyme to be deficient is pancreatic lipase, since gastric lipase is most active on short chain triglycerides, such as those that are found in breast milk.

19.4 **C.** Lactase breaks down lactose into glucose and galactose.

19.5 **B.** Sucrase breaks down sucrose into glucose and fructose.

19.6 **D.** Maltase and isomaltase convert maltose and isomaltose into glucose.

### BIOCHEMISTRY PEARLS

▶ The pancreas is a large exocrine organ that has a role in the digestion of food as well as an endocrine organ that secretes insulin, somatostatin, and glucagon.

▶ Acute pancreatitis occurs from autodigestion of the acinar cells by inappropriate activation of the pancreatic enzymes (especially trypsinogen) within the cell, leading to cellular injury mediated by proinflammatory cytokines.

▶ The 3 major breakdown products of amylase are maltose, maltotriose, and α-dextrins. Enzymes in the brush border of the intestines continue to digest the carbohydrates.

# REFERENCES

Hopfer U. Digestion and absorption of basic nutritional constituents. In: Devlin TM, ed. *Textbook of Biochemistry with Clinical Correlations*. 7th ed. New York: Wiley-Liss; 2010.

Greenberger NJ, Toskes PP. Acute and chronic pancreatitis. In: Fauci AS, Braunwald E, Kasper KL, et al, eds. *Harrison's Principles of Internal Medicine*. 14th ed. New York: McGraw-Hill; 1998.

Kumar V, Cotran RS, Robbins SL. *Robbins Basic Pathology*. 7th ed. Philadelphia, PA: W.B. Saunders; 2003.

Marino CS, Gorelick FS. Pancreatic and salivary glands. In: Boron WF, Boulpaep EL, eds. *Medical Physiology: A Cellular and Molecular Approach*. 2nd ed. Philadelphia, PA: W.B. Saunders; 2011.

# CASE 20

A 21-year-old primigravid woman at 35 weeks gestation presents to the hospital with nausea, vomiting, and malaise over the last several days. Patient has also noticed that her eyes were turning yellow in color. Her prenatal course has otherwise been unremarkable. On examination she is found to have elevated blood pressure, proteinuria, increased liver function tests, prolonged clotting studies, hyperbilirubinemia, hypofibrinogenemia, and hypoglycemia. Pelvic ultrasonography identified a viable intrauterine pregnancy of approximately 35 weeks gestation. After admission, the mother underwent emergent cesarean delivery, and she subsequently developed worsening hypoglycemia and coagulopathy and went into hepatic coma with renal failure. After reviewing all the laboratory results and her clinical picture, the patient was diagnosed with acute fatty liver of pregnancy (AFLP).

▶ What is an associated biochemical disorder?
▶ What is the etiology of the hypoglycemia?

## ANSWERS TO CASE 20:
## Acute Fatty Liver in Pregnancy

*Summary:* 21-year-old woman at 35 weeks gestation with malaise, nausea and vomiting, jaundice, elevated blood pressure, elevated liver function tests, coagulopathy, hypoglycemia, and subsequently hepatic coma and renal failure. She has been diagnosed with AFLP.

- **Associated biochemical defect:** Fetal deficiencies of long chain 3-hydroxyacyl-coenzyme A dehydrogenase (LCHAD).

- **Cause of hypoglycemia:** Decreased liver glycogen after liver undergoes fatty infiltration and subsequent liver failure. Histology reveals swollen hepatocytes in which the cytoplasm is filled with microvesicular fat.

### CLINICAL CORRELATION

AFLP is a poorly understood condition affecting only pregnant women with the clinical manifestations of hypoglycemia, liver failure, metabolic acidosis, renal failure, and coagulopathy. Affected patients may become jaundiced or encephalopathic from liver failure, usually reflected by an elevated ammonia level. Profound hypoglycemia is common. The mortality rate is approximately 10% to 15%. Management is delivery, with supportive measures such as magnesium sulfate to prevent seizures, replacement of blood or clotting factors, and management of blood pressure. The pathophysiology may be related to fetal deficiencies of LCHAD.

## APPROACH TO:
## Glycogen and Carbohydrate Metabolism

### OBJECTIVES

1. Know about glycogen storage, synthesis, and degradation.

2. Be familiar with the regulation of glycogen synthesis and degradation.

3. Understand the role of liver glycogen in carbohydrate metabolism.

### DEFINITIONS

**GLUCOSE TRANSPORTER ISOFORM 2 (GLUT 2):** A facilitative glucose transporter present in the liver, the β-cells of the pancreas, and the basolateral surface of intestinal epithelial cells.

**ADENYLATE CYCLASE:** The enzyme that, when activated by hormones binding to receptors, catalyzes the cyclization of adenosine triphosphate (ATP) to cyclic adenosine monophosphate (cAMP) with the release of pyrophosphate.

**BRANCHING ENZYME:** 1,4-α-Glucan branching enzyme; an enzyme that removes an oligosaccharide of about seven glucosyl residues from the nonreducing end of a glycogen chain and transfers it to another chain, creating an α(1→6) glycosidic bond.

**DEBRANCHING ENZYME:** A bifunctional enzyme that catalyzes 2 reactions in the degradation of glycogen. It transfers a trisaccharide from the nonreducing end of a 4 glucosyl residue branch of the glycogen molecule to the nonreducing end of the same or adjacent glycogen molecule (oligo-1,4–1,4-glucantransferase activity). It also hydrolyzes the α(1→6) linkage of the remaining glucosyl residue of the branch, thus releasing free glucose (amylo-1,6-glucosidase activity).

**GLYCOGEN:** The storage form of glucose in tissues. It is a large polysaccharide composed of glucose residues in primarily α(1→4) glycosidic linkages with some α(1→6) branch points.

**GLYCOGENESIS:** The synthesis of glycogen from glucose 1-phosphate.

**GLYCOGENOLYSIS:** The breakdown of glycogen to glucose 1-phosphate (and some small amount of free glucose).

**GLYCOGEN PHOSPHORYLASE:** The enzyme that causes the release of glucose 1-phosphate from glycogen. It accomplishes this by catalyzing a phosphorolysis of glucosyl residues from glycogen; that is, it breaks the α(1→4) glycosidic bonds by adding inorganic phosphate and releasing glucose 1-phosphate.

**GLYCOGEN SYNTHASE:** The enzyme that causes the addition of glucosyl residues to a growing glycogen molecule using uridine diphosphate (UDP)-glucose and releasing inorganic pyrophosphate.

## DISCUSSION

**AFLP** is a rare (occurring in 1 in 7000 to 16,000 deliveries) but potentially fatal disease that typically develops during the third trimester. Patients most commonly present with clinical and laboratory evidence of acute hepatic failure with decreased hepatic metabolic activity. **Hypoglycemia,** nausea and vomiting, jaundice, general malaise, elevated blood pressure, disseminated intravascular coagulation, hemorrhage, infection, and encephalopathy are the most common clinical findings. The etiology of the syndrome is not clear, although recent reports have linked some cases of AFLP with a **fetal inborn error in fatty acid metabolism.** For the majority of cases in which an inborn error in the fetus does not appear to play a role, the cause of the disease is unknown.

One of the **primary functions of the liver** is to **maintain blood glucose levels.** When blood glucose levels are high following a meal, the liver takes in glucose via the high capacity, insulin-insensitive glucose transporter GLUT 2 and converts it into glycogen for storage, metabolizes it to pyruvate by glycolysis, or uses it to produce NADPH and pentoses for biosynthetic processes via the pentose phosphate pathway. When blood glucose levels drop after fasting or vigorous exercise, the liver mobilizes its glycogen stores in response to glucagon and epinephrine and exports glucose into the blood. As glycogen levels are depleted, the liver begins to synthesize glucose via gluconeogenesis. In addition to a source of carbons to synthesize glucose, which it obtains from either lactate or the breakdown of amino acids, the liver also needs a source of energy in the form of ATP. β-Oxidation of fatty acids provides the reducing equivalents (NADH and $FADH_2$), by which ATP is synthesized through the action of the electron transport system and oxidative phosphorylation.

The **storage form of glucose is glycogen,** which is **stored in both muscle and liver.** However, the function of stored glycogen is different in these 2 tissues. Muscle uses glycogen as a fuel reserve to provide ATP for its own needs, whereas the liver uses stored glycogen as a reservoir for glucose to maintain blood glucose levels. When blood glucose concentrations drop, **glucagon and epinephrine** are released into the bloodstream and bind to glucagon and epinephrine receptors on hepatocytes. The binding of the hormones to the receptors activates **adenylate cyclase** producing **3′,5′-cAMP.** When cAMP binds to cAMP-dependent protein kinase (PKA), it is activated and is able to phosphorylate target proteins. This leads to **activation of glycogen phosphorylase,** the enzyme primarily responsible for mobilizing glucose from glycogen. **Phosphorylase, which is stabilized by pyridoxal phosphate (vitamin B6), catalyzes the phosphorolysis of glycogen;** it **cleaves the 1,4-glycosidic bond** of a terminal glucose residue from the **nonreducing end of the glycogen molecule** using inorganic phosphate (Figure 20-1). The products are glucose 1-phosphate and glycogen that is shorter by 1 glucose residue.

Mobilization of glycogen stores also requires the participation of a **debranching enzyme** because phosphorylase ceases to cleave α-1,4-glycosidic linkages 4 glucosyl residues from an α-1,6-branch site. The debranching enzyme has 2 catalytic activities: a **transferase activity and a glucosidase activity.** The transferase activity of the enzyme removes an oligosaccharide composed of the terminal 3 glucosyl residues from the 4 residue branch and transfers it to a free 4-hydroxyl group of the terminal glucosyl residue of another branch. The remaining glucosyl residue that is in an α-1,6-glucosidic linkage is then hydrolyzed by the glucosidase activity to release free glucose.

**Glucose 1-phosphate** released from glycogen by phosphorylase is converted to **glucose 6-phosphate** by **phosphoglucomutase.** Glucose 6-phosphatase, which is only present in liver and other gluconeogenic tissues, hydrolyzes the phosphate to

**Figure 20-1.** Reactions involved in the synthesis and breakdown of glycogen.

produce free glucose. Glucose is then exported from the liver via the GLUT 2 transporter to increase the blood glucose concentration.

Following a meal, glycogen concentrations within the liver rise rapidly to high levels; this can be up to 10% of the wet weight of the liver. Glucose in the blood is transported into the hepatocyte by the GLUT 2 transporter and is converted to glucose 6-phosphate by glucokinase. **Phosphoglucomutase** then catalyzes the readily reversible reaction that **converts glucose 6-phosphate to glucose 1-phosphate.** The glucose 1-phosphate is further activated to **UDP-glucose** by **glucose 1-phosphate uridylyltransferase** in a reaction that consumes uridine triphosphate (UTP) and produces inorganic pyrophosphate. This reaction is thermodynamically favored by the hydrolysis of pyrophosphate by pyrophosphatase, which also makes the formation of UDP-glucose an irreversible reaction. Glycogen synthase catalyzes the addition of a glucosyl residue to a glycogen molecule using UDP-glucose as the substrate, forming an $\alpha(1{\rightarrow}4)$ glycosidic bond and releasing UDP. Because glycogen synthase cannot create an $\alpha(1{\rightarrow}6)$ linkage, an additional enzyme is required to form branches. When a chain of at least 11 glucosyl residues has been synthesized, 1,4-$\alpha$-glucan branching enzyme removes a chain of about 7 glucosyl residues and transfers it to another chain, creating an $\alpha(1{\rightarrow}6)$ glycosidic bond. This new branch point must be at least 4 glucosyl residues away from another branch point.

Because the **synthesis and mobilization of glycogen** together form a potential futile cycle, the competing processes must be **regulated to prevent waste of ATP/UTP.** This is accomplished by **hormonal as well as allosteric controls.** The enzymatic cascade, which is promulgated when glucagon or epinephrine bind to their respective receptors on the liver cells, is presented in Figure 20-2. The cAMP that is produced by activation of adenylate cyclase binds to PKA and activates it so that it can phosphorylate its target proteins. These include **phosphorylase kinase, glycogen synthase, and inhibitor 1.** Phosphorylation of glycogen synthase converts it to an inactive form, whereas phosphorylation of phosphorylase kinase and inhibitor 1 activate them. The phosphorylated inhibitor 1 strongly binds to protein phosphatase 1, but it is a poor substrate and is slowly hydrolyzed. Although the phosphorylated inhibitor 1 is bound to the phosphatase, it will inhibit it from acting on other phosphorylated proteins. Thus, while protein phosphatase 1 is inhibited, those proteins that are activated by phosphorylation remain active, and those that are inhibited by phosphorylation stay in their inactive form.

Phosphorylation of phosphorylase kinase partially activates it so that it can phosphorylate **phosphorylase b to its active form.** Phosphorylase kinase is also partially activated by $Ca^{2+}$; full activation is obtained when it both binds $Ca^{2+}$ and is phosphorylated. Conversion of phosphorylase b to phosphorylase a enables glucose 1-phosphate to be released from glycogen. Thus, glucagon and epinephrine start a cascade that mobilizes glucose from glycogen and at the same time inhibits the storage of glucose as glycogen.

When blood glucose levels are elevated, **insulin** is secreted from the pancreatic cells. When insulin binds to hepatic insulin receptors, it results in the activation of a **complex series of kinases** that leads to the **activation of protein phosphatase 1. Protein phosphatase 1 dephosphorylates phosphorylase kinase, phosphorylase, and inhibitor 1, thus inactivating them** and inhibiting the phosphorolysis

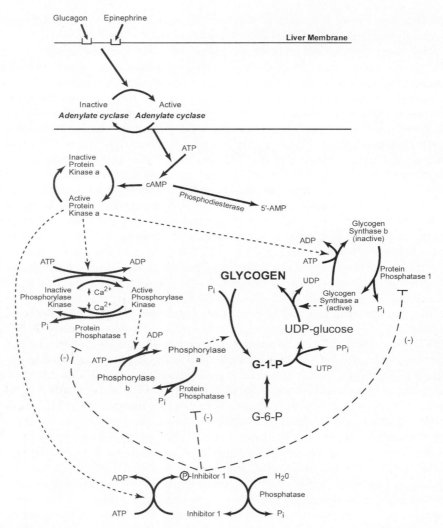

**Figure 20-2.** The mobilization of glycogen in the liver in response to hormonal signals. Binding of the hormones glucagon, epinephrine, or both causes the activation of adenylate cyclase resulting in the production of cyclic adenosine monophosphate, which activates protein kinase A (PKA). By phosphorylation reactions, PKA inactivates glycogen synthase, activates a cascade that results in active glycogen phosphorylase, and produces an active inhibitor of protein phosphatase 1.

of glycogen. It also dephosphorylates glycogen synthase, converting it to its active form and enabling the storage of glucose as glycogen. In addition, the liver form of phosphorylase a is inhibited by elevated intracellular concentrations of glucose. Thus insulin favors the storage of glycogen and inhibits its mobilization.

Although the etiology of the AFLP is unclear, it does appear to be a defect affecting mitochondrial processes. Liver biopsy usually will show mitochondrial disruption and microvesicular fat deposits, indicating decreased β-oxidation of fatty acids. The fatty acids, since they cannot be efficiently oxidized in the mitochondria, are converted to triglycerides, which build up in the hepatocyte. The fat infiltration decreases the amount of glycogen that can be stored and mobilized to maintain blood glucose levels. Gluconeogenesis is also depressed because ATP is not available from the oxidation of fatty acids. Thus, blood glucose levels decline.

As noted above, there have been reports that link some cases of AFLP with a defect in fatty acid metabolism in the fetus. These include **fetal deficiencies of long chain 3-hydroxyacyl-coenzyme A dehydrogenase (LCHAD), carnitine-palmitoyl transferase 1 (CPT 1), and medium chain acylcoenzyme A dehydrogenase (MCAD).** The mechanism by which defective fetal fatty acid oxidation causes maternal illness is not known. However, since the fetus uses primarily glucose metabolism for its energy needs, it is likely that toxic products from the placenta, which does use fatty acid oxidation, cause the maternal liver failure.

## COMPREHENSION QUESTIONS

For questions 20.1 and 20.2 refer to the following case:

A female infant appeared normal at birth but developed signs of liver disease and muscular weakness at 3 months. She had periods of hypoglycemia, particularly on awakening. Examination revealed an enlarged liver. Laboratory analyses following fasting revealed ketoacidosis, blood pH 7.25, and elevations in both alanine transaminase (ALT) and aspartate transaminase (AST) levels. Administration of glucagon following a carbohydrate meal elicited a normal rise in blood glucose, but glucose levels did not rise when glucagon was administered following an overnight fast. Liver biopsy revealed an increase in the glycogen content (6% of wet weight).

20.1 In which of the following enzymes is a genetic deficiency most likely for this patient?

A. Branching enzyme
B. Debranching enzyme
C. Glucose-6-phosphatase
D. Glycogen synthase
E. Muscle phosphorylase

20.2 To prevent the frequent episodes of hypoglycemia, which of the following dietary supplements would be most appropriate for this patient?

A. Casein (milk protein)
B. Fish oil
C. Fructose
D. Lactose
E. Uncooked cornstarch

20.3 A 17-year-old boy presents complaining of an inability to perform strenuous exercise without bringing on painful muscle cramps and weakness. He indicated that mild to moderate exercise resulted in no problems. When he was administered an ischemic exercise test, his serum lactate concentrations did not significantly increase. A deficiency in which of the following enzymes is most likely the cause of the patient's muscle cramps?

A. Carnitine palmityl transferase II
B. Glucose-6-phosphatase
C. Glycogen phosphorylase
D. Glycogen synthase
E. Very long chain acyl-CoA dehydrogenase

20.4 A 23-year-old man has been vigorously working on the yard and begins to feel slightly light-headed from hypoglycemia. He drinks a can of soda and is aware of the competition for the glucose to be stored in his liver as glycogen versus used as energy in his muscles. What is the best explanation regarding the fate of the glucose in the soda?

A. The lower Km of hexokinase compared with the Km of glucokinase will tilt the glucose toward glycolysis.
B. The bolus of glucose via the soda will lead to a higher glucose level, inducing storage of the glucose into glycogen in the liver.
C. The muscle is using high levels of glucose, leading to an increased level of glucose 6-phosphate thus inhibiting glucokinase.
D. The glucose will be equally used by muscle for metabolism and liver for glycogen storage.

## ANSWERS

20.1 **B.** Definitive diagnosis would await analysis of the glycogen structure and enzyme activities, but the hepatomegaly, increased liver glycogen content, fasting hypoglycemia, and muscle weakness are consistent with Cori disease type 3 glycogen storage disease. The increase in glycogen content results from an inability to degrade glycogen beyond the limit dextrin of phosphorylase. A deficiency in the debranching enzyme leaves glycogen with short outer branches.

20.2 **E.** Because fasting hypoglycemia results from an inability to break down glycogen past the limit dextrin of phosphorylase, a patient with type 3 glycogen storage disease should be given frequent meals high in carbohydrates. Uncooked cornstarch is an effective supplement because it is slowly digested, and therefore the glucose is released slowly into the bloodstream, helping to maintain blood glucose concentrations.

20.3 **C.** Although a deficiency in a number of enzymes can result in exercise intolerance, the lack of an increase in serum lactate following ischemic exercise points to an inability to a defect in the breakdown of glycogen in the muscle. The muscle depends on glycogenolysis for intense exercise, and fatigue rapidly ensues when glycogen is depleted. Patients with a deficiency in the muscle isoform of glycogen phosphorylase (McArdle disease) can tolerate mild to moderate exercise, but get muscle cramps with strenuous exercise as a consequence of the lack of glycogenolysis in the muscle cell.

20.4 **A.** Hexokinase is found in most tissues, and because of the very low Km (substrate concentration at which the enzyme achieves half maximal velocity) for glucose, it is designed to work maximally to provide ATP for tissue even at low levels of glucose. Hexokinase is inhibited by glucose 6-phosphate and is most active with low levels of glucose 6-phosphate. Glucokinase found in the liver has a high Km for glucose and is very active after a meal. The glucose in the soda would likely be used for ATP production.

## BIOCHEMISTRY PEARLS

▶ The etiology of the syndrome is not clear, although recent reports have linked some cases of AFLP with a fetal inborn error in fatty acid metabolism.

▶ Following a meal, glycogen concentrations within the liver rise rapidly to high levels; this can be up to 10% of the wet weight of the liver.

▶ Liver insufficiency may be associated with hypoglycemia.

## REFERENCES

Castro M, Fassett MJ, Telfer RB, et al. Reversible peripartum liver failure: A new perspective on the diagnosis, treatment, and cause of acute fatty liver of pregnancy, based on 28 consecutive cases. *Am J Obstet Gynecol.* 1999;181(2):389-395.

Rakheja D, Bennett MJ, Rogers BB. Long-chain L-3-hydroxyacyl-coenzyme A dehydrogenase deficiency: a molecular and biochemical review. *Lab Invest.* 2002;82(7):815-824.

Roe CR, Ding J. Mitochondrial fatty acid oxidation disorders. In: Scriver CR, Beaudet AL, Sly WS, et al, eds. *The Metabolic and Molecular Basis of Inherited Disease.* 8th ed. New York: McGraw-Hill; 2001:2297-2326.

Saudubray J-M, Charpentier C. Clinical phenotypes: diagnosis/algorithms. In: Scriver CR, Beaudet AL, Sly WS, et al, eds. *The Metabolic and Molecular Basis of Inherited Disease.* 8th ed. New York: McGraw-Hill; 2001:1327-1403.

Yang Z, Yamada J, Zhao Y, et al. Prospective screening for pediatric mitochondrial trifunctional protein defects in pregnancies complicated by liver disease. *JAMA.* 2002;288(17):2163-2166.

A 29-year-old man presents to the emergency department with complaints of dark-colored urine, generalized fatigue, myalgias, and weakness after completing a marathon. The patient states that this was his first marathon. He has no significant medical history and denies any medications or drug use. On examination, he appears moderately ill and is afebrile with normal vital signs. Physical examination reveals diffuse musculoskeletal tenderness. Urinalysis revealed large amounts of blood (hemoglobin and myoglobin), and serum creatine phosphokinase (CPK) was significantly elevated, as well as the potassium level on his electrolytes. Serum lactate level was markedly elevated.

▶ What is the most likely diagnosis?
▶ What is the most appropriate treatment?
▶ What is the biochemical basis for the markedly elevated serum lactate level?

# ANSWERS TO CASE 21:
## Rhabdomyolysis

*Summary:* 29-year-old marathon runner with acute episode of generalized myalgias, weakness, fatigue, and dark-colored urine with urine myoglobin/hemoglobin, hyperkalemia, and significantly increased CPK isoenzyme.

- **Most likely diagnosis:** Rhabdomyolysis (skeletal muscle cell lysis) after strenuous exercise.

- **Treatment:** Aggressive intravenous hydration to help clear the excess myoglobin from the serum, and correction of electrolyte abnormalities and treatment of kidney failure if present.

- **Biochemical basis for elevated lactate:** Reduced nicotinamide adenine dinucleotide (NADH) **levels increase because of the relative lack of oxygen for muscle,** adenosine diphosphate (ADP) and adenosine monophosphate (AMP) concentrations rise in the cytoplasm, leading to an increased flux of glucose through the glycolytic pathway in the muscle, causing pyruvate levels to increase. Pyruvate is reduced by NADH to lactate in a reaction catalyzed by lactate dehydrogenase. Lactate is transported out of the muscle cell to the blood.

## CLINICAL CORRELATION

Skeletal muscle has a need for oxygen and fuel (glucose and fatty acids). Short exertion allows for replenishment of these important substrates; however, long, grueling demands on muscle, such as running a marathon, can lead to relative deprivation of oxygen (because of either overexertion or dehydration and insufficient blood flow to the muscles). This lack of oxygen leads to the conversion to the glycolytic pathway versus the tricarboxylic acid (TCA) pathway for adenosine triphosphate (ATP) production. Marathon running has been shown to effect increases in the blood and urinary concentrations of a number of biochemical parameters that result from exertional muscle damage (rhabdomyolysis) and hemolysis. These include increases in serum myoglobin, CPK, as well as an increase in the anionic gap, leading to a metabolic acidosis. In the case of marathon runners, this is usually caused by an increase in the serum lactate concentration. Other causes of rhabdomyolysis include cocaine intoxication, hyperthermia, convulsions, or toxins.

# APPROACH TO:
## Oxidative Phosphorylation and Lactate

### OBJECTIVES

1. Understand how hypoxemia (eg, rhabdomyolysis) leads to reduced oxidative phosphorylation and increased lactic acid production.

2. Be familiar with the pyruvate cycle and the importance of NADH levels.

3. Know about the lactic acid pathway.

## DEFINITIONS

**ANION GAP:** A calculation of the routinely measured cations minus the routinely measured anions. Since in all fluids the sum of the positive charges (cations) must be balanced with the negative charges (anions), the anion gap is an artifact of measurement. Because the $[K^+]$ is small, it is usually omitted from the calculation. The equation most frequently used to calculate the anion gap is

$$AG = [Na^+] - ([Cl^-] + [HCO_3^-])$$

**GLUCONEOGENESIS:** The series of biochemical reactions in which glucose is synthesized in the liver (and other gluconeogenic tissues) from small organic acids such as lactate, pyruvate, and oxaloacetate.

**HEMATIN:** Heme in which the coordinated iron is in the ferric ($Fe^{3+}$) oxidation state.

**MYOGLOBIN:** A large heme-containing protein that is able to bind oxygen and release it in tissues in which the oxygen tension is low.

**β-OXIDATION:** The series of biochemical reactions in which fatty acids are degraded to acetyl-CoA, which then enters the tricarboxylic acid cycle for the production of energy in the form of reducing equivalents and guanosine triphosphate (GTP). Each round of β-oxidation shortens the fatty acid by 2 carbons and, in addition to acetyl-CoA, produces NADH and $FADH_2$, which are fed into the electron transport system for the production of ATP.

## DISCUSSION

The **exercising muscle's sources of energy are primarily glucose and fatty acids.** The muscle obtains glucose from the blood or the breakdown of stored glycogen in the muscle. Fatty acids are acquired as free fatty acids from the blood or from the breakdown of triglycerides that are stored in the muscle. For complete oxidation of these sources of energy, the **metabolic intermediate acetyl coenzyme A (acetyl-CoA) must be oxidized** through the **TCA cycle,** and the reducing equivalents produced (NADH and $FADH_2$) must be transferred to oxygen through the mitochondrial electron transport system. This electron transfer process produces a **proton gradient** across the inner mitochondrial matrix that drives the synthesis of ATP by ATP synthase. For this process to continue, a plentiful supply of oxygen must be supplied to the tissues.

It has been estimated that at the beginning of the marathon, a runner who is running at a reasonable pace consumes energy in a ratio of 75% carbohydrate to 25% fatty acids. This ratio will decrease as glycogen stores in the body diminish. However, as exertion continues and the muscle starts to rely more on the β-oxidation of fatty acids to provide its energy needs, its oxygen demand increases, placing a heavier demand on the heart to provide oxygenated blood. If the runner does not take steps to replace fluids lost through sweat, then dehydration will occur, resulting in decreased perfusion of the muscle with adequately oxygenated blood.

If the muscle uses ATP faster than it can be produced by oxidative phosphorylation either by overexertion or because oxygen uptake is limited, then **NADH levels increase in the mitochondria and in the cytoplasm.** ADP and AMP concentrations in the cytoplasm will rise because ATP is used by the muscle for contraction. This will increase the flux of glucose through the glycolytic pathway in the muscle, causing pyruvate levels to increase. To regenerate the oxidized cofactor NAD$^+$ that is required in the conversion of glyceraldehyde 3-phosphate to 3-phosphoglycerate, **pyruvate is reduced by NADH to lactate** in a reaction catalyzed by lactate dehydrogenase. Lactate is transported out of the muscle cell to the blood.

**Lactate in the blood is taken up by the liver and used as a carbon source in the synthesis of new glucose by the gluconeogenic pathway.** The liver must first reoxidize lactate to pyruvate in a reaction that is catalyzed by lactate dehydrogenase and generates NADH. Pyruvate cannot be directly converted to phosphoenolpyruvate (PEP) by pyruvate kinase because under physiologic conditions; the reaction is thermodynamically irreversible in favor of the formation of pyruvate. Instead, pyruvate must enter the mitochondria and be carboxylated by the enzyme **pyruvate carboxylase** to form **oxaloacetate** in a reaction that requires biotin as a cofactor (Figure 21-1). Oxaloacetate is then reduced to malate by malate dehydrogenase and **malate** then exits the mitochondrion. In the cytosol, malate is reoxidized back to **oxaloacetate** by cytoplasmic malate dehydrogenase. The cytoplasmic **oxaloacetate** is then converted to **PEP by PEP carboxykinase** in a reaction that requires GTP. (In a minor alternate pathway, mitochondrial oxaloacetate can be converted to PEP by the mitochondrial form of the enzyme PEP carboxykinase. PEP then exits the mitochondrion to the cytosol.) The pathway from PEP to

**Figure 21-1.** Interconversion of phosphoenolpyruvate (PEP) and pyruvate. The conversion of PEP to pyruvate is thermodynamically irreversible in the cell. To convert pyruvate back to PEP for gluconeogenesis, pyruvate must enter the mitochondrion, be carboxylated to oxaloacetate (OAA), and reduced to malate. After exiting the mitochondrion, malate is oxidized back to OAA and converted to PEP by the action of phosphoenolpyruvate carboxykinase.

**Figure 21-2.** The reactions that make up the thermodynamically irreversible steps in glycolysis and gluconeogenesis. These steps make up potential "futile" cycles that must be carefully regulated.

glucose is identical to that of glycolysis except for 2 reactions (Figure 21-2). **Fructose 1,6-bisphosphate** is converted to fructose 6-phosphate by hydrolysis of phosphate by the **enzyme fructose-1,6-bisphosphatase.** The final reaction is hydrolysis of glucose 6-phosphate to glucose by glucose-6-phosphatase. Hepatic glucose produced via gluconeogenesis is then delivered to the blood for use by the brain and muscle. This process by which extrahepatic lactate is taken back to the liver, **converted to glucose by gluconeogenesis,** and returned to extrahepatic tissues is called the **Cori cycle.** When the rate of lactate production by muscle exceeds the rate at which the Cori cycle can operate, **lactate accumulates in the blood leading to lactic acidemia.**

During a marathon run, there is constant stretching and tearing of the leg muscle fibers each time the foot hits the ground. This constant shock causes damage to the muscle cells, resulting in a release of cellular contents to the extracellular matrix and the bloodstream. The concentrations of myoglobin, which is in high concentration in slow twitch (red) muscle fibers, and $K^+$, which is concentrated in all cells, therefore rise in the blood. When the concentration of myoglobin increases above 0.5 to 1.5 mg/dL, it is excreted into the urine. Normally myoglobin is not toxic to the kidney; however, when the pH of the urine drops below 5.6, myoglobin undergoes oxidation to produce hematin (porphyrin bound $Fe^{3+}$), which is toxic to the kidneys and can lead to acute renal failure. This toxic effect is exacerbated when the urine is concentrated as a result of dehydration.

## COMPREHENSION QUESTIONS

21.1   During the course of a marathon race a runner expends a large amount of
       energy and must use stored sources of fuel as well as oxygen. Compared with
       the beginning of the race (first mile), which of the following best describes
       the utilization of glycogen and fatty acids as fuels and amount of oxygen
       consumed after running for 26 miles?

|      | Glycogen used | Fatty acids used | Oxygen consumed |
|------|---------------|------------------|-----------------|
| A.   | ↑             | ↑                | ↑               |
| B.   | ↑             | ↓                | ↓               |
| C.   | ↑             | ↓                | ↑               |
| D.   | ↓             | ↑                | ↑               |
| E.   | ↓             | ↑                | ↓               |

21.2   During an extended period of exercise, the enzymes involved in the glyco-
       lytic pathway in muscle tissue are actively breaking down glucose to provide
       the muscle energy. The liver, to maintain blood glucose levels, is synthesiz-
       ing glucose via the gluconeogenic pathway. Which of the following enzymes
       involved in these pathways would be most likely to exhibit Michaelis–Menten
       kinetics (ie, have a hyperbolic curve when plotting substrate concentration
       versus velocity of the reaction)?

   A.   Fructose-1,6-bisphosphatase
   B.   Hexokinase
   C.   Lactate dehydrogenase
   D.   Phosphofructokinase 1
   E.   Pyruvate kinase

21.3   A known person who abuses alcohol is found lying semiconscious at the bot-
       tom of a stairwell with a broken arm by his landlady, who called an ambu-
       lance to take him to the emergency room. Initial laboratory studies showed a
       relatively large anion gap of 34 (normal range: 9-15). His blood alcohol was
       elevated at 245 mg/dL (intoxication level: 150-300 mg/dL), and his blood
       glucose was 38 mg/dL (low normal). The patient's large anion gap and hypo-
       glycemia can best be explained by which of the following?

   A.   Decreased secretion of glucagon
   B.   Increased secretion of insulin
   C.   Increased urination resulting from the diuretic effect of alcohol
   D.   Inhibition of dehydrogenase enzymes by NADH
   E.   Inhibition of glycogenolysis by ethanol

# ANSWERS

21.1 **D.** At the beginning of the race, a runner running at a reasonable pace consumes energy at a ratio of approximately 75% carbohydrate: 25% fatty acids. However, by the end of the race, glycogen stores are for the most part depleted, and the generation of ATP must come from the β-oxidation of fatty acids, which produces reducing equivalents for oxidative phosphorylation. This requires an increase in the amount of oxygen consumed.

21.2 **C.** The activity of regulatory enzymes such as fructose-1,6-bisphosphatase, hexokinase, phosphofructokinase 1, and pyruvate kinase are frequently controlled by binding allosteric effectors. These allosteric enzymes usually exhibit sigmoidal kinetics. Lactate dehydrogenase is not controlled by allosteric effectors and therefore would be expected to exhibit Michaelis–Menten kinetics.

21.3 **D.** People who abuse alcohol frequently do not eat while binge drinking, so it is most likely that his liver glycogen stores became depleted and could not increase his blood glucose levels. The metabolic stress leads to the increase in secretion of epinephrine and other hormones that mobilize fatty acids from stored triglycerides in adipose cells. These fatty acids undergo β-oxidation in the liver but are converted to ketone bodies because of the inhibition of the TCA cycle by high levels of NADH produced by the oxidation of ethanol first to acetaldehyde and acetate. Key gluconeogenic dehydrogenases are also inhibited by the elevated levels of NADH, including lactate dehydrogenase, glycerol 3-phosphate dehydrogenase, and malate dehydrogenase.

## BIOCHEMISTRY PEARLS

▶ The exercising muscle's sources of energy are primarily glucose and fatty acids.

▶ With insufficient oxygen to meet the muscle demands, NADH levels increase in the mitochondria and in the cytoplasm, ADP and AMP concentrations in the cytoplasm will rise, and glucose will be shunted to the glycolytic pathway in the muscle. The pyruvate is converted to lactate, which causes the metabolic acidosis.

▶ Muscle injury can lead to myoglobinemia and myoglobinuria (red urine) and may crystallize in the renal tubules, leading to renal insufficiency.

## REFERENCES

Brady HR, Brenner BM. Acute renal failure. In: Longo D, Fauci AS, Kaspar D, et al, eds. *Harrison's Principles of Internal Medicine*. 18th ed. New York: McGraw-Hill; 2011.

Kratz A, Lewandrowski KB, Siegel AJ, et al. Effect of marathon running on hematologic and biochemical laboratory parameters, including cardiac markers. *Am J Clin Pathol*. 2002;118(12):856-863.

Murakami K. Rhabdomyolysis and acute renal failure. In: Glew RH, Ninomiya Y, eds. *Clinical Studies in Medical Biochemistry*. 2nd ed. New York: Oxford University Press; 1997.

A 50-year-old Hispanic woman presents to your clinic with complaints of excessive thirst, fluid intake, and urination. She denies any symptoms of urinary tract infection and reports no medical problems; however, she has not seen a doctor in many years. On examination, she is an obese woman in no acute distress. Her physical examination is otherwise normal. Urinalysis revealed 4+ glucose, and a serum random blood sugar level was 320 mg/dL.

▶ What is the most likely diagnosis?
▶ What other organ systems can be involved with the disease?
▶ What is the biochemical basis of this disease?

# ANSWERS TO CASE 22:
## Type 2 Diabetes

*Summary:* 50-year-old obese Hispanic woman presents with polydipsia, polyphagia, and urinary frequency and elevated random blood sugar level of 320 mg/dL.

- **Diagnosis:** Type 2 diabetes.

- **Other organ systems involved:** Cardiovascular, eye, peripheral nerves, gastrointestinal, kidney.

- **Biochemical basis:** Insulin resistance as a result of a postinsulin receptor defect. The insulin levels are normal or increased when compared with normal individuals; however, the insulin is not "recognized," and, thus, the glucose levels remain elevated.

## CLINICAL CORRELATION

Diabetes mellitus is characterized by elevated blood glucose levels. It is composed of 2 types depending on the pathogenesis. Type 1 diabetes is characterized by insulin deficiency and usually has its onset during childhood or teenage years. This is also called *ketosis-prone* diabetes. Type 2 diabetes is caused by insulin resistance and usually has elevated insulin levels, and it is diagnosed in the adult years. Type 2 diabetes is far more common than type 1 diabetes. Risk factors include obesity, family history, sedentary life style, and, in women, hyperandrogenic states or anovulation.

Diabetes mellitus is now recognized as one of the most common and significant diseases facing Americans. It is estimated that 1 of 4 children born today will become diabetic in their lifetime because of obesity and inactivity. In addition, diabetes has a severe effect on blood vessels, particularly in the pathogenesis of atherosclerosis (blockage of arteries by lipids and plaque), which can lead to myocardial infarction or stroke. Diabetes mellitus is treated as equivalent to a prior cardiovascular event in its risk for future atherosclerotic disease. Diabetes is also associated with immunosuppression, renal insufficiency, blindness, neuropathy, and other metabolic disorders.

# APPROACH TO:
## Insulin and Glucose

## OBJECTIVES

1. Understand the role of insulin on carbohydrate metabolism.

2. Be aware of the role of glucagon on carbohydrate metabolism.

3. Know about the processes of gluconeogenesis and glycogenolysis.

## DEFINITIONS

**DIABETES MELLITUS:** An endocrine disease characterized by an elevated blood glucose concentration. There are 2 major forms of diabetes mellitus: type 1, or insulin-dependent, and type 2, or non–insulin-dependent. Type 1 is caused by a severe lack or complete absence of insulin. Type 2 is caused by resistance to insulin, that is, an inability to respond to physiologic concentrations of insulin.

**FRUCTOSE 2,6-BISPHOSPHATE:** A metabolite of fructose 6-phosphate produced by the bifunctional enzyme 6-phosphofructokinase-2 (PFK-2)/fructose bisphosphatase-2 (FBPase-2). It serves as an allosteric effector that activates 6-phosphofructokinase-1 and inhibits fructose bisphosphatase-1, thus stimulating the movement of glucose through the glycolytic pathway and inhibiting gluconeogenesis.

**GLUCAGON:** A polypeptide hormone synthesized and secreted by the α-cells of the islets of Langerhans in the pancreas. Glucagon is released in response to low blood glucose levels and stimulates glycogenolysis and gluconeogenesis in the liver.

**INSULIN:** A polypeptide hormone synthesized and secreted by the β-cells of the islets of Langerhans in the pancreas. Insulin is released in response to elevations in blood glucose and promotes the uptake of glucose into cells by increasing the number of GLUT 4 glucose transporters on cell surfaces.

**PROTEIN KINASE A:** An enzyme that will phosphorylate target proteins. It is activated by increased cyclic adenosine monophosphate (cAMP) concentration in the cell that is a response to the activation of adenylate cyclase by binding of certain hormones on cell surfaces.

## DISCUSSION

Every cell in the human body uses **glucose** as an energy source. Indeed, certain cells have an obligate requirement for glucose to meet their energetic demands (eg, erythrocytes). **Neurons,** although can use alternative fuel sources under extreme conditions (eg, **ketone bodies** during prolonged starvation), have a strong preference toward glucose utilization. Therefore, circulating levels of glucose must be maintained sufficiently high to meet the energy demands of the body. Chronic elevations in blood glucose levels are also detrimental, because they are associated with oxidative stress and glycation of cellular proteins. It has been suggested that the latter mediate many of the complications associated with chronic hyperglycemia such as in cases of diabetic microvascular disease and retinopathy.

Despite diurnal variations in meal times, blood glucose levels are normally maintained within a narrow range. This is made possible in large part by the counter regulatory actions of the peptide hormones **insulin and glucagon.** Insulin, secreted by the β-cells of pancreatic islets when blood glucose levels increase, promotes glucose utilization and represses endogenous glucose production (Figure 22-1a). By contrast, **glucagon,** secreted by the α-cells of pancreatic islets when blood glucose levels are low, represses glucose utilization and promotes endogenous glucose production (Figure 22-1b). Therefore, a **careful balance between the actions of insulin and glucagon** helps maintain blood glucose levels within a normal range.

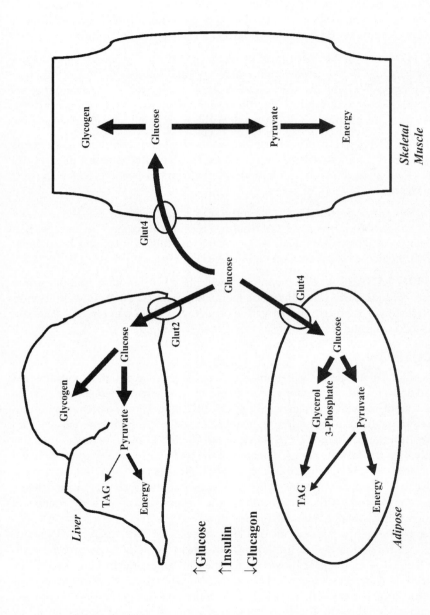

**Figure 22-1a.** The flow of glucose to tissues under conditions of elevated blood glucose concentration. When [glucose]$_{blood}$ is high, the insulin:glucagon ratio is high, leading to the uptake of glucose into the tissues. TAG = triacylglycerol.

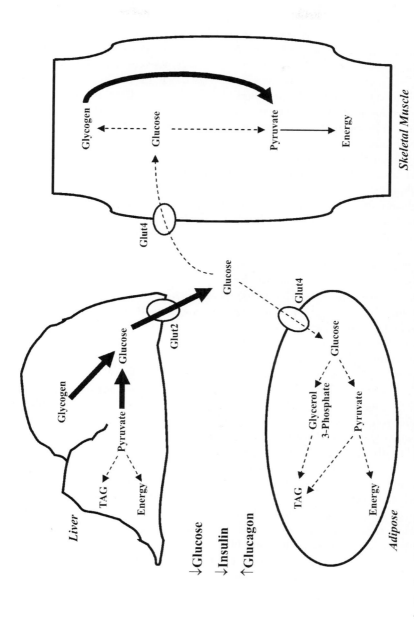

**Figure 22-1b.** The flow of glucose to tissues under conditions of low blood glucose concentration. When [glucose]$_{blood}$ is low, the insulin:glucagon ratio is low, leading to glycogenolysis and gluconeogenesis in the liver. TAG = triacylglycerol.

**Insulin receptors** are essentially expressed ubiquitously, in large part as a result of the mitogenic actions of this peptide hormone. In terms of glucose metabolism, the actions of insulin on the liver, adipose, and skeletal muscle will be the focus of this discussion, although insulin-mediated changes in satiety and blood flow undoubtedly play a role in whole body glucose homeostasis. On binding to its cell surface receptor, insulin elicits a complex cascade of cellular signaling events that have not been elucidated fully to date. This, in turn, increases glucose transport into the cell (skeletal muscle and adipose), promotes storage of excess carbon from glucose as glycogen (skeletal muscle and liver) and triglyceride (TAG; liver and adipose), increases glucose utilization as a fuel source (skeletal muscle, liver, and adipose), and decreases endogenous glucose production (liver; see Figure 22-1a). These actions of insulin can be either acute (affecting activity of preexisting proteins) or chronic (altering protein levels).

Skeletal muscle and adipose express 2 major isoforms of **glucose transports, GLUT 1 and GLUT 4.** GLUT 1, a ubiquitously expressed glucose transporter, resides almost exclusively at the cell surface, where it facilitates a constant "basal" rate of glucose uptake into the cell. By contrast, GLUT 4, whose expression is limited to skeletal muscle, heart, and adipose, can be found both at the cell surface and within specialized intracellular vesicles. Redistribution of GLUT 4 from intracellular vesicles to the cell surface in response to insulin results in increased rates of glucose transport, thereby facilitating insulin-stimulated glucose disposal. By contrast to skeletal muscle and adipose, the liver expresses GLUT 2. This is a freely reversible glucose transporter that resides permanently at the cell surface. GLUT 2 enables glucose to pass down its concentration gradient, allowing increased hepatic glucose uptake when blood glucose levels are high and increased hepatic glucose efflux when blood glucose levels are low.

Once within the cell, glucose undergoes one of several fates. Insulin promotes incorporation of glucose moieties into **glycogen,** the storage form of glucose in mammals. This is driven in large part by insulin-mediated activation of **protein phosphatase 1** (PP1; Figure 22-2a). PP1 dephosphorylates (hydrolytic removal of regulatory phosphate groups from serine/threonine residues on target enzymes) a number of key proteins involved in glycogen metabolism. Dephosphorylation and activation of glycogen synthase (GS), with a concomitant dephosphorylation and inactivation of glycogen phosphorylase (GP), will stimulate net glycogen synthesis (glycogenesis) by liver and muscle, in response to insulin. One way in which insulin promotes PP1-mediated effects on glycogen metabolism is through the targeting of PP1 to the glycogen particle, a subcellular domain comprised of glycogen itself, as well as the enzymes required for glycogen synthesis and degradation. The glycogen binding subunit is a docking protein, allowing PP1 association with the glycogen particle. Insulin induces tyrosine phosphorylation of this glycogen binding subunit, thereby promoting PP1 binding and, therefore, increased glycogenesis.

The glycogen capacity of a cell is of finite size. Once this capacity is reached, excess glucose must undergo alternative metabolic fates. Insulin promotes flux of glucose through the glycolytic pathway (glucose → 2 pyruvate), in part through PP1 activation (see Figure 22-2a). As glycogenolysis is the reciprocal pathway to glycogenesis, gluconeogenesis (the synthesis of glucose) is the reciprocal pathway

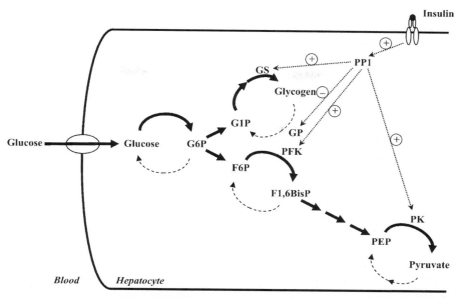

**Figure 22-2a.** Insulin stimulation of the flux of glucose through the glycolytic pathway. Insulin activates protein phosphatase 1, which, in turn, activates glycogen synthase, phosphofructokinase, and pyruvate kinase. Fructose 1,6-bisphosphate = F1,6BisP, fructose 6-phosphate = F6P, glucose 1-phosphate = G1P, glucose 6-phosphate = G6P, glycogen phosphorylase = GP, glycogen synthase = GS, phosphoenolpyruvate = PEP, phosphofructokinase = PFK, pyruvate kinase = PK, protein phosphatase 1 = PP1.

to glycolysis. Gluconeogenesis occurs primarily in the liver and to a lesser extent in the kidney. PP1 increases glycolytic flux in the liver through activation of phosphofructokinase (PFK; indirect effect through dephosphorylation of a bifunctional enzyme, resulting in increased intracellular levels of fructose 2,6-bisphosphate, an allosteric activator of PFK) and pyruvate kinase (PK; direct effect). Glycolytically derived pyruvate could potentially undergo 1 of 2 fates in the liver, namely, full oxidation (via the Krebs cycle and oxidative phosphorylation), entry into the fatty acid synthesis pathway, or both. However, humans on a Western diet, in which excess calories are more often a mixture of carbohydrate and fat, tend to use ingested carbohydrate as a fuel, while fatty acids are stored as triglyceride in adipose tissue. The latter is driven by insulin.

When blood glucose levels begin to decline (eg, during an overnight fast), so too does insulin secretion. By contrast, circulating levels of **glucagon** increase. The latter targets primarily **hepatic glucose metabolism** in humans, increasing glucose production and decreasing glucose utilization. On binding to its cell surface receptors, glucagon increases the activity of **protein kinase A** (PKA; Figure 22-2b). In turn, PKA stimulates net glycogen breakdown (glycogenolysis) through phosphorylation of phosphorylase kinase (increases activity) and glycogen synthase (decreases activity). The former phosphorylates and activates glycogen phosphorylase. PKA further antagonizes the effects of insulin through inactivation of PP1. PKA

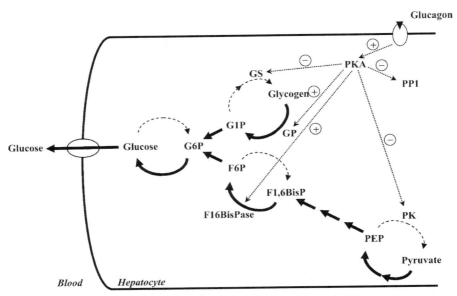

**Figure 22-2b.** Glucagon promotion of glycogenolysis and gluconeogenesis in the liver. Glucagon binding leads to the activation of protein kinase A, which activates glycogen phosphorylase and fructose-1,6-bisphosphatase, while inhibiting glycogen synthase, pyruvate kinase, and protein phosphatase 1. Fructose 1,6-bisphosphate = F1,6BisP, fructose 6-phosphate = F6P, glucose 1-phosphate = G1P, glucose 6-phosphate = G6P, glycogen phosphorylase = GP, glycogen synthase = GS, phosphoenolpyruvate = PEP, phosphofructokinase = PFK, pyruvate kinase = PK, PKA = protein kinase A, protein phosphatase 1 = PP1.

phosphorylates the glycogen binding subunit at specific serine residues, causing the release of PP1 from the glycogen particle. Once released, PP1 binds to inhibitor 1, thus further inactivating PP1 activity. This PP1-inhibitor 1 association is promoted by PKA-mediated phosphorylation of inhibitor 1. Gluconeogenesis is also stimulated by glucagon-induced PKA activation, through activation of fructose 1, 6-bisphosphatase (F1,6BisPase; indirect effect through phosphorylation of a bifunctional enzyme, resulting in decreased intracellular levels of fructose 2,6-bisphosphate, an allosteric inhibitor of F1,6BisPase) and pyruvate kinase (reverse of PP1 effects). Glycogenolysis- and gluconeogenesis-derived glucose is exported out of the liver to help maintain blood glucose levels.

Abnormalities in the above described glucose homeostatic mechanisms arise during diabetes mellitus. **2 major forms of diabetes mellitus** exist, insulin-dependent (type 1) and non–insulin-dependent (type 2) diabetes. **Type 1 diabetes** is caused by a **severe lack or complete absence of insulin.** Also known as early onset diabetes, this disease is often caused by an autoimmune destruction of pancreatic β-cells. In contrast, **type 2 diabetes** is caused by **insulin resistance in the face of insulin insufficiency.** Insulin resistance is defined as an inability to respond to a physiologic concentration of insulin. The pancreas initially compensates by producing more insulin. At this stage, the patient is described as glucose intolerant. As the disease

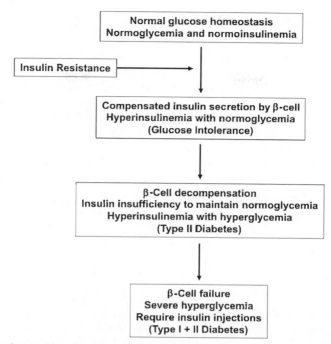

**Figure 22-3.** Schematic diagram showing the effects of insulin resistance leading to diabetes mellitus.

progresses, the degree of insulin resistance often worsens. Type 2 diabetes occurs when insulin secretion is not sufficient to maintain normoglycemia. The disease is thus characterized by both hyperinsulinemia and hyperglycemia (Figure 22-3). The degree at which different organs develop insulin resistance is often not uniform. Skeletal muscle insulin-mediated glucose disposal (which is normally responsible for 60% of whole body glucose disposal) is generally more affected, followed next by insulin suppression of hepatic glucose output. The combination of decreased peripheral glucose utilization and increased hepatic glucose production (driven by hepatic insulin resistance as well as increased circulating glucagon levels in people with type 2 diabetes) together contribute to the hyperglycemia. Insulin signaling in adipose tissue appears least affected in people with type 2 diabetes. **Hyperinsulinemia, in the face of hyperglycemia and dyslipidemia (often associated with type 2 diabetes), drives lipogenesis in adipose tissue** and may therefore contribute to the obesity often associated with this disease.

## COMPREHENSION QUESTIONS

22.1   A 64-year-old man is presented to his family doctor with complaints of frequent episodes of dizziness and of numbness in his legs. During a routine history and physical examination, the doctor finds that the patient leads a sedentary lifestyle, is obese (body mass index of 32 kg/m$^2$), and has hypertension (blood pressure of 200/120 mm Hg). The patient is asked to return to the clinic 1 week later in the fasting state, during which time a blood specimen is obtained, and a glucose tolerance test is performed. Humoral analysis reveals fasting hyperglycemia, hyperinsulinemia, dyslipidemia, and glucose intolerance. The diagnosis is type 2 diabetes mellitus.

Alterations in substrate metabolism within which of the following organs can be a cause for the observed humoral analysis?

A.   Brain
B.   Kidney
C.   Liver
D.   Heart
E.   Spleen

22.2   A mutation, leading to decreased activity, in the gene encoding for which of these proteins is most consistent with this clinical presentation?

A.   Glucagon
B.   Glucose transporter isoform 1
C.   GP
D.   Pyruvate carboxylase
E.   PP1

22.3   Which of the following complications is less likely to occur in people with type 2 diabetes compared with those with type 1 diabetes?

A.   Retinopathy
B.   Weight gain
C.   Cardiovascular disease
D.   Hypoglycemic coma
E.   Neuropathy

## ANSWERS

22.1   **C.** Of the organs listed, changes in hepatic metabolism are most likely to affect circulating glucose and lipids. This in turn influences pancreatic insulin secretion. During type 2 diabetes mellitus, increased hepatic glucose output contributes to the observed hyperglycemia and subsequent hyperinsulinemia, whereas complex alterations in lipid metabolism contribute to dyslipidemia. By contrast, changes in metabolic fluxes within the brain, kidney, heart, and spleen are often a consequence, rather than cause, of their environment. For example, the heart increases further reliance on fatty acids as a fuel in the diabetic milieu.

22.2  **E.** The underlying cause of type 2 diabetes mellitus is insulin resistance (an inability to respond normally to physiologic concentrations of insulin). PP1 is an integral mediator of the metabolic effects of insulin. Failure to activate PP1 adequately in response to insulin would therefore attenuate the metabolic actions of this hormone. Decreased activity of glucose transporter 1, GP, and pyruvate carboxylase would influence basal glucose transport, glycogenolysis, and gluconeogenesis, respectively. Decreased glucagon levels would tend to improve effectiveness of insulin action.

22.3  **D.** Hypoglycemia is a common complication associated with over supplementation of people with type 1 diabetes taking insulin. This is less common in people with type 2 diabetes, because insulin therapy generally occurs only in the later stages of the pathogenesis of this disease. Retinopathy, cardiovascular disease, and neuropathy are common complications associated with both forms of diabetes mellitus. By contrast to type 1 diabetes, patients with type 2 diabetes tend to be overweight. Whether weight gain is a cause or consequence of disease progression is under current debate.

## BIOCHEMISTRY PEARLS

▶ Serum glucose levels are tightly controlled: insulin promotes glucose utilization and represses endogenous glucose production, whereas glucagon represses glucose utilization and promotes endogenous glucose production.

▶ Several types of glucose transport proteins appear on specific tissues, affecting the movement of glucose across cell membranes.

▶ Glucose is converted into glycogen, the storage form of glucose in mammals, in a process regulated by insulin and insulin-mediated activation of PP1.

## REFERENCES

Cohen P. Dissection of the protein phosphorylation cascades involved in insulin and growth factor action. *Biochem Soc Trans.* 1993;21(3):555-567.

Gould GW, Holman GD. The glucose transporter family: structure, function and tissue-specific expression. *Biochem J.* 1993;295(2):329-341.

Newsholme EA, Leech AR. *Biochemistry for the Medical Sciences.* New York: Wiley; 1983.

A 2-year-old black girl is being seen by the hematologist after her pediatrician found her to be severely anemic with splenomegaly and jaundice. Her mother gives a possible history of a "blood problem" in her family but does not know for sure. Hemoglobin electrophoresis was normal, and a complete blood count (CBC) revealed normocytic anemia. The platelet and white blood cell counts are normal. On the peripheral smear, there are many bizarre erythrocytes, including spiculated cells. A diagnosis of pyruvate kinase deficiency is made.

▶ What is the biochemical mechanism for this disorder?
▶ How is this disorder inherited?

# ANSWERS TO CASE 23:
## Hemolytic Anemia

*Summary:* A 2-year-old black girl has normocytic anemia, jaundice, splenomegaly, and peripheral smear showing spiculated cells. A family history of similar symptoms is possible.

- **Biochemical mechanism:** Pyruvate kinase deficiency usually will manifest clinical symptoms on red blood cells (RBCs) with no apparent metabolic abnormalities in other cells. Insufficient adenosine triphosphate (ATP) is produced in the red cell and its membrane is affected, is rigid, and is removed by the spleen.

- **Inheritance:** Autosomal recessive.

## CLINICAL CORRELATION

Hemolytic anemia is not a common cause of anemia, but should be considered in patients with elevated serum bilirubin or urine bilirubin levels. Lysis of the erythrocyte can occur from various mechanisms such as medications, antibodies against red blood cells, infection, coagulopathy, and mechanical processes such as abnormal heart valves, and enzyme deficiencies of the RBC. Patients may notice fatigue, dizziness from the anemia, and dark colored (classically "cola-colored") urine from the bilirubinuria.

Confirmation of hemolysis can be obtained by the peripheral blood smear revealing fragmented RBCs, or increased serum bilirubin or decreased serum haptoglobin. Immunoglobulins can cause RBC lysis by attacking various proteins on the surface of erythrocytes, autoimmune processes (body attacking itself), or alloimmune (immunoglobulins from outside) such as from a blood transfusion or a fetus from the mother. The Coombs tests can assess for immunoglobulin on the RBC or circulating in the serum. Typically, hemolysis of the erythrocyte is associated with increased levels of RBC precursors in the bone marrow and, thus, immature forms of the erythrocytes in the bloodstream; therefore, an increased reticulocyte concentration supports the increased destruction of RBCs.

# APPROACH TO:
## Pyruvate Metabolism

### OBJECTIVES

1. Understand the role of pyruvate kinase in pyruvate metabolism.
2. Be familiar with the Embden-Meyerhof pathway of RBC metabolism.
3. Know how pyruvate kinase deficiency results in anemia.

## DEFINITIONS

**HEMOLYTIC ANEMIA:** A pathologic condition in which there is an abnormally lowered number of circulating RBCs caused by rupture of RBCs as a result of membrane abnormalities or deficient enzyme(s) level within the RBC.

**GLUCOSE 6-PHOSPHATE DEHYDROGENASE:** The enzyme that catalyzes the rate regulating step of the hexose monophosphate shunt, which produces reduced nicotinamide adenine dinucleotide phosphate (NADPH) required for inactivating oxygen radicals and thereby protects the RBC membrane from radical attack and rupture.

**PYRUVATE KINASE:** Last ATP-producing step in glycolysis and critical in the RBC for maintaining energy supply (ATP levels).

**METHEMOGLOBIN REDUCTASE:** RBC enzyme that uses NADH to convert the iron of oxidized hemoglobin (methemoglobin) from the ferric ($Fe^{3+}$) to reduced ferrous state ($Fe^{2+}$) hemoglobin, which alone is capable of binding oxygen.

## DISCUSSION

Hemolytic anemia has many causes, although this case has the marks of undersupply of RBCs caused by an enzyme deficiency within the RBC rather than a membrane abnormality or an environmental factor such as an autoantibody or mechanical trauma.

The RBC in the course of its maturation loses its mitochondria, ribosomes, and nucleus and consequently the functions associated with those organelles such as new enzyme synthesis and mitochondrial energy formation. **Thus, the enzyme endowment present at maturation of the RBC cannot be replaced.** In terms of energy production in the RBC, **only the glycolytic pathway (Embden-Meyerhof pathway) is available.** This pathway, together with the hexose monophosphate shunt (pentose phosphate pathway; Figure 23-1), is the only metabolic pathway that uses glucose in RBCs. As a consequence of this limited metabolic capacity, glucose is the only fuel usable by the RBC to generate ATP. Glucose metabolism is required in the RBC to maintain the ionic milieu within the cell, to maintain the heme cofactor of hemoglobin in its reduced ($Fe^{2+}$) state, to maintain reduced sulfhydryl groups, to maintain the shape of the RBC plasma membrane and to produce 2,3-bisphosphoglycerate, a modulator of hemoglobin affinity for oxygen. To accomplish these tasks approximately 90% of the glucose in the RBC is metabolized directly to pyruvate/lactate while approximately 10% is first metabolized through the hexose monophosphate shunt before reentry into the glycolytic pathway.

**Approximately 90% of all cases of known RBC enzyme deficiencies** involve either altered protein or **decreased protein levels of pyruvate kinase,** whereas **4% are variants of glucose 6-phosphate isomerase, which converts glucose 6-phosphate to fructose 6-phosphate.** Most of these enzyme deficiencies are inherited in an autosomal recessive pattern.

As shown in Figure 23-1, 2 mol of ATP are formed per mole of glucose metabolized by the glycolytic cycle. The primary final product of glucose metabolism by glycolysis in the RBC is not pyruvate, as in other tissues most of the time, but lactate. Because RBCs have no mitochondria, $NAD^+$ cannot be regenerated by

**Figure 23-1.** Metabolism of glucose in erythrocytes. The following abbreviations are used: G6P = glucose 6-phosphate, 6-PG = 6-phosphogluconate, γ-Glu-Cys = γ-glutamyl-cysteine, Gly = glycine, GSH = reduced glutathione, GSSG = glutathione disulfide, ROOH = organic hydroperoxides, F6P = fructose 6-phosphate, R-5-P = rebulose-5-phosphate, F-1,6-BP = fructose 1, 6-bisphosphate, DHAP = dihydroxyacetone phosphate, GAP = glyceraldehyde 3-phosphate, Hb = hemoglobin (Fe$^{+2}$), metHb = hemoglobin (Fe$^{+3}$), 1,3-BPG = 1,3-bisphosphoglycerate, 2,3-BPG, 2,3-bisphosphoglycerate, 3-PG = 3-phosphoglycerate, 2-PG = 2-phosphoglycerate, PEP = phosphoenolpyruvate.

shuttling NADH produced in glycolysis into the mitochondrial electron transport system. Therefore, the only option to continue glycolysis is to regenerate NAD$^+$ from NADH by reducing pyruvate to lactate in the lactate dehydrogenase reaction. But lactate is not the sole product of RBC glycolysis. Methemoglobin reductase uses some of the NADH produced by glycolysis to reduce methemoglobin (Fe$^{3+}$) back to active hemoglobin (Fe$^{2+}$) capable of binding oxygen for transport to the tissues. Thus, the final products are a mixture of lactate and pyruvate with lactate being the primary product.

In tissues other than the RBC, pyruvate has alternative metabolic fates that, depending on the tissue, include gluconeogenesis, conversion to acetyl-CoA by pyruvate dehydrogenase for further metabolism to $CO_2$ in the tricarboxylic acid (TCA) cycle, transamination to alanine or carboxylation to oxaloacetate by pyruvate carboxylase (Table 23-1). However, in the RBC, the restricted enzymatic endowment precludes all but the conversion to lactate. The pyruvate and lactate produced are end products of RBC glycolysis transported out of the RBC to the liver where they can undergo the alternative metabolic conversions described above.

How does compromise of pyruvate kinase activity lead to anemia? Pyruvate kinase lies at the end of the glycolytic pathway in RBCs followed only by lactate dehydrogenase. In any linked pathway where the product of one reaction is the substrate for the next reaction a compromise in one reaction affects the entire pathway. The RBC depends exclusively on glycolysis to produce ATP to discharge all energy-requiring tasks. Pyruvate kinase activity is critical for the pathway and therefore critical for energy production. If ATP is not produced in amounts sufficient to meet the energy demand, then those functions are compromised. Energy is required to maintain the $Na^+/K^+$ balance within the RBC and to maintain the flexible discoid shape of the cell. In the absence of sufficient pyruvate kinase activity and therefore ATP, the ionic balance fails, and the membrane becomes misshapen. Cells reflecting pyruvate kinase insufficiency rather than a change

| Table 23-1 • METABOLIC FATE OF PYRUVATE | | |
|---|---|---|
| **Reaction** | **Enzyme** | **Product** |
| Transamination | Alanine Transaminase | $NH_3^+$<br>$\mid$<br>$CH_3 - CH - COO^-$<br>Alanine |
| Carboxylation | Pyruvate Carboxylase | $O$<br>$\parallel$<br>$^-OOC - C - CH_2 - COO^-$<br>Oxalocetate |
| Decarboxylation | Pyruvate Dehydrogenase | $O$<br>$\parallel$<br>$CH_3 - C - SCoA$<br>Acetyl-CoA |
| Gluconcogencsis | Many | $CH_2\text{-}OH$<br>Glucose |
| Reduction | Lactate Dehydrogenase | $OH$<br>$\mid$<br>$CH_3 - CH - COO^-$<br>Lactate |

in membrane composition are removed from the circulation by the macrophages of the spleen. This results in an increased number of circulating reticulocytes and possibly bone marrow hyperplasia, which is a biologic response to lowered RBC count as a result of hemolysis of erythrocytes.

## COMPREHENSION QUESTIONS

23.1  A young man with normocytic anemia, jaundice, and splenomegaly was diagnosed as having RBC pyruvate kinase deficiency after a peripheral blood smear showed spiculated cells. Because pyruvate kinase is abnormal in this patient, not only is less pyruvate made, but intermediates above pyruvate in the glycolytic pathway also build up, slowing the pathway. Which of the following products may not be made in the appropriate amounts in the RBC because of the deficiency of pyruvate?

A.  Glucose

B.  Oxaloacetate

C.  Acetyl-CoA

D.  Lactate

23.2  In the RBCs of the patient described above, which of the following would be expected?

A.  ADP to ATP ratios would be elevated above normal.

B.  $NADP^+$ would increase relative to NADPH.

C.  Ribulose 5-phosphate levels would decrease.

D.  NADH to $NAD^+$ ratios would decrease.

E.  Methemoglobin levels would increase.

23.3  The glycolytic pathway is a multistep process by which glucose is broken down to a 3-carbon metabolite. Some of the steps are listed below:

1.  Conversion of 3-phosphoglycerate to 2-phosphoglycerate

2.  Conversion of phosphoenolpyruvate to pyruvate

3.  Conversion of glyceraldehyde 3-phosphate to 1,3-bisphosphoglycerate

4.  Conversion of glucose to glucose 6-phosphate

5.  Conversion of fructose 6-phosphate to fructose 1,6-bisphosphate

Which of the following is the correct order of these conversions?

A.  $4 \rightarrow 5 \rightarrow 1 \rightarrow 2 \rightarrow 3$

B.  $4 \rightarrow 3 \rightarrow 1 \rightarrow 2 \rightarrow 5$

C.  $4 \rightarrow 5 \rightarrow 3 \rightarrow 1 \rightarrow 2$

D.  $4 \rightarrow 1 \rightarrow 3 \rightarrow 5 \rightarrow 2$

E.  $4 \rightarrow 5 \rightarrow 3 \rightarrow 2 \rightarrow 1$

# ANSWERS

23.1   **D.** The RBC has no mitochondria so glucose cannot be made from pyruvate or acetyl-CoA or oxaloacetate. The RBC does have lactate dehydrogenase and conversion to lactate depends on pyruvate levels.

23.2   **A.** In the RBC a deficiency of pyruvate kinase would tend to shunt glucose toward the hexose monophosphate pathway increasing ribulose 5-P levels, and the ratio of $NADP^+$ to NADPH would decrease. NADH to $NAD^+$ ratios would increase as a result of lower pyruvate levels making more NADH available to reduce methemoglobin and regenerate $NAD^+$. Because pyruvate kinase is deficient, the last ATP formation site is compromised, and so is the formation of ATP in the RBC, elevating the ADP to ATP ratio.

23.3   **C.** Glucose to glucose 6-phosphate → fructose 6-phosphate → fructose 1,6-bisphosphate → glyceraldehyde 3-phosphate → 1,3-bisphosphoglycerate → 3-phosphoglycerate → 2-phosphoglycerate → phosphoenolphosphate → pyruvate.

## BIOCHEMISTRY PEARLS

▶ The enzyme endowment present at maturation of the RBC cannot be replaced, and only the glycolytic pathway (Embden-Meyerhof pathway) is available for energy production in the RBC.

▶ Glucose metabolism is required in the RBC to maintain the ionic milieu within the cell, the vast majority via conversion to lactate.

▶ The vast majority of RBC enzyme deficiencies involves either altered protein or decreased protein levels of pyruvate kinase.

▶ Insufficient pyruvate kinase activity compromises erythrocyte ATP production, leading to ionic imbalance and misshaped cell membranes. These cells are removed from the circulation by the macrophages of the spleen.

▶ Pyruvate kinase catalyzes 1 of the 3 irreversible steps in the glycolytic pathway, the others being the phosphorylation of glucose to glucose 6-phosphate and the phosphorylation of fructose 6-phosphate to fructose 2,6-bisphosphate.

# REFERENCE

Longo D, Fauci AS, Kaspar D, et al, eds. *Harrison's Principles of Internal Medicine*. 18th ed. New York: McGraw-Hill; 2011.

A 3-year-old boy is brought to the emergency department after several episodes of vomiting and lethargy. His pediatrician has been concerned about his failure to thrive and possible hepatic failure, along with recurrent episodes of the vomiting and lethargy. After a careful history is taken, you observe that these episodes occur after ingestion of certain types of food, especially those high in fructose. His blood sugar was checked in the emergency department and was extremely low.

▶ What is the most likely diagnosis?
▶ What is the biochemical basis for the clinical symptoms?
▶ What is the treatment of the disorder?

# ANSWERS TO CASE 24:
## Fructose Intolerance

*Summary:* A 3-year-old boy with failure to thrive and possible hepatic failure. He presents with hypoglycemia and recurrent episodes of nausea and vomiting after ingestion of foods high in fructose.

- **Diagnosis:** Fructose intolerance.

- **Biochemical basis of disorder:** Because of a genetic disorder, the hepatic aldolase B enzyme is defective, normally functioning in glycolysis but not in fructose metabolism. Glucose production is inhibited by elevated fructose 1-phosphate. When fructose is ingested, severe hypoglycemia results.

- **Treatment:** Avoid dietary fructose.

## CLINICAL CORRELATION

Individuals with a deficiency in aldolase B have the condition known as fructose intolerance. As with most enzyme deficiencies, this is an autosomal recessive disease; it does not cause difficulty as long as the patient does not consume any foods with fructose or sucrose. Frequently, children with fructose intolerance avoid candy and fruit—behavior that should cause concern. Likewise, they usually do not have many dental caries. However, if chronically exposed to fructose-containing foods, infants and small children may have poor weight gain and abdominal cramping or vomiting.

# APPROACH TO:
## Disaccharide Metabolism

### OBJECTIVES

1. Describe the metabolism of disaccharides, specifically fructose.

2. Explain the role of aldolase B in fructose metabolism.

### DEFINITIONS

**DISACCHARIDE:** Two sugar molecules (monosaccharides) linked together by a glycosidic bond. The major disaccharides obtained in the diet are maltose [4-(α-d-glucosido)-d-glucose], sucrose [β-d-fructofuranosyl-α-d-glucopyranoside], and lactose [4-(β-d-galactosido)-d-glucose].

**ESSENTIAL FRUCTOSURIA:** A rare, benign genetic condition in which fructose spills over to the urine because the liver, kidney, and intestine lack the enzyme fructokinase.

**FRUCTOKINASE:** An enzyme present in the liver, kidney, and intestine that will phosphorylate fructose to fructose 1-phosphate at the expense of adenosine triphosphate (ATP).

**FRUCTOSE INTOLERANCE:** A genetic deficiency in the liver enzyme aldolase B. The absence of this enzyme leads to a build up of fructose 1-phosphate and depletion of liver ATP and phosphate stores.

**GLUT 5:** A facilitative glucose transporter isoform present in the small intestine and other tissues that will transport fructose (and glucose to a lesser extent) across the plasma membrane.

**β-GLYCOSIDASE:** A bifunctional, membrane-bound enzyme located on the brush-border membrane of the small intestine. This single polypeptide enzyme has 2 activities, lactase and glucosylceramidase, located in different domains of the protein. It will hydrolyze lactose to glucose and galactose.

**SGLT1:** A sodium-dependent glucose transporter located on the luminal side of the intestinal epithelial cells. It will transport glucose and galactose across the intestinal cell using a sodium ion gradient.

**SGLT2:** A sodium-dependent glucose transporter that has a high specificity for glucose and is specific to the kidney.

**SUCRASE-ISOMALTASE COMPLEX:** An enzyme complex comprised of 2 enzyme units. Both units have high α-1,4-glucosidase activity and will hydrolyze maltose and maltotriose to glucose. The sucrase unit will also hydrolyze sucrose to fructose and glucose, whereas the isomaltase unit will hydrolyze α-1,6 bonds found in isomaltose and the limit dextrins of starch.

## DISCUSSION

The **major disaccharides** obtained in the diet are **maltose, sucrose, and lactose. Maltose** is primarily obtained from the consumption of the **plant storage polysaccharide starch.** Starch is degraded to glucose and small-branched oligosaccharides called limit dextrins by exhaustive digestion by α-amylase. The limit dextrins are further enzymatically hydrolyzed to a branched tetrasaccharide by glucoamylase and to maltotriose and maltose and ultimately to glucose by the sucrase-isomaltase complex. Both of these enzyme complexes are located on the **brush-border membrane of the small intestine. Sucrose,** or table sugar, is hydrolyzed to **glucose and fructose by the sucrase** subunit of the sucrase-isomaltase complex. **Lactose,** or milk sugar, is enzymatically converted to **glucose and galactose by β-glycosidase,** also located on the brush-border membrane of the small intestine. This membrane-bound enzyme is a single polypeptide that has lactase and glucosylceramidase activities located in different domains of the protein.

   **Glucose and galactose** are absorbed from the lumen of the intestine by the **sodium-dependent glucose transporter (SGLT1),** which is located on the luminal side of the intestinal epithelial cells. **Fructose** absorption is not dependent on a sodium gradient. It is transported into the intestinal cell by **facilitative diffusion** by a glucose transporter isoform, **GLUT 5.** Fructose transport is less rapid than glucose transport, and GLUT 5 does not have a high capacity. Thus, in most individuals, ingestion of fructose in amounts higher than 0.5 to 1.0 g/kg body weight can result in malabsorption. Fructose enters the bloodstream, along with glucose and galactose, via the **GLUT 2 transporter.** Fructose is taken up by the liver by the same GLUT 2 transporter, along with glucose and galactose. There is a large gradient between the extracellular and intracellular concentrations of fructose in the liver cells, indicating that the rate for fructose uptake by the hepatocyte is low.

In the liver, kidney, and intestine, **fructose** can be converted to glycolytic/gluconeogenic intermediates by the actions of 3 enzymes—**fructokinase, aldolase B, and triokinase** (also called triose kinase)—as shown in Figure 24-1. In these tissues, fructose is rapidly phosphorylated to fructose 1-phosphate (F1P) by fructokinase at the expense of a molecule of ATP. This has the effect of trapping fructose inside the cell. A deficiency in this enzyme leads to the rare but benign condition known as *essential fructosuria*. In other tissues such as muscle, adipose, and red blood cells, hexokinase can phosphorylate fructose to the glycolytic intermediate fructose 6-phosphate (F6P).

**F1P** is further metabolized to dihydroxyacetone phosphate (DHAP) and glyceraldehyde by the hepatic isoform of the enzyme aldolase, which catalyzes a reversible aldol condensation reaction. **Aldolase** is present in 3 different isoforms. Aldolase A is present in greatest concentrations in the **skeletal muscle,** whereas the B isoform predominates in the liver, kidney, and intestine. Aldolase C is the brain isoform. Aldolase B has similar activity for either fructose 1,6-bisphosphate (F16BP) or F1P; however, the A or C isoforms are only slightly active when F1P is the substrate.

**Glyceraldehyde** may be converted to the glycolytic intermediate, **glyceraldehyde 3-phosphate (GAP),** by the action of the enzyme triokinase. This enzyme phosphorylates glyceraldehyde at the expense of another molecule of ATP. The GAP can then enter into the glycolytic pathway and be further converted to pyruvate, or recombine with DHAP to form F16BP by the action of aldolase.

A **deficiency in aldolase B** leads to the condition known as **fructose intolerance.** This inherited condition is benign as long as the patient does not consume any foods with fructose or sucrose. Patients with this condition usually develop an aversion to sweets early in life and as a result frequently are without any caries. However, infants and small children if chronically exposed to fructose-containing foods usually exhibit periods of vomiting and poor feeding as well as failure to thrive. A defect in the aldolase B gene results in a decrease in activity that is 15 percent or less than that of normal controls. This results in a buildup of F1P levels in the hepatocyte.

**Figure 24-1.** The metabolic pathway for the entrance of fructose into the glycolytic pathway. Fructokinase rapidly converts fructose to fructose 1-phosphate, which in the liver is cleaved by aldolase B to dihydroxyacetone phosphate (DHAP) and glyceraldehyde.

**Figure 24-2.** The inhibition of AMP deaminase by inorganic phosphate ($P_i$). A decrease in $[P_i]$ increases the activity of AMP deaminase and leads to increased production of uric acid.

Because the maximal rate of fructose phosphorylation by fructokinase is so high (almost 1 order of magnitude greater than that of glucokinase), intracellular levels of both ATP and inorganic phosphate ($P_i$) are significantly decreased. The drop in ATP concentration adversely affects a number of cellular events, including detoxification of ammonia, formation of cyclic AMP (cAMP), and RNA and protein synthesis. The decrease in intracellular concentrations of $P_i$ leads to a hyperuricemic condition as a result of an increase in uric acid formation. AMP deaminase is inhibited by normal cellular concentrations of $P_i$. When these levels drop, the inhibition is released and AMP is converted to IMP and, ultimately, uric acid (Figure 24-2).

The toxic effects of F1P can also be exhibited in patients that do not have a deficiency in aldolase B if they are parenterally fed with solutions containing fructose. Parenteral feeding with solutions containing fructose can result in blood fructose concentrations that are several times higher than can be achieved with an oral load. Because the rate of entry into the hepatocyte is dependent on the fructose gradient across the cell, intravenous loading results in increased entry into the liver and increased formation of F1P. Because the rate of formation of F1P is much faster than its further metabolism, this can lead to hyperuricemia and hyperuricosuria by the mechanisms described above.

## COMPREHENSION QUESTIONS

24.1  A 22-year-old soldier collapses from dehydration during maneuvers in the desert and is sent to a military hospital. Prior to enlisting, a physician observed a high level of glucose in his urine during an examination. At first, he was not allowed to enlist because he was suspected of having diabetes. However, further tests determined that his insulin level was normal. A glucose tolerance test exhibited a normal pattern. Laboratory tests following his dehydration episode repeat the previous findings, but further testing of the urine reveals that only d-glucose is elevated. Other sugars were not elevated. This patient's elevated urinary glucose and his dehydration episode are caused by a deficiency in which of the following?

A. GLUT 2

B. GLUT 4

C. Insulin receptor

D. SGLT1

E. SGLT2

24.2 Your patient is a 7-month-old baby girl, the second child born to unrelated parents. She did not respond well to breast-feeding and was changed entirely to a formula based on cow's milk at 4 weeks. Between 7 and 12 weeks of age, she was admitted to the hospital twice with a history of screaming after feeding, but was discharged after observation without a specific diagnosis. Elimination of cow's milk from her diet did not relieve her symptoms; her mother reported that the screaming bouts were worse after the child drank juice and that she frequently had gas and a distended abdomen. Analysis of a liver needle biopsy did not reveal any liver enzyme deficiencies. Overall, the girl is thriving (weight > 97th percentile) with no abnormal findings on physical examination.

24.3 If biopsy of intestinal tissue were obtained from your patient and analyzed, which of the following would most likely be deficient or defective?

A. GLUT 2

B. GLUT 5

C. Isomaltase

D. Lactase

E. SGLT1

24.4 A 24-year-old African-American woman presents with complaints of intestinal bloating, gas, cramps, and diarrhea following a meal including dairy products. A lactose-tolerance test confirms your suspicion that she had a deficiency of lactase in her intestine. Which of the following dairy products could you recommend that would be least likely to cause her difficulties in the future?

A. Condensed milk

B. Cottage cheese

C. Ice cream

D. Skim milk

E. Yogurt

## ANSWERS

24.1 **E.** The patient has normal levels of blood insulin and exhibits a normal glucose tolerance test. This indicates that glucose absorption from the intestine is normal as is clearance of glucose from the blood. The presence of glucose in the urine is most likely a kidney problem. Because the defect seems to involve only D-glucose and no other sugar, this points to a transporter with high specificity. The kidney has the GLUT 2, SGLT1, and SGLT2 transporters. GLUT 2 and SGLT1 are present in other tissues, and a defect in these would be expected to result in more serious sequelae. SGLT2 is a sodium-dependent glucose transporter specific to the kidney that has a high specificity for glucose. The glucose is present in the urine because of a failure to reabsorb it as a consequence of a defect in SGLT2. This also leads to a loss of water because it is reabsorbed with glucose.

24.2  **B.** Because the patient's liver enzymes are normal and her symptoms seem to correlate with her intake of fruit juices, most likely her problem stems from an inability to absorb fructose. Since removal of cow's milk from her diet did not eliminate the problem, a lactase deficiency can be ruled out. GLUT 5 is the primary transporter of fructose in the intestine and a deficiency in this transporter would lead to an inability to absorb fructose in the gut, making it a substrate for bacterial metabolism that produces various gases, including hydrogen, as well as organic acids.

24.3  **E.** The microorganisms that convert milk to yogurt (*Streptococcus salivarius thermophilus* and *Lactobacillus delbrueckii bulgaricus*) metabolize most of the lactose in the milk, thus removing the source of this patient's intestinal disquietude. Yogurt is also a good source of dietary calcium.

## BIOCHEMISTRY PEARLS

▶ The major disaccharides obtained in the diet are maltose, sucrose, and lactose.

▶ Sucrose, or table sugar, is hydrolyzed to glucose and fructose.

▶ Lactose, or milk sugar, is enzymatically converted to glucose and galactose by β-glycosidase, also located on the brush-border membrane of the small intestine.

▶ A deficiency in aldolase B leads to the condition known as fructose intolerance.

## REFERENCES

Gitzelmann R, Steinmann B, Van den Berghe G. Disorders of fructose metabolism. In: Ludueña RF. *Learning Biochemistry: 100 Case-Oriented Problems.* New York: Wiley-Liss; 1995.

Scriver CR, Beaudet AL, Sly WS, et al., eds. *The Metabolic and Molecular Bases of Inherited Disease.* 7th ed. New York: McGraw-Hill; 1995.

Semenza G, Auricchio S. Small-intestinal disaccharidases. In: Scriver CR, Beaudet AL, Sly WS, et al., eds. *The Metabolic and Molecular Bases of Inherited Disease.* 7th ed. New York: McGraw-Hill; 1995.

A 38-year-old woman presents to the clinic with complaints of alternating diarrhea and constipation. She reports some abdominal discomfort and bloating that are relieved with her bowel movement. She states that her episodes are worse in times of stress. She denies any blood in her diarrhea. She denies any weight loss or anorexia. Her physical examination is all within normal limits. She has been prescribed a cellulose-containing dietary supplement, which her doctor says will increase the bulk of her stools.

▶ What is the most likely diagnosis?
▶ What is the biochemical mechanism of the effect of the dietary supplement on the intestines?

# ANSWERS TO CASE 25:
## Irritable Bowel Syndrome

*Summary:* A 38-year-old woman complains of alternating constipation and diarrhea associated with times of stress and abdominal cramping and bloating relieved with bowel movements. She is prescribed a cellulose dietary supplement.

- **Diagnosis:** Irritable bowel syndrome.

- **Biochemical mechanism:** Cellulose-containing foods are not digestible but swell up by absorbing water and correlate with larger softer stools. The increase in dietary fiber also increases the intestinal transit time and decreases the intracolic pressure, thereby decreasing the symptoms of irritable bowel.

## CLINICAL CORRELATION

Irritable bowel syndrome affects many individuals in Western countries, and it manifests as abdominal cramping and bloating in the absence of disease. It is thought to be caused by increased spasms of the intestines. Constipation with or without episodes of diarrhea may be seen. Weight loss, fever, vomiting, bloody stools, or anemia would be worrisome and should not be attributed to irritable bowel syndrome. Typically, affected patients are anxious and may be under stress. After ruling out other disease processes, a trial of fiber-containing foods, stress reduction, and avoidance of aggravating foods are effective therapies. Patients should be advised to avoid the use of laxatives. Rarely, antispasmodic or antiperistaltic agents can be used. Notably, increased fiber in the diet may also decrease the absorption of fats and may lower the risk of colon cancer.

# APPROACH TO:
## Indigestible Polysaccharides

### OBJECTIVES

1. Know about the indigestible polysaccharides.

2. Be aware of β-1,4 cellulose bonds.

3. Know about the major types of fiber.

### DEFINITIONS

**CELLULOSE:** A polysaccharide composed of β-D-glucopyranose units joined by a β(1→4) glycosidic bond, which is not hydrolyzed by enzymes in the digestive tracts of humans.

**GUMS:** Complex polysaccharides composed of arabinose, fucose, galactose, mannose, rhamnose, and xylose. Gums are soluble in water and, because of their muciaginous nature, slowly digestible.

**HEMICELLULOSE:** Polysaccharides with a random, amorphous structure that are components of plant cell walls. Unrelated to cellulose structurally, they are composed of a variety of monosaccharides, including some acidic sugars, with xylose being the most prevalent.

**INSOLUBLE FIBERS:** Components of plant cell walls that are insoluble in water and not broken down by the digestive enzymes of the body.

**LIGNINS:** Aromatic polymers formed by the irreversible dehydration of sugars. Because of their structure, they cannot be broken down by the digestive enzymes and make up part of the stool bulk.

**MUCILAGINOUS:** Having a characteristic that is like the viscous and sticky nature of glue.

**PECTINS:** One of the soluble fibers in the diet composed primarily of polymers of galacturonic acid with varying amounts of other hexose and pentose residues.

**SOLUBLE FIBERS:** Mucilaginous fibers such as pectin and true plant gums that are soluble in water and digestible by the enzymes of the intestinal tract. By absorbing water and forming viscous gels, they decrease the rate of gastric emptying.

## DISCUSSION

Simply stated, dietary fiber is that part of food that remains intact and not absorbed following the digestive process in humans. It consists of all of the components of the cell walls of plants that are not broken down by the body's digestive enzymes. Dietary fiber can be grouped into 2 main categories, those that are soluble and those that are insoluble in water. The soluble fibers include pectins, gums, some hemicelluloses, and storage polysaccharides (starch and glycogen). The insoluble fibers include cellulose, most hemicelluloses, and lignins.

Cellulose is a major structural component of plant cell walls. Cellulose is a long, linear polymer of glucose ($\beta$-D-glucopyranose) units that are joined by $\beta(1{\rightarrow}4)$ glycosidic bonds (Figure 25-1a). Cellulose molecules have an extended, rigid structure

**Figure 25-1a.** The molecular structure of cellulose, indicating the repeating disaccharide unit, cellobiose.

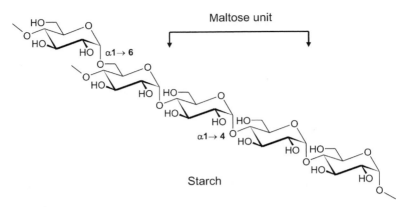

**Figure 25-1b.** The molecular structure of starch, indicating the repeating disaccharide unit, maltose, as well as the α-1,6-glycosidic bond present in the branch points of amylopectin.

that is stabilized by interchain hydrogen bonds. Starch, the plant storage polysaccharide, which is also a polymer of glucose, differs in its structure in that the glucose monomer units are joined by α(1→4) glycosidic bonds (Figure 25-1b). Starch is composed of 2 types of polymers, amylose, which has a nonbranched helical structure, and amylopectin, which is branched with α(1→6) glycosidic bonds joining the branches to the main polymer chain. Although starch is easily digested by salivary and pancreatic amylase and the disaccharidases present on the brush border of intestinal mucosal cells, cellulose cannot be hydrolyzed. The β(1→4) glycosidic bonds of the cellulose chain cannot be cleaved by the amylases present in the digestive tract.

Hemicelluloses are also polysaccharides that are structural components of plant cell walls. However, unlike what their name implies, they are unrelated to cellulose. They are polymers made up of a variety of sugar monomers that include glucose, galactose, mannose, arabinose, and xylose, as well as acidic forms of these monosaccharides. Xylose is the monosaccharide that is most abundant. Hemicelluloses have a random, amorphous structure that is suitable for their location in the plant cell wall matrix. Depending on their molecular structure, hemicelluloses are partially digestible.

Lignins are formed by the irreversible dehydration of sugars that result in aromatic structures. The remaining alcohol or phenol OH groups can react with each other and with aldehyde and ketone groups to form polymers. An example of a lignin molecule in the early stage of condensation is shown in Figure 25-2. These polymers cannot be broken down by the digestive enzymes and, like cellulose and the indigestible portion of hemicelluloses, form the stool bulk.

The soluble fibers such as pectin and true plant gums are mucilaginous and are digestible. Pectins are predominantly polygalacturonic acids with varying amounts of other hexose or pentose residues. True plant gums are complex polysaccharides composed of primarily arabinose, fucose, galactose, mannose, rhamnose, and xylose. The gums are soluble in water and are digestible by the enzymes in the intestinal tract. Both pectins and gums are mucilaginous; they absorb water to form viscous gels in the stomach that decrease the rate of gastric emptying.

Lignin

**Figure 25-2.** A lignin molecule in an early stage of condensation. The aromatic rings are a result of irreversible dehydration of sugar residues.

Although cellulose and hemicellulose are insoluble, they absorb water to swell and increase the stool bulk. This results in larger, softer stools. It has been shown that diets plentiful in insoluble fiber also increase the transit time of food in the digestive tract and decrease intracolonic pressure. In addition to increasing stool bulk, lignins also bind organic molecules such as cholesterol and many potential carcinogens. The mucilaginous nature of the soluble fibers, pectins, and gums tends to decrease the rate at which carbohydrates are digested and absorbed, thus decreasing both the rise in blood glucose levels and the ensuing increase in insulin concentration.

## COMPREHENSION QUESTIONS

25.1 A patient with type 1 diabetes mellitus has fasting and postprandial blood glucose levels frequently above the normal range despite good compliance with his insulin therapy. He was referred to a dietician that specialized in diabetic patients. The patient was recommended to incorporate foods high in dietary fiber. Which of the following dietary fibers would be most helpful in maintaining a normal blood glucose level?

A. Cellulose

B. Hemicellulose

C. Lignins

D. Pectins

25.2  Some individuals complain of flatulence following a meal plentiful in beans, peas, soybeans, or other leguminous plants. All legumes contain the oligosaccharides raffinose and stachyose that contain glycosidic linkages that are poorly hydrolyzed by intestinal enzymes but are good sources of energy for intestinal bacteria that convert these sugars to $H_2$. Which of the following glycosidic bonds are contained in raffinose and stachyose and are not hydrolyzed by our intestinal enzymes but can be by intestinal flora?

A.  Galactose ($\alpha1\rightarrow6$) glucose

B.  Galactose ($\beta1\rightarrow4$) glucose

C.  Glucose ($\beta1\rightarrow2$) fructose

D.  Glucose ($\alpha1\rightarrow4$) glucose

E.  Glucose ($\beta1\rightarrow4$) glucose

25.3  Cellulose is the most abundant polysaccharide and is an important structural component of cell walls. Strict vegetarians consume a large amount of cellulose, but it is not a source of energy because it is indigestible by the human intestinal tract. Cellulose is indigestible because it contains which of the following glycosidic bonds?

A.  Galactose ($\beta1\rightarrow4$) glucose

B.  Galactose ($\beta1\rightarrow6$) galactose

C.  Glucose ($\alpha1\rightarrow4$) glucose

D.  Glucose ($\beta1\rightarrow2$) fructose

E.  Glucose ($\beta1\rightarrow4$) glucose

## ANSWERS

25.1  **D.** Pectins and gums are soluble dietary fibers that absorb water and form mucilaginous gels. In doing so, they delay gastric emptying and decrease the rates at which monosaccharides, such as glucose and fructose, and disaccharides are absorbed by the intestinal tract. By decreasing the rate of sugar absorption, postprandial spikes in blood glucose concentration are avoided.

25.2  **A.** Raffinose and stachyose are sucrose molecules that have 1 and 2 galactose residues in an $\alpha1\rightarrow6$ glycosidic linkage. These bonds are not hydrolyzed by intestinal enzymes, but can be broken down by intestinal bacteria to produce $CO_2$ and $H_2$. Although they contain the glucose ($\beta1\rightarrow2$) fructose link, sucrase can hydrolyze that bond. The galactose ($\beta1\rightarrow4$) glucose, glucose ($\alpha1\rightarrow4$) glucose, and glucose ($\beta1\rightarrow4$) glucose linkages are not found in these oligosaccharides.

25.3  **E.** Cellulose is a polymer of glucose in $\beta1,4$ glycosidic linkages. This bond is not hydrolyzed by intestinal enzymes or the flora of the human intestine. It makes up the bulk of the stool.

## BIOCHEMISTRY PEARLS

▶ Dietary fiber comprises those components that are not digestible, which can be grouped into 2 main categories, those that are soluble, and those that are insoluble in water.

▶ The soluble fibers include pectins, gums, some hemicelluloses, and storage polysaccharides (starch and glycogen). The insoluble fibers include cellulose, most hemicelluloses, and lignins.

▶ Cellulose is a long, linear polymer of glucose (β-d-glucopyranose) units that are joined by **β(1→4) glycosidic bonds, which cannot be broken by human enzymes**.

▶ Starch, the plant storage polysaccharide, which is also a polymer of glucose, differs in its structure in that the glucose monomer units are joined by α(1→4) glycosidic bonds.

## REFERENCES

Chaney SG. Principles of nutrition I: macronutrients. In: Devlin TM, ed. *Textbook of Biochemistry with Clinical Correlations*. 7th ed. New York: Wiley-Liss; 2010.

Mayes PA. Nutrition. In: Murray RK, Granner KK, Mayes PA, et al., eds. *Harper's Illustrated Biochemistry*. 26th ed. New York: Lange Medical Books/McGraw-Hill; 2003:656-657.

Pettit JL. Fiber. *Clin Rev*. 2002;12(9):71-75.

A 56-year-old man presents to your clinic for follow-up on his diabetes. He has had diabetes since the age of 12 years and has always required insulin for therapy. He reports feeling very tremulous and diaphoretic at 2 AM with the blood sugars in the range of 40 mg/dL, which is very low. However, he notes that his morning fasting blood sugar level is high without taking any carbohydrates. His physician describes the morning high sugars as a result of biochemical processes in response to the nighttime hypoglycemia.

► What are the biochemical processes that govern the response to the nighttime hypoglycemia?

## ANSWER TO CASE 26:
## Somogyi Effect

*Summary:* A 56-year-old man with a long history of insulin diabetes with evening hypoglycemia and fasting morning hyperglycemia.

- **Biochemical mechanism of hypoglycemia:** The low nighttime serum blood sugar stimulates the counter-regulatory hormones to try to raise the glucose level. These include epinephrine, glucagon, cortisol, and growth hormone, which affect the glucose level and raise it by the time morning comes around.

## CLINICAL CORRELATION

This individual has a classic manifestation of the Somogyi effect, which is fasting morning hyperglycemia in response to hypoglycemia in the early morning and late night hours. The danger is that if nighttime blood glucose levels are not measured, the physician may interpret the patient as having hyperglycemia and require even higher doses of insulin. This would be exactly the wrong treatment, because the hypoglycemia is leading to counter-regulatory hormone reaction, and a very low sugar level bound to the high level in the morning. The diagnosis is established by measuring a 2 am glucose level, and when confirmed, then the bedtime neutral protamine Hagedorn (NPH) insulin (intermediate to long-acting) must be decreased.

## APPROACH TO:
## Glucose and Counter-Regulatory Hormones

### OBJECTIVES

1. Describe the regulation of glycogen and glucose production.
2. Explain how insulin and epinephrine affect glucose levels.
3. Summarize the regulation of glucagons.
4. Describe diabetic ketoacidosis and its biochemical mechanism.

### DEFINITIONS

**EPINEPHRINE:** Adrenaline; a catecholamine hormone derived from the amino acids phenylalanine or tyrosine that is synthesized and secreted by the adrenal medulla in response to stress.

**GLUT 2:** Glucose transporter isoform 2; a transport protein located on the plasma membrane of liver, pancreas, intestine, and kidney that will allow glucose to cross the membrane depending on the concentration gradient. GLUT 2 is the transporter that enables export of glucose from the liver.

**KETOACIDOSIS:** An elevation of the ketone body concentration that decreases the pH of the arterial blood to a pathologic condition.

**KETOGENESIS:** The production of ketone bodies by the liver in response to increased β-oxidation with a decreased rate of the Krebs cycle as a result of shuttling $C_4$ acids from the mitochondrion for the synthesis of glucose via gluconeogenesis.

**KETONE BODIES:** Acetoacetate, β-hydroxybutyrate, and acetone. Acetoacetate and β-hydroxybutyrate are formed by liver enzymes that condense molecules of acetyl-CoA, thus regenerating CoA for continual use in β-oxidation of fatty acids. Acetone is a spontaneous decomposition product of acetoacetate. Ketone bodies are exported from the liver and can be used by some extrahepatic tissues for energy generation.

**OXIDATIVE PHOSPHORYLATION:** The process by which adenosine triphosphate (ATP) is synthesized from a hydrogen ion gradient across the mitochondrial inner membrane. The hydrogen ion gradient is formed by the action of protein complexes in the mitochondrial membrane that sequentially transfer electrons from the reduced cofactors nicotinamide adenine dinucleotide (NADH) and $FADH_2$ to molecular oxygen. Movement of hydrogen ions back into the mitochondrion via ATP synthase drives the synthesis of ATP.

**PROTEIN PHOSPHATASE 1:** An enzyme that will hydrolyze phosphate groups from target proteins such as glycogen synthase, phosphorylase, phosphorylase kinase, and the phosphorylated form of inhibitor 1. The phosphorylated inhibitor 1 is a substrate that binds well but is hydrolyzed slowly. While bound to protein phosphatase 1, the phosphorylated inhibitor 1 serves as an inhibitor of the enzyme.

## DISCUSSION

The **liver is a highly specialized organ** that plays a central role in whole body **glucose metabolism.** During periods of increased glucose availability, the liver increases uptake, storage, and utilization of glucose. By contrast, when exogenous glucose availability declines (eg, during an overnight fast), the liver increases glucose production, thereby helping to maintain blood glucose levels. The liver uses 2 mechanisms for **endogenous glucose production,** the mobilization of intracellular glycogen (glycogenolysis) and the **synthesis of glucose from noncarbohydrate precursors (gluconeogenesis;** Figure 26-1). These pathways converge at **glucose 6-phosphate.** The latter is hydrolyzed to free glucose by glucose-6-phosphatase, the enzyme unique to gluconeogenic tissues, such as the liver. Once generated, glucose passes down its concentration gradient (eg, from the cytosol of the liver cell to the blood during periods of decreased blood glucose levels), via glucose transporter isoform 2 (GLUT 2).

During periods of increased glucose availability (eg, postprandially), glucose in excess of the energetic demands of the organism is stored as **glycogen** (the storage form of glucose in mammals). Although found within the cytosol of virtually every cell, glycogen is primarily concentrated in muscle (cardiac and skeletal) and liver. The purpose of glycogen synthesis (glycogenesis) is to anticipate subsequent periods of decreased glucose availability (eg, overnight fast). During the latter period of time,

**Figure 26-1.** Schematic diagram showing events that will lead to the export of glucose from the liver cell during times of low blood glucose.

glycogen will be mobilized as a readily available source of glucose. In the case of muscle, glycogen is selfishly used as an energy source by the myocyte alone. By contrast, liver glycogen will be mobilized to help maintain blood glucose levels. The biochemical pathways of glycogenesis and glycogenolysis are illustrated in Figure 26-2.

As glycogenesis is the reciprocal pathway to glycogenolysis, gluconeogenesis is the reciprocal pathway to glycolysis. Glycolysis, the "lysis" of glucose to 2 pyruvate molecules, is a ubiquitous metabolic pathway, whereas gluconeogenesis occurs in only a select number of tissues, including the liver. During periods of increased

**Figure 26-2.** The biochemical pathways of the synthesis of glycogen (glycogenesis) and its breakdown to glucose 6-phosphate (glycogenolysis).

glucose availability, flux through the glycolytic pathway increases, thereby utilizing this readily available fuel source. By contrast, during periods of decreased glucose availability, rates of gluconeogenesis increase, in an attempt to maintain blood glucose levels. The sources of carbon for gluconeogenesis depend on the given metabolic situation (eg, exercise, starvation, diabetes mellitus), and include glycerol, amino acids, and lactate. Although the majority of fatty acid–derived carbon cannot be used for the net synthesis of glucose, fatty acid metabolism plays a central role in gluconeogenesis. Gluconeogenesis is an energetically demanding process, which is driven by the β-oxidation of fatty acids. When the rate of acetyl-CoA generation through fatty acid β-oxidation exceeds the rate of acetyl-CoA oxidation via the Krebs cycle and oxidative phosphorylation (ox phos), acetyl-CoA accumulates. This acetyl-CoA is shunted into the pathway of ketone body synthesis (ketogenesis), allowing continued β-oxidation of fatty acids and therefore maintenance of high rates of gluconeogenesis. The interplay between glycolysis, gluconeogenesis, β-oxidation, and ketogenesis is illustrated in Figure 26-3.

Flux of carbon through the pathways of hepatic glucose metabolism described above is strongly influenced by the hormones insulin, glucagon, and epinephrine. Insulin is secreted from the β-cells of pancreatic islets during periods of increased glucose availability. This peptide hormone helps to lower blood glucose back within the normal range by stimulating glycogenesis and glycolysis, and simultaneously inhibiting glycogenolysis and gluconeogenesis. The effects of insulin on hepatic glucose metabolism are mediated in large part by the enzyme protein phosphatase 1 (PP1). For a more detailed discussion of the mechanism by which PP1 affects glucose metabolism, see case 22.

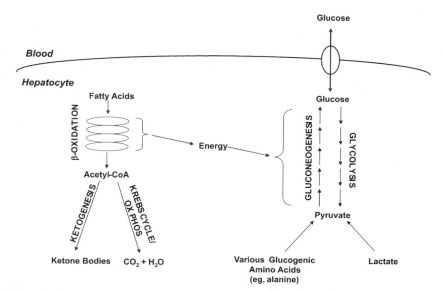

**Figure 26-3.** Schematic diagram of the interplay of fatty acid breakdown and ketone body formation with the synthesis (gluconeogenesis) and degradation of glucose (glycolysis). The β-oxidation of fatty acids provides the energy that drives the formation of glucose.

When blood glucose levels begin to decline (eg, during an overnight fast), so too does insulin secretion. By contrast, the secretion of glucagon from α-cells of pancreatic islets is stimulated. The latter targets primarily hepatic glucose metabolism, increasing glucose production (via gluconeogenesis and glycogenolysis), and decreasing glucose utilization. **Glucagon** acts in larger part by reversing the effects of insulin-mediated PP1 activation. On binding to its cell surface receptor, glucagon increases the activity of protein kinase A (PKA), which phosphorylates many of the proteins/enzymes that PP1 dephosphorylates. For a detailed discussion, of the mechanism by which PKA acts, see case 22.

Like glucagon, **epinephrine** secretion increases during periods of decreased glucose availability. Binding of epinephrine to β-adrenergic receptors on the surface of the hepatocyte results in activation of PKA, thereby increasing further hepatic glucose production through glycogenolysis and gluconeogenesis (Figure 26-4). Epinephrine is also able to bind to a second receptor on the surface of the hepatocyte, the β-adrenergic receptor, causing elevation of intracellular $Ca^{2+}$ levels. The latter allosterically activates a kinase called phosphorylase kinase, which, in turn, augments activation of glycogenolysis.

Abnormalities in the above described glucose homeostatic mechanisms arise during diabetes mellitus. Two major forms of diabetes mellitus exist, insulin-dependent (type 1) and insulin-independent (type 2) diabetes. Type 1 diabetes is caused by a severe lack or complete absence of insulin. Also known as early onset diabetes, this disease is often caused by an autoimmune destruction of pancreatic β-cells. Lack of insulin, in the face of elevated glucagon and epinephrine, leads to high rates of

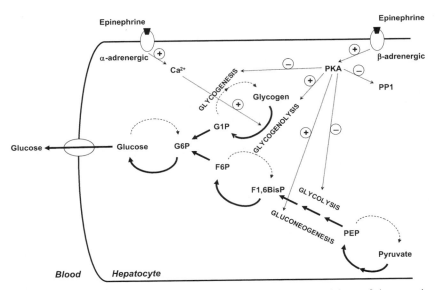

**Figure 26-4.** Schematic diagram showing how epinephrine leads to the breakdown of glycogen, the synthesis of glucose and export of glucose to the bloodstream. Epinephrine binds to both α- and β-adrenergic receptors on the plasma membrane of hepatocytes, leading to increased release of $Ca^{2+}$ and activation of adenylate cyclase and protein kinase A.

hepatic glucose output, being driven by β-oxidation of fatty acids. The latter results in an excessive production of ketone bodies and subsequent ketoacidosis. Treatment of type 1 diabetes involves regular monitoring of blood glucose levels and insulin administration as required. Insulin therapy associated with an evening meal will lower blood glucose levels. The latter triggers release of the counter-regulatory hormones glucagon and epinephrine, thereby stimulating hepatic glucose production. This inadvertently results in elevated glucose levels in the morning (the Somogyi effect). By contrast to type 1 diabetes, type 2 diabetes is caused by insulin resistance in the face of insulin sufficiency. Thus, the disease is characterized by both hyperglycemia and hyperinsulinemia. Ketoacidosis is a less common complication of type 2 diabetes.

## COMPREHENSION QUESTIONS

26.1 A 27-year-old man has been rushed to the emergency department following his sudden collapse and entry into a state of unconsciousness. Examination of personal belongings revealed the patient is an insulin-dependent diabetic. A rapid decline in which of the following humoral factors likely triggered the sudden collapse of the patient?

    A. Insulin

    B. Glucagon

    C. Fatty acids

    D. Glucose

    E. Triglyceride

26.2 Which of the following is the *least likely* to contribute to the hyperglycemia associated with uncontrolled type 1 diabetes?

    A. Decreased skeletal muscle glucose uptake

    B. Decreased adipose lipogenesis

    C. Increased adipose lipolysis

    D. Increased hepatic gluconeogenesis

    E. Increased skeletal muscle glycogenolysis

26.3 Which of the following changes in hepatic metabolism best explains the increased incidence of ketoacidosis observed in type 1 diabetes?

    A. Increased glucose uptake

    B. Increased protein synthesis

    C. Increased lipoprotein synthesis

    D. Increased β-oxidation

    E. Increased glycogen breakdown

## ANSWERS

26.1  **D.** Glucose is the primary source of energy for the central nervous system. A sudden decrease in circulating glucose levels will therefore impair ATP generation, in turn impeding cognitive function. If hypoglycemia persists, then the patient will slip into a coma and eventually die. This unfortunately common complication in people with type 1 diabetes is a consequence of oversupplementation with insulin. By contrast, a sudden decrease in circulating insulin, glucagon, fatty acids, or triglyceride would have little immediate effect on cognitive function.

26.2  **E.** Unlike the liver, skeletal muscle cannot export glucose into the circulation. Once glucose enters the myocyte, it is destined for use by that cell. Thus, intramyocellular glycogen is used as a fuel source by skeletal muscle and therefore cannot contribute to the hyperglycemia observed in uncontrolled type I diabetes. In contrast decreased insulin-mediated glucose utilization by skeletal muscle and adipose will contribute to hyperglycemia, as will decreased insulin-mediated suppression of hepatic glucose output. Decreased insulin-mediated suppression of lipolysis will indirectly contribute to hyperglycemia, by providing alterative, nonglucose fuels (fatty acids and ketone bodies) for organs such as skeletal muscle and the liver.

26.3  **D.** Decreased circulating insulin signals a need to increase hepatic glucose production. This is an energetically demanding process, driven by β-oxidation of fatty acids. However, acetyl-CoA, the major end product of β-oxidation, cannot be used for glucose production. Instead, acetyl-CoA is shunted into the pathway of ketone body synthesis (ketogenesis). By contrast, carbon from intrahepatic glycogen will contribute less to ketone body synthesis in uncontrolled type 1 diabetes mellitus. Net glucose uptake, protein synthesis, and lipoprotein synthesis are decreased, as opposed to increased, during uncontrolled type 1 diabetes.

## BIOCHEMISTRY PEARLS

▶ The liver uses 2 mechanisms for endogenous glucose production, the mobilization of intracellular glycogen (glycogenolysis) and the synthesis of glucose from noncarbohydrate precursors (gluconeogenesis).

▶ Flux of carbon through the pathways of hepatic glucose metabolism described above is strongly influenced by the hormones insulin, glucagon, and epinephrine.

▶ Lack of insulin, in the face of elevated glucagon and epinephrine, leads to high rates of hepatic glucose output, driven by β-oxidation of fatty acids. The latter results in an excessive production of ketone bodies and subsequent ketoacidosis.

# REFERENCES

Cohen P. Dissection of the protein phosphorylation cascades involved in insulin and growth factor action. *Biochem Soc Trans.* 1993;21:555.

Newsholme EA, Leech AR. *Biochemistry for the Medical Sciences.* New York: Wiley; 1983.

A 51-year-old man presents to the emergency department with chest pain. He states that he has had chest discomfort or pressure intermittently over the last year especially with increased activity. He describes the chest pain as a pressure behind his breastbone that spreads to the left side of his neck. Unlike previous episodes, he was lying down, watching television. The chest pain lasted approximately 15 minutes then subsided on its own. He also noticed that he was nauseated and sweating during the pain episode. He has no medical problems that he is aware of and has not been to a physician for several years. On examination, he is in no acute distress with normal vital signs. His lungs were clear to auscultation bilaterally, and his heart had a regular rate and rhythm with no murmurs. Electrocardiography (ECG) revealed ST segment elevation and peaked T waves in leads II, III, and aVF. Serum troponin I and T levels are elevated.

▶ What is the most likely diagnosis?
▶ What biochemical shuttle may be active to produce more adenosine triphosphate (ATP) per glucose molecule?

# ANSWERS TO CASE 27:
## Myocardial Infarction

*Summary:* A 51-year-old man with a history of chest pain with exertion presents with retrosternal chest pressure that radiates to the neck. He has nausea and diaphoresis while at rest. The patient has ST segment elevation and peaked T waves in the inferior ECG leads. The troponin I and T levels are elevated.

- **Likely diagnosis:** Acute myocardial infarction.

- **Biochemical shuttle:** The malate-aspartate shuttle is primarily seen in the heart, liver, and kidney. This shuttle requires cytosolic and mitochondrial forms of malate dehydrogenase and glutamate-oxaloacetate transaminase and 2 antiporters, the malate-α-ketoglutarate antiporter and the glutamate-aspartate antiporter, which are both localized in the mitochondrial inner membrane. In this shuttle cytosolic nicotinamide adenine dinucleotide (NADH) is oxidized to regenerate cytosolic $NAD^+$ by reducing oxaloacetate to malate by cytosolic malate dehydrogenase.

## CLINICAL CORRELATION

The most common cause of death of Americans is coronary heart disease. The patient's symptoms in this case are very typical of myocardial infarction, that is, chest pressure or chest pain, often radiating to the neck or to the left arm. The pain is usually described as deep and "squeezing chest pain." Cardiac muscle is perfused by coronary arteries with very little redundant or shared circulation; thus, occlusion of one coronary artery usually leads to ischemia or necrosis of the corresponding cardiac muscle. Laboratory confirmation of myocardial infarction (death of cardiac muscle) includes ECG showing elevation of the ST segment, an increase in cardiac enzymes, or both. When there is insufficient oxygen available for the cardiac muscle, then the glycolytic pathway must be used, which leads to a very small amount of ATP per glucose molecule. The malate-aspartate shuttle can offer 2 or 3 more times the ATP by oxidizing NADH to regenerate cytosolic $NAD^+$ by reducing oxaloacetate to malate by cytosolic malate dehydrogenase.

# APPROACH TO:
## Glycolysis and the Malate-Aspartate Shuttle

## OBJECTIVES

1. Be familiar with glycolysis.

2. Know the role of glycerol 3-phosphate and the malate-aspartate shuttle.

3. Be aware of the role of mitochondria in glycolysis.

## DEFINITIONS

**MYOCARDIAL INFARCTION:** An area of heart muscle is inadequately perfused as a result of cardiac vessel occlusion resulting in ischemia, cell death, and loss of cell constituents including enzymes into the circulation. Electrocardiographic changes occur as a result of damaged heart tissue.

**ANGINA:** Transient disruption of adequate blood flow to a portion of heart muscle leading to pain and a temporary shift to anaerobic glycolysis producing pyruvate and lactate that are released into the circulation.

**AEROBIC GLYCOLYSIS:** Metabolism of glucose to pyruvate. Pyruvate in the presence of sufficient oxygen can be metabolized to $CO_2$ via the tricarboxylic acid cycle in the mitochondrion-producing NADH and $FADH_2$, which contribute electrons through the electron transfer chain to molecular oxygen producing $H_2O$ and ATP.

**ANAEROBIC GLYCOLYSIS:** Metabolism of glucose to lactate in the absence of sufficient oxygen. When oxygen is lacking, pyruvate is converted to lactate, and no further oxidative pathway is available.

**ELECTRON SHUTTLES:** Enzymatic processes whereby electrons from NADH can be transferred across the mitochondrial barrier. The **glycerol 3-phosphate shuttle** uses the reduction of dihydroxyacetone phosphate to glycerol 3-phosphate and reoxidation to transfer electrons from cytosolic NADH to coenzyme Q in the electron transport chain. The **malate-aspartate shuttle** uses malate and aspartate in a 2-member transfer exchange to transfer electrons from cytosolic NADH to mitochondrial NADH (Figures 27-1 and 27-2).

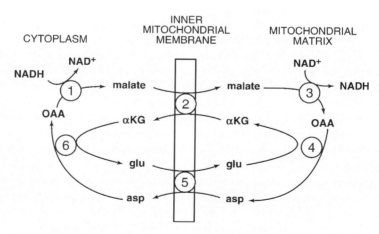

| | |
|---|---|
| 1 Malate dehydrogenase (cytosolic) | 4 Glutamate - OAA transaminase (mitochondrial matrix) |
| 2 Malate - KG antiporter (mitochondrial inner membrane) | 5 Glutamate - aspartate antiporter (mitochondrial inner membrane) |
| 3 Malate dehydrogenase (mitochondrial matrix) | 6 Glutamate - OAA transaminase (cytosolic) |

**Figure 27-1.** Malate-aspartate shuttle.

Figure 27-2. Glycerol 3-phosphate shuttle.

## DISCUSSION

**Myocardial infarction** arises when perfusion of cardiac muscle is inadequate, result-ing in insufficient oxygen delivery to that portion of cardiac muscle. This causes the affected muscle to rely on anaerobic metabolism for its energy supply with con-comitant production of lactic acid. Even transient ischemia can lead to changes in muscle tissue, but prolonged ischemia leads to breakdown of muscle cells and release of cellular proteins such as **creatine kinase, lactic acid dehydrogenase, and troponin I.** Reperfusion by thrombolytic treatment or mechanical means can restore oxygen levels and return the metabolic processes to aerobic metabolism. A second-ary consequence of reperfusion is reperfusion injury in which the highly reduced state of injured cells meets increased oxygen concentration and produces reactive oxygen radicals. Most notable of these is the hydroxyl radical ($OH^{\bullet}$), which attacks tissue components such as lipids and protein sulfhydryl groups. Myocardial infarc-tion causes changes in the pathways of energy generation triggered by oxygen insuf-ficiency in the affected heart muscle.

The **glycolytic pathway** for all cells under conditions of adequate tissue oxygen-ation is shown in Figure 27-3. **Two molecules of ATP** are required to initiate the pathway—one at the **hexokinase** step to phosphorylate glucose to glucose 6-phos-phate and a second to **phosphorylate fructose 6-phosphate to fructose 1,6-bispho-sphate.** Cleavage of fructose 1,6-bisphosphate by aldolase yields 2 triose phosphates, glyceraldehyde 3-phosphate, and dihydroxyacetone phosphate, which is isomerized to glyceraldehyde 3-phosphate by triose phosphate isomerase. The oxidation of the aldehyde group to the acid level through the reduction of $NAD^+$ to NADH with the concomitant binding of inorganic phosphate to produce 1,3-bisphosphoglyc-erate is catalyzed by 3-phosphoglyceraldehyde dehydrogenase. This step requires

**Figure 27-3.** Glycolytic pathway.
*From glyceraldehyde 3-phosphate onward, 2,3-carbon molecules/glucose proceed through the pathway requiring a total of 2NAD⁺ and 4ADP producing a total of 4ATP, 2NADH, and 2H₂O.

NAD⁺ regeneration to continue. Inorganic phosphate is present in tissues at such a high concentration (typically 25 mM) as not to be limiting. The first substrate level phosphorylation occurs next, wherein phosphoglycerate kinase catalyzes the transfer of the acyl phosphate group of 1,3-bisphosphoglycerate to adenosine diphosphate (ADP), yielding ATP and 3-phosphoglycerate. Phosphoglucomutase shifts the phosphate of 3-phosphoglycerate to carbon position 2 producing 2-phosphoglycerate. Enolase catalyzes the removal of the elements of water between carbon positions 2 and 3 to produce phosphoenolpyruvate. Pyruvate kinase then catalyzes the second substrate level phosphorylation of ADP to produce ATP and pyruvate, the end product of aerobic glycolysis. Because fructose 1,6-bisphosphate is cleaved to 2 triose phosphate moieties and each triose phosphate produces 2 ATP molecules, the total produced by substrate level phosphorylation is 4 ATP molecules. But 2 ATP molecules are consumed in the activation of hexose leaving 2 ATP molecules as the net gain from glycolytic substrate level phosphorylation.

As noted above, however, NAD⁺ must be regenerated from the NADH produced or the glycolytic cycle would cease. Under aerobic conditions regeneration of cytosolic NAD⁺ from cytosolic NADH is accomplished by transferring electrons across the mitochondrial membrane barrier to the electron transfer chain where the electrons are transferred to oxygen. There are **2 different shuttle mechanisms** whereby this transfer of electrons across the membrane to regenerate cytosolic

$NAD^+$ can be accomplished: the glycerol 3-phosphate shuttle and the malate-aspartate shuttle.

The **glycerol 3-phosphate shuttle** functions primarily in **skeletal muscle and brain** (Figure 27-2). The shuttle takes advantage of the fact that the enzyme glycerol-3-phosphate dehydrogenase exists in 2 forms, a cytosolic form that uses $NAD^+$ as cofactor and a mitochondrial FAD-linked form. Cytosolic glycerol-3-phosphate dehydrogenase uses electrons from cytosolic NADH to reduce the glycolytic intermediate dihydroxyacetone phosphate to glycerol 3-phosphate, thereby regenerating cytosolic $NAD^+$. The newly formed glycerol 3-phosphate is released from the cytosolic form of the enzyme and crosses to and is bound to the mitochondrial FAD-linked glycerol-3-phosphate dehydrogenase, which is bound to the cytosolic side of the mitochondrial inner membrane. There the mitochondrial glycerol-3-phosphate dehydrogenase reoxidizes glycerol 3-phosphate to dihydroxyacetone phosphate (preserving mass balance), reducing its FAD cofactor to $FADH_2$. Electrons are then passed to coenzyme Q of the electron transport chain and on to oxygen generating 2 additional ATP molecules per electron pair and therefore per glycerol 3-phosphate.

However, the **malate-aspartate shuttle** functions primarily in the **heart, liver, and kidney** (Figure 27-3). This shuttle requires cytosolic and mitochondrial forms of malate dehydrogenase and glutamate-oxaloacetate transaminase and 2 antiporters, the malate-$\alpha$-ketoglutarate antiporter and the glutamate-aspartate antiporter, which are both localized in the mitochondrial inner membrane. In this shuttle cytosolic NADH is oxidized to regenerate cytosolic $NAD^+$ by reducing oxaloacetate to malate by cytosolic malate dehydrogenase. Malate is transported into the mitochondrial matrix while $\alpha$-ketoglutarate is transported out by the malate-$\alpha$-ketoglutarate antiporter, seemingly a mass imbalance. Next malate is oxidized back to oxaloacetate producing NADH from $NAD^+$ in the mitochondrial matrix by mitochondrial malate dehydrogenase. Oxaloacetate cannot be transported per se across the mitochondrial membrane. It is instead transaminated to aspartate from the $NH_3$ donor glutamate by mitochondrial glutamate-oxaloacetate transaminase. Aspartate is transported out of the matrix whereas glutamate is transported in by the glutamate-aspartate antiporter in the mitochondrial membrane, obviating the apparent mass unbalance noted above. The last step of the shuttle is catalyzed by cytosolic glutamate-oxaloacetate transaminase regenerating cytosolic oxaloacetate from aspartate and cytosolic glutamate from $\alpha$-ketoglutarate both of which were earlier transported in opposing directions by the malate-$\alpha$-ketoglutarate antiporter. The net effect of this shuttle is to transport electrons from cytosolic NADH to mitochondrial $NAD^+$. Therefore, those electrons can be presented by the newly formed NADH to electron transport system complex I, thereby producing 3 ATP molecules by oxidative phosphorylation. Note that depending on which shuttle is used (ie, which tissue is catalyzing glycolysis) either 2 or 3 extra ATP molecules are produced by oxidative phosphorylation per triose phosphate going through the latter steps of glycolysis.

In nonaerobic glycolysis, as in the case when a tissue is subjected to an ischemic episode (ie, myocardial infarction), neither the extra ATP molecule produced by the shuttle nor the ATP molecules produced by normal passage of electrons through glucose    glucose-6-P    fructose-6-P    fructose-1,6-bisP

dihydroxyacetone-P

glyceraldehyde-3-P

lactate    pyruvate    P-enolpyruvate    2-P-glycerate    3-P-glycerate    1,3-bisP-glycerate

1  Hexokinase
2  Glucose-6-P isomerase
3  6-Phosphofructokinase
4  Fructose 1,6-bisphosphate aldolase
5  Triosephosphate isomerase

6  3-Phosphoglyceraldehyde dehydrogenase
7  Phosphoglycerate kinase
8  Phosphoglyceromutase
9  Enolase
10  Pyruvate kinase
11  Lactate dehydrogenase

**Figure 27-4.** Glycolytic pathway under conditions of insufficient oxygen.

the electron transport chain are produced because of oxygen insufficiency. There-fore, glycolysis must increase in rate to meet the energy demand. In damaged tissue this increased rate is compromised. Moreover, the shuttle mechanisms to regenerate $NAD^+$ from NADH formed by glycolysis are unavailable, as shown in Figure 27-4. Glycolysis under ischemic conditions satisfies the requirement for $NAD^+$ by reduc-ing pyruvate, the glycolytic end product under normative conditions, to lactate with the reducing equivalents of NADH.

The new end product lactate accumulates in muscle cells under ischemic condi-tions and damages cell walls with its low pH causing rupture and loss of cell contents such as myoglobin and troponin I. These compounds as well as other end products combine to cause increased cell rupture and pain.

Reopening vasculature by reperfusion as rapidly as possible is a first step in treat-ment. Thrombolysis within an hour after infarction gives best results. Supportive measures, regulation of heart rate and pressure are required following the infarction to allow recovery from the ischemic episode and repair of tissue damage. Nutritional monitoring is required both for tissue repair and prevention of recurrence.

## COMPREHENSION QUESTIONS

27.1 Following an episode of retrosternal chest pressure with radiation to the neck and associated nausea and diaphoresis while at rest, a middle-aged man was diagnosed with unstable angina and possibly myocardial infarction. Subsequent laboratory findings of increased serum levels of troponin I and cardiac enzymes were consistent with the diagnosis.

If the patient described above did indeed have angina, which of the following change(s) in metabolism in the affected area would occur?

A. Increased oxidative phosphorylation

B. Increased rate of fatty acid oxidation

C. Increased conversion of pyruvate to acetyl-CoA

D. Increased formation of lactate

E. Increased use of ketone bodies

27.2 In the case described in question 27.1, an ischemic episode very likely occurred. What changes in glucose metabolism would be observed?

A. The overall rate of glucose utilization would decrease.

B. Pyruvate kinase is allosterically inhibited.

C. The rate of ATP production in the cytosol increases.

D. NADH is reoxidized to $NAD^+$ via the glycerol 3-phosphate shuttle.

27.3 If the patient described in question 27.1 does indeed have angina, his is a focal lesion wherein only one portion of heart muscle is affected while other portions still receive adequate oxygen, enabling the malate-aspartate shuttle to function. Which of the following is involved in this shuttle to transfer electrons across the mitochondrial barrier?

A. Malate-aspartate antiporter

B. Malate-α-ketoglutarate antiporter

C. Glutamate-α-ketoglutarate antiporter

D. Aspartate-α-ketoglutarate symporter

E. Malate-glutamate symporter

## ANSWERS

27.1 **D.** In this case the problem is insufficient oxygen reaches an area of cardiac muscle. In the absence of sufficient oxygen, the use of the electron transfer chain to generate ATP from ADP is severely compromised, and therefore all products feeding into that chain accumulate reducing the formation of tricarboxylic acid products. Fatty acid oxidation, formation of acetyl-CoA from pyruvate oxidation of ketone bodies, and oxidative phosphorylation are all decreased. In glycolysis under reduced oxygen conditions, one pyruvate is converted to lactate to reoxidize NADH to $NAD^+$ to meet the requirement for glycolysis to continue. Therefore, there is increased formation of lactate.

27.2  **C.** The rates of both glucose utilization and ATP generation by glycolysis increase to compensate for the absence of sufficient ATP production from oxidative phosphorylation as a result of oxygen deprivation. Under these circumstances, ATP is used as rapidly as it is made so it is not present in sufficient concentration to inhibit pyruvate kinase. Furthermore, fructose 1,6-bisphosphate tends to stimulate pyruvate kinase activity.

27.3  **B.** The malate-α-ketoglutarate antiporter carries malate from the cytosol, where it is oxidized to oxaloacetate by mitochondrial malate dehydrogenase, forming NADH. In order for the malate-α-ketoglutarate antiporter to function, a molecule of α-ketoglutarate must be transported from the mitochondrial matrix to the cytosol. The only other transporter involved in this shuttle mechanism is the aspartate-glutamate antiporter. None of the other suggested transporters is required in this shuttle mechanism.

## BIOCHEMISTRY PEARLS

▶ Coronary heart disease is the most common cause of mortality in Americans.

▶ Myocardial infarction is suspected with typical chest pain, ECG findings of ST segment elevation, and increased cardiac enzymes.

▶ When oxygen is unavailable, the anaerobic glycolytic pathway is used.

▶ Two shuttles allow for more ATP to be generated under aerobic conditions: the glycerol 3-phosphate shuttle, which functions primarily in skeletal muscle and brain, and the malate-aspartate shuttle, primarily in the heart, liver, and kidney.

## REFERENCES

Devlin TM, ed. *Textbook of Biochemistry with Clinical Correlations*. 7th ed. New York: Wiley-Liss; 2010.

Longo D, Fauci AS, Kaspar D, et al, eds. *Harrison's Principles of Internal Medicine*. 18th ed. New York: McGraw-Hill; 2011.

A Jewish couple of Eastern European descent presents to the clinic for prenatal counseling after their only child died early in childhood. The family could not remember the name of the disorder but said it was common in their ancestry. Their first child was normal at birth, a slightly larger than normal head circumference, an abnormal "eye finding," and a severe progressive neurologic disease with decreased motor skills and eventually death. The results of the autopsy are consistent with Tay-Sachs disease.

▶ What type of inheritance is this disorder?
▶ What is the biochemical cause of the disorder?

# ANSWERS TO CASE 28:
## Tay-Sachs Disease

*Summary:* A Jewish couple of Eastern European descent presents for prenatal counseling after having a child die with a progressive neurologic disorder with loss of motor skills and abnormally large head and an abnormal eye examination. Autopsy shows Tay-Sachs disease.

- **Inheritance:** Autosomal recessive; 1:30 carrier rate in Ashkenazi Jews.

- **Molecular basis of disorder:** Lysosomal storage disorder with deficiency of hexosaminidase A enzyme resulting in $G_{M2}$ gangliosides accumulating throughout the body.

## CLINICAL CORRELATION

Tay-Sachs disease is a fatal genetic disorder where harmful amounts of lipids called ganglioside $G_{M2}$ accumulate in the nerve cells and brains of those affected. Infants with this disorder appear normal for the first several months of life, and then as the lipids distend the nerve cells and brain cells, progressive deterioration occurs; the child becomes blind, deaf, and eventually unable to swallow. Tay-Sachs disease mainly occurs in Jewish children of Eastern European descent, and death from bronchopneumonia usually occurs by 3 to 4 years of age. A reddish spot on the retina also develops, and symptoms first appear around 6 months of age. It is a lysosomal storage disorder with insufficient activity of the enzyme hexosaminidase A, which catalyzes the biodegradation of the gangliosides. The diagnosis is made by clinical suspicion and serum hexosaminidase level. Currently, no treatment is available for this disease.

# APPROACH TO:
## Lysosomal Storage

### OBJECTIVES

1. Describe the enzymatic defects that lead to the lysosomal storage disorders.

2. Describe the synthesis and degradation of sphingolipids.

### DEFINITIONS

**CERAMIDE:** A component of all sphingolipids that is composed of a long-chain fatty acyl group in an amide linkage to sphingosine.

**GANGLIOSIDE:** Complex carbohydrate-rich glycosphingolipids containing 3 or more monosaccharides esterified to ceramide with at least one of the sugars being N-acetylneuraminic acid (sialic acid). Gangliosides are membrane components found on nerve endings.

**GANGLIOSIDOSES:** The build-up of gangliosides in the lysosome as a result of the deficiency of one or more enzymes involved in the degradation of gangliosides.

**I-CELL DISEASE:** A disease in which there is a buildup of a number of different biomolecules that are normally degraded in the lysosome as a result of a deficiency in an enzyme that modifies lysosomal enzymes so that they are targeted to the lysosome.

**LYSOSOMAL STORAGE DISORDERS:** Genetic diseases that are a result of a deficiency of 1 or more enzymes present in the lysosome. This leads to a buildup of the biomolecules that are normally degraded in the lysosome.

**SPHINGOLIPID:** Any of a number of lipid molecules that contain sphingosine as part of its molecular structure. These include ceramide, sphingomyelin, cerebrosides, sulfatides, and gangliosides.

**TAY-SACHS DISEASE:** A genetic disease that is a result of a deficiency in hexosaminidase A (β-N-acetylhexosaminidase), an enzyme involved in the degradation of gangliosides in the lysosome. The disease is prevalent in Jewish children of Eastern European descent and leads to a buildup of ganglioside $G_{M2}$ in nerve cells of the brain and neuronal dysfunction.

## DISCUSSION

**Sphingolipids** are a class of **lipids** found in **biologic membranes** in which the **backbone of the lipid molecule is sphingosine, an 18-carbon amino alcohol.** This is in contrast to the glycerol backbone found in lipids such as phospholipids. The precursor molecules for the synthesis of sphingosine are palmitoyl-CoA and serine, which condense to form 3-dehydrosphinganine (3-ketodihydrosphingosine; Figure 28-1). This is followed by a reduction reaction using NADPH to form sphinganine (dihydrosphingosine). Ceramide is formed in a 2-step reaction by the formation of an amide bond between sphinganine and a long-chain fatty acid (usually behenic acid, a saturated C-22 fatty acid). This is followed by an oxidation reaction using FAD that introduces a transdouble bond into the sphinganine backbone.

Ceramide is a building block for all other sphingolipids. Figure 28-2 shows the synthesis of some of these sphingolipids from ceramide. The reaction of phosphatidyl choline and ceramide (via esterification) yields sphingomyelin, a phosphate-containing subclass of sphingolipids found in the nervous tissue of higher animals. The addition of 1 or more sugar residues to ceramide yields the glycosphingolipids. The glycosphingolipid cerebroside contains one residue of glucose or galactose.

**Gangliosides are complex carbohydrate-rich sphingolipids containing 3 or more sugar residues** esterified to ceramide with one of the sugars being sialic acid (N-acetylneuraminic acid). Gangliosides are synthesized by the stepwise addition of nucleoside-activated sugar residues to ceramide. Ganglioside nomenclature is a bit unusual. The ganglioside is represented by the letter G followed by a subscript letter and a number. The subscript letter indicates the number of sialic acid residues present in the molecule (M = 1, D = 2, T = 3), and the number is equal to 5 minus the number of neutral sugars. More than 60 gangliosides have been characterized, and the structure of one of these, ganglioside $G_{M1}$, is schematically represented in Figure 28-3. Glycosphingolipids function in cell–cell recognition and

$$\text{Palmitoyl CoA} + {}^-O - \overset{\overset{\displaystyle O}{\|}}{C} - \underset{\underset{\displaystyle NH_3^+}{|}}{CH} - CH_2 - OH$$

**Serine**

⤷ $CO_2 + CoA$

$$CH_3 - (CH_2)_{14} - \overset{\overset{\displaystyle O}{\|}}{C} - \underset{\underset{\displaystyle NH_3^+}{|}}{CH} - CH_2OH$$

**3-Dehydrosphinganine**

⤷ NADPH
⤷ $NADP^+$

$$CH_3 - (CH_2)_{14} - \overset{\overset{\displaystyle OH}{|}}{CH} - \underset{\underset{\displaystyle NH_3^+}{|}}{CH} - CH_2OH$$

**Sphinganine**

⤷ Acyl-CoA (Behenyl CoA)
⤷ CoA

$$CH_3 - (CH_2)_{14} - \overset{\overset{\displaystyle OH}{|}}{CH} - \underset{\underset{\displaystyle NH}{|}}{CH} - CH_2OH$$

$$R - \overset{\displaystyle C}{\underset{\displaystyle O}{\diagup}}$$

**Dihydroceramide**

⤷ FAD
⤷ $FADH_2$

Addition of various hydrophilic groups

$$CH_3 - (CH_2)_{12} - CH = CH - \overset{\overset{\displaystyle OH}{|}}{CH} - \underset{\underset{\displaystyle NH}{|}}{CH} - CH_2OH$$

$$R - \overset{\displaystyle C}{\underset{\displaystyle O}{\diagup}}$$

|⎣ Hydrophobic ⎦|⎣ Hydrophilic ⎦|

**Ceramide**

Figure 28-1. Biosynthesis of ceramide.

tissue immunity. Gangliosides are found at nerve endings and may be important in nerve impulse transmission.

Sphingolipids are constantly being turned over in the lysosomes of cells by specific hydrolytic enzymes that remove the sugars in a stepwise fashion. Defects in these enzymes can occur and result in disease states resulting from the accumulation of undegraded sphingolipids. Lysosomal storage diseases are a group of approximately 40 different diseases that occur in approximately 1 in 5000 live births. Many of these diseases are characterized by a deficiency in a specific lysosomal enzyme, but some

**Figure 28-2.** The formation of sphingomyelin and cerebrosides from ceramide.

diseases can be caused by the inability of enzymes to be translocated to the lysosome (I-cell disease), defective transport of small molecules out of the lysosome (cystinosis), or a deficiency in sphingolipid activator proteins, which are small molecular weight proteins that participate in the degradation of sphingolipids. The net result in all of these diseases is a lack of the ability of the cell to breakdown sphingolipids in the lysosome. The accumulation of these macromolecules or partial derivatives of these molecules in the lysosome results in the pathologic conditions associated with the lysosomal storage diseases known as sphingolipidoses.

Proteins destined for the lysosome must contain certain carbohydrate signals. In I-cell disease, the enzyme that catalyzes the addition of a mannose-6-phosphate moiety to the protein is defective. Without the addition of this mannose residue the proteins cannot be transported to the lysosome.

Tay-Sachs disease results from a deficiency in the **enzyme hexosaminidase A** ($\beta$-N-acetylhexosaminidase). The human gene for this enzyme is found at **chromosome position 15q23-q24.** The deficiency in hexosaminidase A leads to the accumulation of ganglioside $G_{M2}$ in the nerve cells of the brain. Hexosaminidase A removes a terminal N-acetylgalactosamine residue from ganglioside $G_{M2}$ to form ganglioside $G_{M3}$ (Figure 28-4). The inability of patients with Tay-Sachs disease to remove these sugar residues results in the accumulation of gangliosides in the lysosome. This results in swelling of the neurons containing these lipid-filled lysosomes and the disruption of neuronal function.

Other lysosomal storage disorders include $G_{M1}$ gangliosidoses, $G_{M2}$ gangliosidoses, Gaucher disease, Niemann-Pick disease, Fabry disease, fucosidosis, Schindler disease, metachromatic leukodystrophy, Krabbe disease, multiple sulfatase deficiency, Farber disease, and Wolman disease. Table 28-1 illustrates the enzyme deficiencies found in some of these disorders.

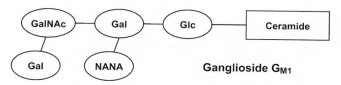

**Figure 28-3.** The schematic structure of ganglioside $G_{M1}$. The nomenclature is as follows: G stands for ganglioside; the subscript letter indicates the number of sialic acid residues; the numeral is equal to 5 minus the number of neutral sugars. Gal = galactose, GalNAc = N-acetylgalactosamine, Glc = glucose, NANA = N-acetylneuraminic acid (sialic acid).

**Figure 28-4.** The reaction catalyzed by hexosaminidase A, the enzyme deficient in patients with Tay-Sachs disease.

| Table 28-1 • LYSOSOMAL STORAGE DISORDERS | | |
|---|---|---|
| **DISEASE** | **DEFICIENT ENZYME** | **CONSEQUENCE** |
| Tay-Sachs disease | β-N-acetylhexosaminidase | Increased ganglioside $G_{M2}$ |
| Gaucher disease | β-Glucosidase | Increased glucocerebrosides |
| Fabry disease | α-Galactosidase A | Accumulation of glycosphingolipids with α-Galactosyl moieties |
| Farber disease | Ceramidase | Increased ceramide |
| Niemann-Pick disease | Sphingomyelinase | Accumulation of sphingomyelin |
| I-cell disease | N-Acetylglucosaminyl-1-phosphotransferase | Incorrect packaging of lysosomal enzymes impairing lysosome function |

# COMPREHENSION QUESTIONS

28.1 A couple is seen in your office for genetic counseling regarding Tay-Sachs disease. They are very knowledgeable and request more information about the specific enzyme that is defective in this disease. You explain that Tay-Sachs results from the lack of an enzyme activity necessary for which of the following?

A. Removal of N-acetylgalactosamine from ganglioside $G_{M2}$

B. Addition of N-acetylgalactosamine to ganglioside $G_{M2}$

C. Removal of the disaccharide galactose-N-acetylgalactosamine from ganglioside $G_{M2}$

D. Addition of the disaccharide galactose-N-acetylgalactosamine to ganglioside $G_{M2}$

E. Removal of a galactose residue from ganglioside $G_{M2}$

28.2 Tay-Sachs disease involves the metabolism of gangliosides. Gangliosides are composed of a ceramide backbone with at least which one of the following?

A. Phosphorylated sugar residue

B. Glucose residue

C. Galactose residue

D. Sialic acid residue

E. Fructose residue

28.3 The genetic disease which results from a mutation in the gene coding for the enzyme hexosaminidase ($\beta$-N-acetylhexosaminidase) is called what?

A. Huntington disease

B. Lesch-Nyhan syndrome

C. Tay-Sachs disease

D. Amyotrophic lateral sclerosis

E. Neurofibromatosis

# ANSWERS

28.1 **A.** Tay-Sachs disease is the result of the lack of the enzyme $\beta$-N-acetylhexosaminidase. This enzyme hydrolyzes a terminal N-acetylgalactosamine from the ganglioside $G_{M2}$. This ganglioside is found in high concentrations in the nervous system and is normally degraded in the lysosome by the sequential removal of terminal sugars. The lack of $\beta$-N-acetylhexosaminidase results in the accumulation of the partially degraded ganglioside in the lysosome leading to significant swelling of the lysosome. The abnormally high level of lipid in the lysosome of the neuron affects its function resulting in the disease.

28.2  **D.** Gangliosides are carbohydrate-rich lipids in which an oligosaccharide chain is attached to ceramide. The oligosaccharide chain must contain at least one acidic sugar such as N-acetylneuraminate or N-glycosylneuraminate. These sugars are commonly referred to as sialic acid residues. Gangliosides are synthesized by the stepwise addition of sugar residues to ceramide.

28.3  **C.** Tay-Sachs disease is the result of the lack of the enzyme β-N-acetylhexosaminidase. Affected infants show weakness and retarded motor skills before 1 year of age. Other abnormalities follow, and death usually occurs before 3 years of age.

## BIOCHEMISTRY PEARLS

▶ Sphingolipids are a class of lipids found in biologic membranes in which the backbone of the lipid molecule is sphingosine, an 18-carbon amino alcohol.

▶ Sphingolipids are constantly being turned over in the lysosomes of cells by specific hydrolytic enzymes that remove the sugars in a stepwise fashion. Defects in these enzymes can result in accumulation of undegraded sphingolipids.

▶ This disease results from a deficiency in the enzyme hexosaminidase A (β-N-acetylhexosaminidase). The deficiency in hexosaminidase A leads to the accumulation of ganglioside $G_{M2}$ in the nerve cells of the brain.

▶ Other lysosomal storage disorders include $G_{M1}$ gangliosidoses, $G_{M2}$ gangliosidoses, Gaucher disease, Niemann-Pick disease, Fabry disease, fucosidosis, Schindler disease, metachromatic leukodystrophy, Krabbe disease, multiple sulfatase deficiency, Farber disease, and Wolman disease.

## REFERENCES

Berg JM, Tymoczko JL, Stryer L. *Biochemistry*. 5th ed. New York: Freeman; 2002:721-722.

Devlin TM, ed. *Textbook of Biochemistry with Clinical Correlations*. 7th ed. New York: Wiley-Liss; 2010.

A 6-year-old boy is brought to his pediatrician with profound mental retardation. Upon questioning the mother, several members of the parents' families have had mental retardation. She also has noticed that he appears very active and restless, frequently getting into trouble in school. On examination, the boy appears restless and his speech is significantly delayed and incomprehensible. The boy has coarse facial features but otherwise has a normal examination. Laboratory tests reveal an elevated level of heparan sulfate.

▶ What is the most likely diagnosis?
▶ What is the inheritance pattern of this disorder?
▶ What are some other causes of mucopolysaccharidoses (MPS)?

# ANSWERS TO CASE 29:
## Sanfilippo Syndrome

*Summary:* A 6-year-old boy with severe mental retardation, family history of mental retardation, language delays, and behavioral problems.

- **Diagnosis:** Sanfilippo syndrome
- **Inheritance pattern:** Autosomal recessive
- **Other causes:** Hunter syndrome, Hurler syndrome, or Morquio syndrome

## CLINICAL CORRELATION

Excessive accumulation of proteins, nucleic acids, carbohydrates, and lipids can result from deficiency of 1 or more lysosomal hydrolases. Lysosomal storage diseases are classified by the stored material. Accumulation of glycosaminoglycans results in MPS. Common causes of this disorder include Hunter syndrome, Hurler syndrome, and Sanfilippo syndrome. Sanfilippo syndrome is inherited in an autosomal recessive pattern and clinically evident by profound mental retardation, lack of normal developmental milestones, and significant language delay. Sanfilippo syndrome results in an excess of heparan sulfate and can be caused by a variety of enzyme deficiencies.

# APPROACH TO:
## Lysosomal Degradation of Glycosaminoglycans

### OBJECTIVES

1. Understand the structural roles of glycosaminoglycans and proteoglycans.

2. Describe how glycosaminoglycans and proteoglycans are synthesized.

3. Describe the biochemical pathways needed for glycosaminoglycan catabolism.

4. Explain why lysosomal enzyme deficiencies and glycosaminoglycan accumulation result in clinical signs/symptoms.

### DEFINITIONS

**ENDOGLYCOSIDASE:** An enzyme that hydrolyzes an interior glycosidic bond between 2 sugars in a polysaccharide or oligosaccharide to produce 2 smaller oligosaccharides.

**EXOGLYCOSIDASE:** An enzyme that hydrolyzes the glycosidic bond between the terminal 2 sugars of an oligosaccharide or polysaccharide releasing the terminal sugar from the nonreducing end of the polymer, thus leaving it 1 sugar shorter.

**GLYCOSAMINOGLYCAN (GAG):** Formerly known as mucopolysaccharide; a heteropolysaccharide composed of a repeating disaccharide of an N-acetylated hexosamine (glucosamine or galactosamine) and an acidic hexose (glucuronic acid or iduronic acid); this repeating disaccharide unit is frequently sulfated in 1 or more positions; most glycosaminoglycans are covalently linked to a core protein in structures known as proteoglycans.

**HYALURONAN:** Formerly known as hyaluronic acid; a glycosaminoglycan composed of alternating residues of glucuronic acid and N-acetylglucosamine. Hyaluronan is not sulfated nor is it covalently linked to a protein.

**MUCOPOLYSACCHARIDOSIS:** A genetic disorder involving a lack of a lysosomal enzyme required for the degradation of glycosaminoglycans leading to buildup of glycosaminoglycans in the lysosome and increased excretion of glycosaminoglycan fragments in urine.

**SULFATASE:** An enzyme that catalyzes the hydrolysis of sulfate ester bond releasing free inorganic sulfate from the substrate.

## DISCUSSION

The extracellular matrix that surrounds and binds certain types of cells is composed of numerous components, including fibrous structural proteins, such as various collagens, adhesive proteins like laminin and fibronectin, and proteoglycans that form the gel into which the fibrous structural proteins are embedded. Proteoglycans are very large macromolecules consisting of a core protein to which many long polysaccharide chains called glycosaminoglycans are covalently bound. Due to the high negative charge of the glycosaminoglycans, the proteoglycans are very highly hydrated, a property that allows the proteoglycans to form a gel-like matrix that can expand and contract. The proteoglycans are also effective lubricants.

The glycosaminoglycans (GAGs; formerly called mucopolysaccharides) are long, linear polymers of repeating disaccharide units containing an acidic sugar (glucuronic acid or iduronic acid) and a hexosamine (glucosamine or galactosamine, both usually N-acetylated). The exception to this general structure is keratan sulfate, which has galactose in place of the acidic hexose. Table 29-1 lists the various types of GAGs and the structures of their repeating disaccharide units. The GAGs are often highly sulfated, which increases their negative charge and their ability to bind water molecules. All of the GAGs except hyaluronan are covalently linked to one of approximately 30 different core proteins to form proteoglycans. The core protein is synthesized on the rough endoplasmic reticulum and transferred to the Golgi where nucleoside diphosphate–activated acidic and amino sugars are alternately added to the nonreducing end of the growing polysaccharide by glycosyltransferases, resulting in the characteristic repeating disaccharide structure common to the GAGs. Hyaluronan, which is not sulfated nor covalently linked to a core protein, is synthesized at the plasma membrane by hyaluronan synthases. Hyaluronan synthases are integral membrane proteins that catalyze the alternate addition of UDP-glucuronate and UDP-N-acetylglucosamine to the reducing end of the growing hyaluronan polymer at the inner surface of the plasma membrane as it extrudes

## Table 29-1 • GLYCOSAMINOGLYCAN COMPOSITION

| Glycosaminoglycan | Repeating Disaccharide Unit* |
|---|---|
| Hyaluronan | <br>GlcA β(1→3) GlcNAc β(1→4) |
| Chondroitin sulfate | <br>GlcA β(1→3) GalNAc β(1→4) |
| Dermatan sulfate | <br>IdoA β(1→3) GalNAc β(1→4) |
| Heparan sulfate / Heparin ** | <br>GlcA β(1→4) GlcNAc α(1→4)<br><br>IdoA α(1→4) GlcNAc α(1→4) |
| Keratan sulfate I & II | <br>Gal β(1→4) GlcNAc β(1→3) |

* Dashed ellipses indicate possible site of sulfation
** Heparan sulfate contains primarily GlcA; heparin contains primarily IdoA
Abbreviations used: Gal = galactose; GalNAc = N-acetylgalactosamine; Glc A = glucuronic acid;
GlcNAc = N-acetylglucosamine; IdoA = iduronic acid

the nonreducing end of the GAG into the extracellular space. Hyaluronan can then assemble into large macromolecular complexes with other proteoglycans, which are noncovalently attached to hyaluronan by link proteins.

Degradation of proteoglycans during normal turnover of the extracellular matrix begins with proteolytic cleavage of the core protein by proteases in the extracellular matrix, which then enters the cell via endocytosis. The endosomes deliver their content to the lysosomes, where the proteolytic enzymes complete the degradation of the core proteins and an array of glycosidases and sulfatases hydrolyze the GAGs to monosaccharides. The lysosomes contain both endoglycosidases, which hydrolyze the long polymers into shorter oligosaccharides, and exoglycosidases that cleave individual acidic- or aminosugars from the GAG fragments.

Lysosomal catabolism of GAGs proceeds in a stepwise manner from the nonreducing end, as is shown with the degradation of heparan sulfate in Figure 29-1. If the terminal sugar is sulfated, then the sulfate bond must be hydrolyzed by a specific sulfatase before the sugar can be removed. When the sulfate has been removed, a specific exoglycosidase then hydrolyzes the terminal sugar from the nonreducing end of the oligosaccharide, thus leaving it 1 sugar shorter. Degradation continues in this stepwise fashion, alternating between removal of sulfates by sulfatases and cleavage of the terminal sugars by exoglycosidases. If removal of a sulfate leaves a terminal glucosamine residue, then it must first be acetylated to N-acetylglucosamine because the lysosome lacks the enzyme required to remove glucosamine. This is accomplished by an acetyltransferase that uses acetyl-CoA as the acetyl group donor. When the glucosamine residue has been N-acetylated it can be hydrolyzed by $\alpha$-N-acetylglucosaminidase, allowing the continuation of the stepwise degradation of the GAG.

Disease states known as Mucopolysaccharidoses (MPS) occur when there is a genetic deficiency of the enzymes involved in the lysosomal breakdown of the GAGs. A deficiency of any of these enzymes can lead to the accumulation of partially degraded GAGs in lysosomes and increased urinary excretion of GAG fragments. Histologic examination of affected cells shows large vacuoles, which are lysosomes engorged with partially degraded GAGs. Because GAGs are present throughout the body, deficiencies of enzymes that degrade them affect bone, connective tissues, and other organs.

MPS is classified into 7 clinical types and all are transmitted by autosomal recessive inheritance except for Hunter syndrome (MPS II, iduronate sulfatase deficiency), which is an X-linked disorder. Diagnosis of the specific disorder is made by measuring the specific enzyme activities in leukocytes or cultured skin fibroblasts. Because it takes some time for the GAGs to accumulate, individuals with a mucopolysaccharidosis usually have a period of normal development before symptoms appear. Depending on the type and severity of the disorder, physical symptoms can include coarse facial features, dwarfism and deformities of the skeleton, cardiovascular impairments, hepatosplenomegaly, neurologic deficits, and mental retardation. As shown in Figure 29-1, Sanfilippo syndrome can be caused by a deficiency of 1 of 4 different enzymes that degrade heparan sulfate. Although the facial coarsening is mild in individuals with Sanfilippo syndrome, the accumulation of heparan sulfate in lysosomes leads to severe neurologic and mental impairment that result in death usually by the end of the second decade of life.

**Figure 29-1.** Lysosomal degradation of heparan sulfate. Dark arrows indicate the site of action of the enzyme, which is listed in italics. Mucopolysaccharidoses (MPS) due to a deficiency of the indicated enzymes are listed in bold to the right of the enzyme.

## COMPREHENSION QUESTIONS

29.1  A 5-year-old boy is seen by a pediatrician because his parents are concerned about his aggressive behavior, hyperactivity, and loss of language skills. He also has recently become increasingly unsteady on his feet and has experienced a recent seizure. Slight facial feature coarsening is noted. In which of the following processes is this child most likely to have a disorder?

A.  Mobilization of glycogen

B.  Gluconeogenesis

C.  Salvage of purine bases

D.  Degradation of glycosaminoglycans

E.  Cholesterol metabolism

29.2  A 15-month-old white girl is brought to the pediatrician because of recurrent upper-respiratory tract infection. During the physical examination, the girl is noted to have a short stature, some clouding of the corneas, coarse facial features, and an enlarged tongue. She also appears to have some hearing loss and other developmental delays. The pediatrician suspects the child has a mucopolysaccharidosis. Which of the following is she least likely to have?

A.  Hurler syndrome (MPS I)

B.  Hunter syndrome (MPS II)

C.  Morquio syndrome (MPS IV)

D.  Sly syndrome (MPS VI)

E.  Sanfilippo syndrome (MPS III)

29.3  A 3-year-old boy with coarse facial features, progressive loss of motor skills, hepatosplenomegaly and chronic diarrhea is suspected of having Hunter syndrome (MPS II). Which of the following monosaccharide residues would be expected to be found at the nonreducing end of glycosaminoglycans in this patient's urine?

A.  N-Acetylglucosamine

B.  N-Acetylgalactosamine

C.  Glucuronate

D.  Iduronate

E.  Iduronate 2-sulfate

## ANSWERS

29.1  **D.** The patient is exhibiting the classic symptoms of Sanfilippo syndrome, which is a deficiency in 1 of 4 different lysosomal enzymes that breakdown glycosaminoglycans leading to the buildup of heparan sulfate and dermatan sulfate in lysosomes.

29.2  **B.** All the types of MPS are transmitted by autosomal recessive inheritance except Hunter syndrome (MPS II), a deficiency in iduronate sulfatase that is X-linked recessive. Because Hunter syndrome is X-linked, it is almost exclusively seen in males. Because this patient is female, she would not be expected to have an X-linked disorder.

29.3  **E.** Because this patient is suspected of having Hunter syndrome, a deficiency in iduronate sulfatase, iduronate 2-sulfate would be expected to be present at the nonreducing end of glycosaminoglycans found in this patient's urine. A deficiency of iduronate sulfatase would prevent the sulfate ester bond of iduronate 2-sulfate residues from being hydrolyzed and further degradation of the glycosaminoglycan would be halted.

## BIOCHEMISTRY PEARLS

▶ Often enzyme deficiencies are inherited as autosomal recessive disorders, so that both chromosomes are defective for the individual to be affected.

▶ MPS occur when there is a genetic deficiency of the enzymes involved in the lysosomal breakdown of the glycosaminoglycans.

▶ In Sanfilippo syndrome, the accumulation of heparan sulfate in lysosomes leads to severe neurologic and mental impairment that result in death usually by the end of the second decade of life.

## REFERENCES

Bittar T, Washington ER III. Mucopolysaccharidosis. http://emedicine.medscape.com/article/1258678-overview.

Baloghova J, Schwartz RA, Baranova Z. Mucopolysaccharidoses Types I-VII. http://emedicine.medscape.com/article/1115193-overview.

Neufeld EF, Muenzer J. The mucopolysaccharidoses. In: Scriver CR, Beaudet AL, Sly WS, et al, eds. *The Metabolic and Molecular Bases of Inherited Disease.* 8th ed. New York: McGraw-Hill; 2001.

A 48-year-old man presents to the clinic because of concerns about heart disease. He reports that his father died from a heart attack at 46 years of age, and his older brother has also had a heart attack at 46 years of age but survived and is on medications for elevated cholesterol. The patient reports chest pain occasionally with ambulation around his house and is not able to climb stairs without significant chest pain and shortness of breath. The physical examination findings are normal, and the physician orders electrocardiography (ECG), an exercise stress test, and blood work. The patient's cholesterol level comes back as 350 mg/dL (normal 200). The physician prescribes medication, which he states is directed at the rate-limiting step of cholesterol biosynthesis.

▶ What is the rate-limiting step of cholesterol metabolism?
▶ What is the class of medication prescribed?

# ANSWERS TO CASE 30:

## Hypercholesterolemia

*Summary:* A 48-year-old man with strong family history of heart disease and now angina and exertional dyspnea presents with a significantly elevated cholesterol level. A medication is prescribed that is directed at the rate-limiting step of cholesterol biosynthesis.

- **Rate-limiting step:** The enzyme hydroxymethylglutaryl-CoA reductase (HMG-CoA reductase) catalyzes an early rate-limiting step in cholesterol biosynthesis.

- **Likely medication:** HMG-CoA reductase inhibitor, otherwise known as "statin" medications.

## CLINICAL CORRELATION

Hyperlipidemia is one of the most treatable risk factors of atherosclerotic vascular disease. In particular, the level of the low-density lipoprotein (LDL) cholesterol correlates with the pathogenesis of atherosclerosis. Exercise, dietary adjustments, and weight loss are the initial therapy of hyperlipidemia. If these are not sufficient, then pharmacologic therapy is required. The exact LDL targets depend on the patient's risk of cardiovascular disease. For example, if an individual has had a cardiovascular event previously (heart attack or stroke), then the LDL target is 100 mg/dL; 1 to 2 risk factors without prior events = 130 mg/dL; and no risk factors = 160 mg/dL.

# APPROACH TO:

## Lipid Metabolism

### OBJECTIVES

1. Describe cholesterol metabolism.

2. Explain the role of serum lipoproteins.

3. List the types of hereditary hyperlipidemias.

4. Explain why the LDL cholesterol level is increased with familial hypercholesterolemia.

### DEFINITIONS

**APOLIPOPROTEIN:** The protein component of a lipoprotein; in addition to being a structural component of a lipoprotein, apolipoproteins also serve as activators of enzymes and ligands for receptors.

**CHYLOMICRON:** A lipoprotein synthesized by the intestine to transport dietary lipids to peripheral tissues and the liver.

**HDL:** High-density lipoprotein; synthesized in the liver, the HDL serves as a source of apolipoproteins for other lipoproteins, as the site of action for the conversion of cholesterol to cholesterol ester in the plasma by the enzyme lecithin-cholesterol acyltransferase (LCAT), and delivers cholesterol esters derived from peripheral membranes to the liver. It is commonly called the "good cholesterol."

**LDL:** Low-density lipoprotein; a product of the degradation of very-low-density lipoproteins (VLDLs) by the action of lipoprotein lipase. LDLs are taken up by a receptor-mediated endocytosis by both peripheral tissues and the liver. It is commonly called the "bad cholesterol."

**LIPOPROTEIN:** A macromolecular particle composed of varying quantities of protein, triacylglycerol, phospholipids, cholesterol, and cholesterol esters. The lipoprotein structure has a phospholipid and free cholesterol skin surrounding a core composed of triacylglycerol and cholesterol esters, with the proteins imbedded on the surface. They serve as carriers of lipid in the circulation.

**VLDL:** Very-low-density lipoprotein; synthesized by the liver to transport triacylglycerol from the liver to peripheral tissues.

## DISCUSSION

**Although cholesterol can be synthesized in almost all cells,** the **liver, intestine, and the steroidogenic tissues such as the adrenal glands and reproductive tissues** are the **primary sites.** In the **liver,** cholesterol is synthesized in the **endoplasmic reticulum** along with phospholipids, triacylglycerides, and apoproteins. Prelipoprotein particles are assembled in the endoplasmic reticulum and then transferred to the Golgi. Further processing and addition of **cholesterol esters occur in the Golgi,** culminating in the formation of secretory granules containing **lipoprotein particles.** These vesicles then fuse with the plasma membrane and export cholesterol from the cell via exocytosis in the form of VLDLs (see below), which then enter the circulation. As the lipoprotein complexes are transported through the bloodstream they are converted from VLDL to intermediate density lipoproteins (IDL) to LDL by the removal of triacylglycerides by lipoprotein lipase, which is located on the surface of capillary epithelial cells.

    **Cholesterol and triacylglycerides (TAGs)** are transported as complexes in the form of lipoprotein particles. These **lipoprotein particles** contain a core of TAGs and cholesteryl esters surrounded by a monolayer of phospholipids, cholesterol, and specific proteins called apoproteins. The **apoproteins,** specific to each type of lipoprotein, enable the hydrophobic lipids to be transported in the aqueous environment of the bloodstream. They also contain signals that target the lipoprotein particles to the cells or activate enzymes. The lipoprotein particles vary in density depending on the lipid/protein ratio and are named based on these densities. The higher the lipid–protein ratio, the lower the density of the particle.

    The major classes of lipoproteins (Table 30-1) and some of their properties are:

- Chylomicrons
  – Lowest density
  – Transport dietary lipids from the intestine to target tissues

| Table 30-1 • MAJOR APOPROTEINS INVOLVED IN LIPID TRANSPORT BY LIPOPROTEINS | | |
|---|---|---|
| APOPROTEIN | LOCATION | FUNCTION |
| A | HDL | Activates lecithin-cholesterol acyltransferase |
| B-48 | Chylomicrons, chylomicron remnants | Structural, binds to B-48:E receptor in liver |
| B-100 | VLDL, IDL, LDL | Structural, binds to LDL receptor in liver and extrahepatic tissues |
| C-II | Chylomicrons, VLDL, (IDL), HDL | Binds to and activates lipoprotein lipase |
| E | Chylomicrons, chylomicron remnants, VLDL, (IDL), HDL | Structural, binds to B-48:E receptor in liver |

- VLDLs
  - Produced by liver cells to transport endogenously synthesized lipids to target cells
  - Production controlled by lipid availability
  - Contain 5 different apoproteins

- IDLs

- LDLs
  - Primarily cholesteryl esters
  - Apoprotein B-100

- HDLs
  - Secreted by liver and intestine
  - Contains apoprotein A-1
  - "Good cholesterol," high levels associated with low incidence of atherosclerosis

The LDLs (containing cholesteryl esters) are taken up by cells by a process known as **receptor-mediated endocytosis.** The LDL receptor mediates this endocytosis and is important to cholesterol metabolism. LDLs bind to these receptors, which recognize apoprotein B-100. After LDL binding to the LDL receptor, the ligand-receptor complexes cluster on the plasma membrane in coated pits, which then invaginate, forming coated vesicles. These coated vesicles are internalized, and clathrin, the protein composing the lattice in membrane-coated pits, is removed. These vesicles are now called endosomes and these endosomes fuse with the lysosome. The LDL receptor–containing membrane buds off and is recycled to the plasma membrane. Fusion of the lysosome and endosome releases lysosomal proteases that degrade the apoproteins into amino acids. Lysosomal enzymes also hydrolyze the cholesteryl esters to free cholesterol and fatty acids. The free cholesterol is released into the cytoplasm of the cell, and this free cholesterol is then available to be used by the cell. Excess cholesterol is reesterified by acyl-CoA:cholesterol acyltransferase (ACAT), which uses fatty acyl-CoA as the source of activated fatty acid. Free cholesterol affects cholesterol metabolism by inhibiting cholesterol biosynthesis. Cholesterol inhibits the enzyme β-hydroxy-β-methylglutaryl-CoA reductase (HMG-CoA reductase), which catalyzes an early rate-limiting step in cholesterol biosynthesis. HMG-CoA reductase is the target of the statin drugs in wide use for treating patients with elevated cholesterol levels. In addition, free cholesterol inhibits the synthesis of the LDL receptor, thus limiting the amount of LDLs that are taken up by the cell.

**Hyperlipidemia** is defined as elevated lipoprotein levels in the plasma, which may be primary or secondary. Several different types of hereditary hyperlipidemias have been defined.

- Type 1: A relatively rare inherited deficiency of either lipoprotein lipase activity or the lipoprotein lipase-activating protein apo C-II. This results in the inability to effectively remove chylomicrons and VLDL triglycerides from the blood.

- Type 2: Includes familial hypercholesterolemia described in detail below.

- Type 3: Associated with abnormalities of apolipoprotein E (apo E) and defective conversion and removal of VLDL from the plasma.

- Type 4: A common disorder characterized by variable elevations of plasma triglycerides contained predominantly in VLDL. This leads to a possible predisposition to atherosclerosis and often has a familial distribution.

- Type 5: An uncommon disorder, sometimes familial, associated with defective clearance of exogenous and endogenous triglycerides and the risk of life-threatening pancreatitis.

The disease *familial hypercholesterolemia* results from a mutation in the LDL-receptor gene found on **chromosome 19.** The overall phenotype of the inability to internalize the LDL receptor can be caused by 3 different types of defects. In the first type, the LDL receptor is not produced. The second type is a result of a mutation in the terminal region of the receptor that results in an LDL receptor unable to bind LDL. The third type is caused by a mutation in the C-terminal region that prevents the LDL-receptor complex from undergoing endocytosis. In the absence of a functioning LDL receptor, LDL cholesterol levels are greatly elevated in individuals with this disease. This elevation results in premature atherosclerosis of the coronary arteries. Genetic defects in apoprotein B-100, the protein in the LDL recognized by the LDL receptor, also exist and lead to elevated LDL because the LDL complex is not recognized by the LDL receptor. A diet low in fat and cholesterol, an exercise regimen, and anticholesterol medications are used in the treatment of this disease.

## COMPREHENSION QUESTIONS

30.1  A patient presents in your office with very high levels of serum cholesterol. After a series of tests, you conclude that the patient has high circulating levels of LDL cholesterol, but has normal levels of the liver LDL receptor. One possible explanation for this observation is which of the following?

   A.  The patient has a mutated form of apoprotein B-100
   B.  The inability to selectively remove cholesterol from the LDL complex
   C.  The absence of the enzyme lipoprotein lipase
   D.  Decreased levels of acyl-CoA: cholesterol acyltransferase
   E.  Altered phosphorylation of the LDL receptor

30.2  A patient with hereditary type 1 hyperlipidemia presents with elevated levels of chylomicrons and VLDL triglycerides in the blood. The main function of the chylomicrons in circulation is to do which of the following?

   A.  Transport lipids from the liver
   B.  Transport dietary lipids from the intestine to target tissues
   C.  Transport cholesterol from IDL to LDL
   D.  Act as a receptor for triacylglycerols in the liver
   E.  Bind cholesterol esters exclusively

30.3  Free cholesterol can affect cholesterol metabolism in the body by inhibiting cholesterol biosynthesis. The step at which free cholesterol inhibits its biosynthesis is by inhibiting which of the following processes?

   A.  Cyclizing of squalene to form lanosterol
   B.  Reduction of 7-dehydrocholesterol to form cholesterol
   C.  Formation of mevalonate from hydroxymethylglutaryl-CoA
   D.  Kinase that phosphorylates hydroxymethylglutaryl-CoA reductase
   E.  Condensation of acetyl-CoA and acetoacetyl-CoA to form hydroxymethylglutaryl-CoA

30.4  A patient presents in your office with very high levels of serum cholesterol. He states that he has tried to follow the diet and exercise regimen you gave him last year. You decide that this patient would benefit from a drug such as atorvastatin. This class of drugs is effective in treating hypercholesterolemia because it has what effect?

   A.  Stimulates phosphorylation of the β-hydroxy-β-methylglutaryl-CoA reductase enzyme
   B.  Decreases the stability of the β-hydroxy-β-methylglutaryl-CoA reductase protein
   C.  Binds cholesterol preventing it from being absorbed by the intestine
   D.  Directly prevents the deposition of cholesterol on artery walls
   E.  Inhibits the enzyme β-hydroxy-β-methylglutaryl-CoA reductase

# ANSWERS

30.1  **A.** A common genetic mutation leading to high-circulating LDL cholesterol levels is caused by mutations in the LDL receptor. The lack of a functional receptor prevents the removal of LDL cholesterol from circulation. Apoprotein B-100 is found in the LDL-cholesterol complex and is the protein recognized by the LDL receptor. In this patient, the LDL receptor is normal so it is reasonable to conclude that the reason that the LDL cholesterol remains in circulation is because it is not recognized by the normal LDL receptor. A mutation in the apoprotein B-100 such that it is not recognized by the receptor would lead to elevated LDL-cholesterol levels.

30.2  **B.** The liver and intestine are the main sources of circulating lipids. Chylomicrons carry triacylglycerides and cholesterol esters from the intestine to other target tissues. VLDLs carry lipids from the liver into circulation. Lipoproteins are a mix of lipids and specific proteins and these complexes are classified based on their lipid–protein ratio. Lipoprotein lipases degrade the triacylglycerides in the chylomicrons and VLDLs with a concurrent release of apoproteins. This is a gradual process that converts the VLDLs into IDLs and then LDLs.

30.3  **C.** The major regulatory enzyme of cholesterol metabolism, β-hydroxy-β-methylglutaryl-CoA reductase, is regulated by 3 distinct mechanisms. The first is phosphorylation by a cAMP-dependent protein kinase. Phosphorylation of β-hydroxy-β-methylglutaryl-CoA reductase inactivates the enzyme. The other 2 mechanisms involve the levels of cholesterol. The degradation of the enzyme is controlled by cholesterol levels. The half-life of β-hydroxy-β-methylglutaryl-CoA reductase is regulated by cholesterol levels with high concentrations of cholesterol leading to a shorter half-life. The final regulatory mechanism involves control of the expression of the β-hydroxy-β-methylglutaryl-CoA reductase gene. High levels of cholesterol lead to a decrease in the mRNA levels coding for β-hydroxy-β-methylglutaryl-CoA reductase.

30.4  **E.** The statin class of drugs—atorvastatin, lovastatin, and simvastatin—is used to treat hypercholesterolemia. This class of drugs lowers cholesterol levels by inhibiting the biosynthesis of cholesterol. Specifically, these drugs inhibit the enzyme β-hydroxy-β-methylglutaryl-CoA (HMG-CoA) reductase, which catalyzes the reaction that converts HMG-CoA to mevalonate. This is the rate-limiting step of cholesterol biosynthesis.

In addition to the statin drugs, which inhibit HMG-CoA reductase, numerous other drugs are used to lower cholesterol levels. The first are resins, which are also referred to as bile acid sequestrants such as cholestyramine. The resins work by binding to the bile acids followed by excretion of the resin–bile complex. To make up for the loss of the bile acids the body converts cholesterol into bile acids, thus reducing the cholesterol levels.

Another type of drug used is the fibrates such as gemfibrozil. These compounds work by lowering the levels of triglycerides and increasing the levels of the "good" HDLs. Niacin is also effective in lowering cholesterol levels when used in large doses (more than that required for niacin as a vitamin). Niacin acts to lower levels of triglycerides and LDLs and increasing the levels of the "good" HDLs.

Drugs, such as ezetimibe, which inhibits the absorption of cholesterol in the intestine, are effective in lowering cholesterol levels. This drug is often given in combination with a statin and this combination therapy is very effective in lowering cholesterol levels.

## BIOCHEMISTRY PEARLS

▶ Cholesterol can be synthesized in almost all cells, but the liver, intestine, and steroidogenic tissues, such as the adrenal glands and reproductive tissues, are the primary sites.

▶ The major classes of lipoproteins are chylomicrons (lowest density), VLDLs, IDLs, LDLs, and HDLs (considered the "good cholesterol").

▶ Familial hyperlipidemia is subdivided into 5 types, with type 5 being most common, characterized by variable elevations of plasma triglycerides contained predominantly in VLDL.

▶ The rate-limiting step in cholesterol biosynthesis is the enzyme HMG-CoA reductase, which is the target of the statin drugs.

## REFERENCES

Berg JM, Tymoczko JL, Stryer L. *Biochemistry.* 5th ed. New York: Freeman; 2002:722-731.

Devlin TM, ed. *Textbook of Biochemistry with Clinical Correlations.* 7th ed. New York: Wiley-Liss; 2010.

A 45-year-old woman presents to the clinic with concerns over occasional midepigastric discomfort and nausea/vomiting after eating "greasy meals." The symptoms gradually disappear, and she has no further discomfort. She denies any hematemesis, and pain is worse after eating. She further mentions that she had elevated cholesterol levels in the past and was on an exercise program, but not anymore. On examination, she is afebrile with normal vital signs. Her physical examination is completely normal with no evidence of abdominal pain. Abdominal ultrasonography is performed and revealed a few gallstones in the gallbladder but no thickening of the gallbladder wall.

- What factors would you need to consider to assess the need for cholecystectomy?
- What are gallstones made of?
- Can gallstones be seen on abdominal radiography?

# ANSWERS TO CASE 31:
## Gallstones

*Summary:* A 45-year-old woman presents with hypercholesterolemia, ultrasonographic evidence of gallstones, and recurrent symptoms of gallbladder disease.

- **Surgical candidates:** Frequent and severe attacks, previous complications from gallstones, presence of underlying condition predisposing the patient to increased risk of gallbladder disease.

- **Components of gallstones:** Cholesterol, calcium bilirubinate, and bile salts.

- **Abdominal radiography and diagnosis:** Mixed stones are easier to see on plain film secondary to calcifications, which make up approximately 10% of gallstones.

## CLINICAL CORRELATION

This individual fits the "classic" patient with gallbladder disease (ie, a middle-aged woman who is overweight). The gallbladder acts to store bile salts produced by the liver. The gallbladder is stimulated to contract when food enters the small intestine; the bile salts then travel through the bile duct to the ampulla of Vater into the duodenum. The bile salts act to emulsify fats, helping with the digestion of fat. Gallstones form when the solutes in the gallbladder precipitate. The 2 main types of stones are cholesterol stones and pigmented stones. Cholesterol stones are usually yellow-green in appearance and account for approximately 80% of gallstones. Pigmented stones are usually made of bilirubin and appear dark in color. Patients may have pain from the gallstones, usually after a fatty meal. The pain is typically epigastric or right upper quadrant and perhaps radiating to the right shoulder. If the gallbladder becomes inflamed or infected, then cholecystitis can result. The stones can also travel through the bile duct and obstruct biliary flow leading to jaundice (yellow color of the skin), or irritate the pancreas and cause pancreatitis.

# APPROACH TO:
## Bile Salt Metabolism

## OBJECTIVES

1. Know about bile salt metabolism.
2. Be able to identify where bile salts are synthesized.
3. Know where bile salts emulsify dietary fats.

# DEFINITIONS

**BILE SALTS:** Cholesterol derivatives with detergent-like properties used to solubilize cholesterol, assist in intestinal absorption of fat-soluble vitamins, and emulsify dietary lipids passing through the intestine to enable fat digestion and absorption by exposing fats to pancreatic lipases.

**BILE ACIDS:** Neutral, protonated form of bile salts.

**PRIMARY BILE ACIDS:** Synthesized from cholesterol as cholic acid and chenodeoxycholic acid. They are secreted as taurine and glycine conjugates.

**SECONDARY BILE ACIDS:** Products of deconjugated and reduced primary acids. Bacteria in the intestine remove the $7\alpha$-hydroxyl group, leaving the secondary bile acids.

**CHOLESTEROL $7\alpha$-HYDROXYLASE (CYP7A1):** The mixed-function oxidase cytochrome P450 enzyme catalyzing the initial, rate-limiting step for conversion of cholesterol to bile acids.

**$\beta$-HYDROXY-$\beta$-METHYLGLUTARYL-COENZYME A (HMG-COA) REDUCTASE:** The rate-limiting enzyme in cholesterol biosynthesis.

# DISCUSSION

Bile salts are derivatives of cholesterol that make up the major component of bile. They are very efficient detergents when conjugated to amino acids because of the presence of both polar and nonpolar regions. This property helps to emulsify dietary lipids in the intestine, which aids in fat digestion and absorption by making fat vulnerable to pancreatic lipases. Other functions of **bile salt** (ionized, deprotonated form) and **bile acid** (neutral, protonated form) are to solubilize cholesterol thus preventing precipitation of cholesterol crystals and facilitating cholesterol excretion. The only significant removal of excess cholesterol from the body is achieved through the excretion of bile salts. Finally, they assist in intestinal absorption of fat-soluble vitamins.

The conversion of cholesterol to bile acids is a multienzyme process. **The initial and rate-limiting step of bile acid synthesis is oxidation of cholesterol to $7\alpha$-hydroxycholesterol by a mixed function oxidase from the cytochrome P450 superfamily, cholesterol $7\alpha$-hydroxylase (CYP7A1;** Figure 31-1). The remaining steps include reduction of the $\Delta^5$-double bond, side chain shortening, and oxidation. The products of this pathway, cholic acid and chenodeoxycholic acid, are termed the primary bile acids because they have been synthesized de novo from cholesterol. To increase the pH range over which the bile salts remain ionized and serve as good detergents, they may be conjugated via amide bonds with either of the amino acids glycine or taurine (Figure 31-2).

**Bile salts/acids are synthesized in the liver, stored and concentrated in the gallbladder,** and **secreted into the intestine** where they may undergo **deconjugation** and reduction by intestinal bacteria to produce secondary bile acids (see Figure 31-1). Once formed in the liver, the bile salts/acids are secreted through the bile ducts, which are made up of the bile canaliculi and bile ductules, and passed on to the

**Figure 31-1.** Simplified biosynthetic pathway of bile salts.

gallbladder for storage as bile. Ultimately, they are passed on to the intestine. Most of the bile acids/salts are deconjugated in the intestinal ileum and reduced to secondary bile acids by bacteria, which remove the 7α-hydroxyl group by a dehydroxylation reaction. Although some are lost by excretion, approximately 90% of the bile

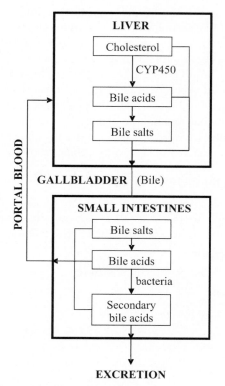

**Figure 31-2.** Conjugation of bile salts.

acids and salts are reabsorbed in the terminal ileum and returned to the liver. The liver cannot provide sufficient amounts of newly synthesized bile acids for the body's daily needs; therefore, the body relies on enterohepatic circulation (Figure 31-3) to sustain necessary bile acid levels. The portal vein transports bile acids from the intestine back to the liver as complexes with serum albumin.

The synthesis of bile salts is under very tight regulatory control to maintain cholesterol homeostasis and supply sufficient amounts of detergent to the intestine.

**Figure 31-3.** The enterohepatic circulation of bile acids.

This is controlled in part by a feedback mechanism on cholesterol 7α-hydroxylase, the rate-limiting enzyme in the synthetic pathway. Increased concentrations of bile acids inhibit cholesterol 7α-hydroxylase, while low levels relieve the inhibition. Elevated cholesterol levels, however, activate the enzyme, thus increasing bile acid biosynthesis. Levels of both cholesterol and bile acids affect the concentration of cholesterol 7α-hydroxylase and this regulation appears to be controlled at the transcriptional level via nuclear receptors. Therefore, binding of bile acids or cholesterol to a given nuclear receptor in turn regulates the expression of the CYP7A1 gene, activating expression in the case of binding to cholesterol and repressing it when bile acids are bound. Thus, the proper maintenance of bile acid levels can prevent accumulation of cholesterol.

A total of 80% of gallstones in the Western world are a result of cholesterol precipitation from the bile, a condition known as cholelithiasis. The pathogenetic mechanism of gallstone formation usually involves a culmination of deleterious events involving the metabolic pathways of cholesterol or the bile acids/salts. First, the cholesterol concentration in bile becomes supersaturated. Bile is a controlled mixture of cholesterol, bile acids, and phospholipids (with small amounts of bile pigments), and if cholesterol levels are elevated or bile acids/salts lowered, the ratio of the 3 major components changes leaving cholesterol less protected against the aqueous environment and more likely to precipitate. Elevated cholesterol levels can occur by having excess HMG-CoA reductase activity, the rate-limiting enzyme in cholesterol biosynthesis; this condition is typically seen in the obese. Alternatively, reduced levels of acyl-CoA: cholesterol acyltransferase (ACAT), the enzyme that esterifies cholesterol within cells, or reduced levels of cholesterol 7α-hydroxylase can cause elevation of cholesterol. Deoxycholate, a secondary bile acid synthesized by intestinal bacteria, inhibits CYP7A1. Therefore, high levels of deoxycholate resulting from prolonged exposure of bile acids to intestinal bacteria may result in high levels of cholesterol in bile. In addition to elevated cholesterol levels in bile, there must be adequate time for cholesterol crystal nucleation, which will ultimately form macroliths. Similar to overnight sleeping, fasting allows for long-term storage of bile in the gallbladder and could give ample time for crystal nucleation.

## COMPREHENSION QUESTIONS

31.1 The modification to bile salts that increases the working pH range and amphipathic nature of bile salts is which of the following?

  A. 7α-Hydroxylation

  B. Dehydroxylation by intestinal bacteria

  C. Esterification

  D. Conjugation to taurine or glycine

31.2   A new drug called CT2033, a corticosteroid, has reached the clinical trial stage. This drug was designed to treat inflammation but seems to also cause an undesired side effect where there is disturbance of cholesterol and bile acid homeostasis. Which of the following is *least likely* to explain the adverse events caused by CT2033?

A.   It downregulates the expression of a hepatobiliary bile acid transporter gene.

B.   It inhibits a hepatobiliary transporter protein decreasing bile acid secretion.

C.   It competes with cholesterol for CYP7A1 binding.

D.   It binds and inhibits pancreatic lipases.

31.3   A 53-year-old man with elevated levels of low-density lipoprotein (LDL) cholesterol, signs of premature cholesterol gallstone disease, and substantially elevated triglycerides visited his physician for a follow-up to check his current status. The patient had received various statin and HMG-CoA-reductase inhibitors therapies for the last 2 years. However, after blood work done at this follow-up visit, complications had still not subsided. This patient has similar problems as 2 of his siblings. Which of the following best explains this patient's dyslipidemia?

A.   Influx of abnormal phospholipids in the gallbladder as a result of ileal disease

B.   Loss of HMG-CoA reductase function

C.   Loss of CYP7A1 (cholesterol 7$\alpha$-hydroxylase) function

D.   Elevated levels of ACAT

## ANSWERS

31.1   **D.** Conjugation of bile acids to these 2 amino acids through amide linkages is important for maintaining the detergent properties of bile salts over the wide pH range of the intestinal tract. Conjugation decreases the pKa of the bile salts assuring ionization and solubility in the intestines.

31.2   **D.** Any of the situations in answers A through C could directly alter cholesterol and bile acid homeostasis. Many of the bile acid transporters are regulated by nuclear receptors. Therefore, a nuclear receptor ligand such as CT2033 could change the expression levels of the transporters, which could then result in problems with secretion of bile acids and probable accumulation of cholesterol. If the new drug were to directly bind and inhibit the transporter, then the same result would occur. Because corticosteroids are derivatives of cholesterol, it could be reasonable for CT2033 to fit in the same CYP7A1 binding pocket and compete with cholesterol. This could cause accumulation of cholesterol because CYP7A1 is needed to convert cholesterol into bile salts. The drug could act to effectively lower active CYP7A1 levels. However, answer D is least likely to affect cholesterol and bile acids because pancreatic lipases are involved in the breakdown of fat. Bile acids simply emulsify fats and allow pancreatic lipases to degrade the fat. Therefore, inhibiting pancreatic lipases should not have much of an effect on cholesterol and bile acid homeostasis.

31.3 **C.** A loss in function of *CYP7A1* prevents the catabolism of cholesterol to bile salts. Elevated levels of LDL cholesterol, signs of premature cholesterol gallstone disease, and substantially elevated triglycerides are all complications that can result from blocking the enzyme that breaks down cholesterol. Therefore, high levels of cholesterol accumulate in the bile and, with decreased production of bile salts to help dissolution of cholesterol, the formation of cholesterol gallstones. Statin therapy is not as effective because it inhibits the enzyme that controls the rate of cholesterol synthesis but does nothing with respect to the degradation of cholesterol. The increase in blood triglyceride levels when *CYP7A1* is deficient is not well understood, but triglyceride levels appear to have a reciprocal relationship to bile acid synthesis. Finally, this appears to be a genetic disorder because other siblings showed the same phenotype, which would point to a possible mutated gene and likely prevent function of *CYP7A1*.

## BIOCHEMISTRY PEARLS

▶ Bile salts are the major component of bile and are very efficient "detergents" when conjugated to amino acids because of the presence of both polar and nonpolar regions, aiding in fat digestion.

▶ The initial and rate-limiting step of bile acid synthesis is oxidation of cholesterol to 7α-hydroxycholesterol by a mixed function oxidase from the cytochrome P450 superfamily, cholesterol 7α-hydroxylase (*CYP7A1*).

▶ The synthesis of bile salts is under very tight regulatory control, mainly by a feedback mechanism on cholesterol 7α-hydroxylase, the rate-limiting enzyme in the synthetic pathway.

## REFERENCES

Chiang JYL. Regulation of bile acid synthesis. *Front Biosci.* 1998;3:D176-D193.

Pullinger CR, Eng C, Salen G, et al. Human cholesterol 7α-hydroxylase (CYP7A1) deficiency has a hypercholesterolemic phenotype. *J Clin Invest.* 2002;110(1):109-117.

Russell DW. The enzymes, regulation, and genetics of bile acid synthesis. *Annu Rev Biochem.* 2003;72:137-174.

Trauner M, Boyer JL. Bile salt transporters: molecular characterization, function, and regulation. *Physiol Rev.* 2003;83(2):633-671.

A 63-year-old woman presents to the clinic with recurrent midepigastric pain during the last 3 months. She reports some relief shortly after eating, but then the discomfort returns. She has tried various over-the-counter medications without relief. She also reports feeling tired and has had to increase the amount of ibuprofen needed for relief of her arthritis. She denies nausea, vomiting, and diarrhea. On examination she is found to have mild midepigastric tenderness and guaiac positive stool. A complete blood count revealed a microcytic anemia and normal white blood cell count, consistent with iron deficiency. The patient was referred to a gastroenterologist who performed an upper gastrointestinal (GI) endoscopy that identified gastric ulcers. He stated that he suspected that the ibuprofen, a nonsteroidal anti-inflammatory drug (NSAID) was the causative agent and suggested switching from ibuprofen to a coxib, such as celecoxib.

▶ What is the likely biochemical etiology of the disorder?
▶ Why do coxibs generally have a lower incidence of upper GI problems than other NSAIDs?
▶ What is the major difference between aspirin and other NSAIDs with regard to platelet function?

# ANSWERS TO CASE 32:
## NSAID-Associated Gastritis

*Summary:* A 63-year-old woman with arthritis taking an NSAID with recent onset of epigastric pain relieved with food, guaiac positive stools, and iron deficiency anemia. Endoscopic examination reveals gastric ulcers.

- **Biochemical etiology:** Primarily, NSAID inhibition of a gastric enzyme (cyclooxygenase [COX]-1) required for synthesis of prostaglandins that have a protective effect on the gastric mucosa. A contributory factor is direct mucosal damage due to the acidic chemistry of NSAIDs.

- **Decreased gastric side effects with coxibs:** Traditional NSAIDs, such as ibuprofen and aspirin, inhibit both COX-1 and COX-2. The coxibs are selective inhibitors of COX-2, allowing continued production of protective prostaglandins by gastric COX-1.

- **Difference between aspirin and other NSAIDs:** Aspirin covalently modifies platelet COX-1, thus irreversibly blocking thromboxane formation and reducing platelet function for the lifespan of the affected platelet (platelets cannot synthesize new proteins). The inhibitory action of other NSAIDs on platelet COX-1 is not covalent and is eventually reversed when the agents' blood levels decline.

## CLINICAL CORRELATION

NSAIDs, also known as prostaglandin synthesis inhibitors or COX inhibitors, can induce upper GI irritation or ulcers. The NSAIDs include a wide variety of medications including aspirin, ibuprofen, naproxen, and indomethacin. These medications are used for pain, inflammation, dysmenorrhea, headache, arthritis, or fever. These compounds act as anti-inflammatory and antipyretic agents by inhibiting COX catalysis by prostaglandin H synthase (PGHS). PGHS has 2 isoenzymes: PGHS-1 (or COX-1) is generally a basal enzyme found in various tissues including platelets and gastric mucosa, while PGHS-2 (or COX-2) is an inducible enzyme typically expressed in response to cytokines and mitogens at sites of inflammation or cell proliferation.

Older NSAIDs, such as aspirin and ibuprofen, inhibit both COX-1 and -2, but a newer class of NSAIDs, called coxibs, is selective for COX-2 inhibition. By sparing production of cytoprotective prostaglandins by mucosal COX-1, coxibs have fewer problems with irritation and ulceration in the upper GI tract.

Thromboxane produced by platelet COX-1 in concert with a downstream enzyme is prothrombotic, so aspirin and other NSAIDs cause platelet dysfunction and increase bleeding time. Aspirin is unusual in that it causes covalent, irreversible inhibition of the COX protein, whereas other NSAIDs have noncovalent, reversible actions. Thus, because they cannot synthesize more COX protein, platelets are irreversibly affected by aspirin but only temporarily affected by other NSAIDs. Low-dose aspirin is often used in antithrombotic prophylaxis.

The prothrombotic and vasoconstrictive actions of COX-1-derived thromboxane in the vasculature are opposed by an antithrombotic and vasodilative prostaglandin, prostacyclin, that originates from COX-2 in vascular endothelial cells. Thus, the COX-2 selective coxibs tend to decrease prostacyclin levels in the vasculature without reducing the thromboxane levels. This tendency is thought to explain the small but significant increase in cardiovascular risk that led to withdrawal of 2 coxibs from the US market.

## APPROACH TO:
## Prostaglandin Metabolism

## OBJECTIVES

1. Describe the biosynthetic and cell signaling pathways involving prostanoids.

2. Distinguish between the pathophysiologic roles of the 2 PGHS isoforms.

3. Cite the pharmacologic targets of NSAIDs and the characteristics that distinguish coxibs and aspirin from other NSAIDs.

## DEFINITIONS

**EICOSANOIDS:** Oxygenated lipid-signaling molecules containing 20 carbons derived from polyunsaturated fatty acids released from membrane phospholipids by the action of phospholipase $A_2$. These include the prostanoids produced by the cyclooxygenase pathway and the leukotrienes produced by the lipoxygenase pathway.

**PROSTANOIDS:** Oxygenated lipid signaling molecules derived from polyunsaturated fatty acids released from membrane phospholipids by the action of phospholipase $A_2$. Prostanoids include prostaglandins, prostacyclin, and thromboxanes.

**PROSTAGLANDIN:** An oxygenated lipid-signaling molecule that has a 5-member ring system that is derived from arachidonic acid and other 20-carbon polyunsaturated fatty acids. The prostaglandins are hormone-like molecules that regulate cellular events near the area in which they are synthesized.

**THROMBOXANE:** An oxygenated lipid-signaling molecule that has a 6-member ring system derived from arachidonic acid and other 20-carbon polyunsaturated fatty acids. Thromboxanes are involved in platelet aggregation as well as vasoconstriction and bronchoconstriction and lymphocyte proliferation.

**PGH SYNTHASE:** Prostaglandin H synthase; the enzyme that catalyzes the formation of prostaglandin H from $C_{20}$ polyunsaturated acids. PGH synthase has 2 activities; the cyclooxygenase activity introduces the 5-membered ring into the polyunsaturated fatty acid while also introducing an endoperoxide between carbons 9 and 10 and a hydroperoxide at carbon 15. The peroxidase activity reduces the hydroperoxide to a hydroxyl group using glutathione as the source of reducing equivalents. PGH synthase exists in 2 isoforms, PGHS-1 and PGHS-2. PGHS-1 is the "basal" isoform and is expressed constitutively, whereas PGHS-2 is the inducible isoform and has been implicated in cell proliferation and inflammation.

**NSAID:** Nonsteroidal anti-inflammatory drug; NSAIDs inhibit the COX activity of PGH synthase, thus inhibiting the production of prostaglandins and thromboxanes.

**COXIBS:** A class of NSAIDs that is selective for inhibition of the cyclooxygenase activity of PGHS-2, with weaker action against the PGHS-1 cyclooxygenase.

## DISCUSSION

**Prostanoids are oxygenated lipid-signaling molecules** derived from **polyunsaturated fatty acids.** The major prostanoids synthesized from the prototypical polyunsaturated fatty acid, arachidonic acid, are prostaglandin (PG) $D_2$, $PGE_2$, $PGF_{2a}$, $PGH_2$, $PGI_2$ (also known as **prostacyclin**), and thromboxane (TX) $A_2$. The prostanoid-signaling cascade begins with an external stimulus, most often the binding of a ligand to a cell surface receptor that activates one or more phospholipases $A_2$. The latter are enzymes that release arachidonic acid from its esterified form in membrane phospholipids such as phosphatidylethanolamine and phosphatidylinositol. Arachidonate is converted to $PGH_2$ by one of the isoforms of PGH synthase (PGHS-1 or -2), enzymes localized to the endoplasmic reticulum membrane and the nuclear envelope.

In turn, $PGH_2$ is metabolized to the prostanoid lipid signals ($PGD_2$, $PGE_2$, $PGF_{2a}$, $PGH_2$, $PGI_2$, or $TXA_2$) by one of the secondary enzymes named for the individual prostanoid produced (Figure 32-1). The type of prostanoid produced is determined

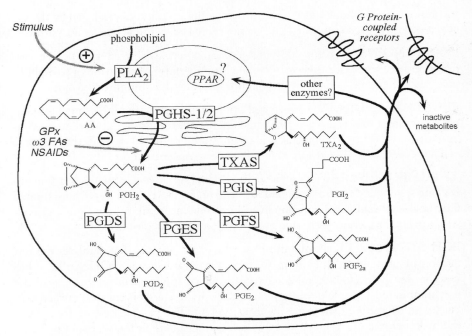

**Figure 32-1.** Diagram illustrating cell-signaling pathways involving prostanoids.

by which downstream enzyme is present; usually one downstream enzyme predominates in a given cell. For example, **the prominent secondary enzyme in platelets is thromboxane synthase,** whereas **vascular endothelial cells feature prostacyclin (PGI) synthase.** Prostanoid signaling molecules usually exit the cell that produces them to act on G-protein coupled receptors on the surface of the same cell or cells nearby (termed autocrine or paracrine actions). Some prostanoids may be further metabolized to ligands for a subset of nuclear receptors, the peroxisome proliferator-activated receptors (PPARs). The active prostanoids are rapidly converted to inactive metabolites by enzymes present in a variety of cells. As a result, prostanoid signaling molecules have very short half-lives in the circulation and are not hormones in the conventional sense.

Conversion of arachidonate to $PGH_2$ **is a key regulatory step in prostanoid biosynthesis.** Each PGHS isoform catalyzes 2 separate reactions (Figure 32-2). The first reaction (**arachidonate** $\rightarrow PGG_2$) involves insertion of 2 molecules of oxygen and cyclization of the fatty acid backbone. This step is catalyzed by the **COX** activity of PGHS-1 or -2; it is these COX activities (also called COX-1 and COX-2) that are **inhibited by** NSAIDs. The **second step** ($PGG_2 \rightarrow PGH_2$) involves the **reduction of the hydroperoxide** on C15 to an alcohol and is **catalyzed by the peroxidase activity of PGHS-1 or -2.**

Although both PGHS isoforms have cyclooxygenase and peroxidase activities and are structurally similar proteins, they have very distinct pathophysiologic

**Figure 32-2.** Steps in conversion of arachidonic acid to $PGH_2$ by PGH synthase. A cosubstrate, indicated by e⁻, is required to furnish 2 reducing equivalents for the peroxidase reaction.

**Figure 32-3.** Structures of some cyclooxygenase inhibitors.

functions. Many cells, including platelets and gastric mucosal cells, have moderate levels of the "basal" isoform, PGHS-1. Functions attributed to PGHS-1 include regulating hemostasis and vascular tone, renal function, and maintaining gastric mucosal integrity. A smaller number of cells, such as macrophages, vascular endothelial cells, and fibroblasts, dramatically upregulate levels of the "inducible" isoform, PGHS-2, in response to cytokines or mitogens. PGHS-2 has been implicated in cell proliferation, inflammation, carcinogenesis, and parturition.

Many COX inhibitors have been developed and their structures are quite varied (Figure 32-3). All known inhibitors compete with fatty-acid substrate for binding to the cyclooxygenase site on the enzyme. **Aspirin** was one of the earliest NSAIDs discovered and is now widely used as an analgesic and antiinflammatory agent. More recently, aspirin has emerged as a very useful **antithrombotic agent** because of its action against **platelet COX activity.** Aspirin shows both archetypal modes of COX inhibition. The first mode involves rapid reversible binding of inhibitor (I) at the COX site of the enzyme (E) to form an EI complex; the second mode involves a slower conversion of EI to a higher affinity complex, EI' (Equation 1).

$$E + I \leftrightarrow EI \rightarrow EI' \qquad \text{Equation 1}$$

EI and EI' cannot bind fatty acid and thus neither can catalyze the cyclooxygenase reaction. For **aspirin, conversion of EI to EI' is accompanied by covalent modification of the protein, making the transition irreversible.** Formation of the EI' complex produces a more powerful COX inhibition because the inhibitor is not readily displaced by substrate and because inhibition persists even when free inhibitor is removed. **Flurbiprofen and indomethacin** form EI' complexes with both PGHS-1 and -2, although they do not covalently modify either protein. Ibuprofen forms only EI complexes with both PGHS isoforms. The coxibs (such as celecoxib and rofecoxib) derive their exquisitely selective inhibition of PGHS-2 cyclooxygenase from their ability to form noncovalent EI' complexes with PGHS-2 and not with PGHS-1. This selectivity has made coxibs useful for anti-inflammatory and antiproliferative therapy with reduced GI adverse events, but it also makes them ineffective as antiplatelet agents and, consequently, can increase cardio-vascular risks.

## COMPREHENSION QUESTIONS

32.1 The coxibs, including celecoxib, are a recently developed class of NSAIDs. The coxibs show anti-inflammatory actions without affecting platelet function. These effects of the coxibs are best attributed to selective inhibition of which of the following?

A. The cytosolic isozyme of phospholipase $A_2$ ($cPLA_2$)

B. The COX activity of the "basal" prostaglandin H synthase isozyme (PGHS-1)

C. The COX activity of the "inducible" PGHS-2

D. The microsomal isozyme of prostaglandin E synthase (mPGES-1)

32.2 Prostaglandins comprise a family of oxygenated lipid signaling molecules derived from polyunsaturated fatty acids such as arachidonic acid. They are involved in regulating a number of cellular processes. Some of the prostaglandins act to increase vasodilation and levels of cAMP in cells, whereas others increase vasoconstriction and bronchoconstriction and smooth-muscle contraction. In the conversion of arachidonic acid to prostaglandins, the oxygenation step is accomplished by the enzyme that synthesizes which of the following compounds?

A. Prostaglandin $D_2$

B. Prostaglandin $E_2$

C. Prostaglandin $F_{2\alpha}$

D. Prostaglandin $H_2$

E. Prostaglandin $I_2$

32.3 Signaling via prostanoids begins by interaction of the prostanoid with its receptor. The receptor involved is usually located in which part of the cell?

A. Plasma membrane of a cell near the cell making the prostanoid

B. Nucleus of a cell in a different organ from the cell making the prostanoid

C. Endoplasmic reticulum of the cell making the prostanoid

D. Lysosomes of a cell circulating in the blood

E. Golgi of a cell circulating in the blood

# ANSWERS

32.1 **C.** The coxibs were designed to inhibit the activity of the inducible form of PGH synthase so as not to inhibit the constitutive production of prostaglandins and thromboxanes. They inhibit the first step in the process, which is catalyzed by the COX activity of PGH synthase-2.

32.2 **D.** The first step in the synthesis of prostaglandins and thromboxanes is the reaction catalyzed by the cyclooxygenase activity of PGHS. This reaction causes the cyclization of the fatty acid while at the same time introducing an unstable endoperoxide between carbons 9 and 10 and a hydroperoxide at carbon 15 to produce $PGG_2$, which is rapidly reduced to $PGH_2$ by the peroxidase activity of PGHS.

32.3 **A.** The prostanoids have a wide variety of physiologic effects, but they regulate these processes locally by binding to a receptor on the plasma membrane of a cell close to where the prostanoid was synthesized. Binding of the prostanoid to the receptor usually activates a GTP-binding protein, which acts to activate (or inhibit) adenylate cyclase or the phosphatidylinositol cascade.

## BIOCHEMISTRY PEARLS

▶ Conversion of arachidonate to $PGH_2$ via COX catalysis is a key regulatory step in prostanoid biosynthesis.

▶ Aspirin has emerged as a very useful antithrombotic agent because of its action against platelet COX activity.

▶ The coxibs (such as celecoxib) derive their exquisitely selective inhibition of COX-2 cyclooxygenase from their ability to form noncovalent EI′ complexes with COX-2 and not with COX-1.

▶ The selectivity of coxibs for COX-2 over COX-1 gives them anti-inflammatory and antiproliferative actions with reduced GI adverse events, but it also makes them ineffective as antiplatelet agents, thus increasing the risks of myocardial infarction and stroke.

## REFERENCES

Blobaum AL, Marnett LJ. Structural and functional basis of cyclooxygenase inhibition. *J Med Chem.* 2007;50(7):1425-1441.

Funk CD. Prostaglandins and leukotrienes: advances in eicosanoid biology. *Science.* 2001;294(5548):1871-1875.

Grosser T, Fries S, FitzGerald GA. Biological basis for the cardiovascular consequences of COX-2 inhibition: therapeutic challenges and opportunities. *J Clin Invest.* 2006;116(1):4-15.

Parfitt JR, Driman DK. Pathological effects of drugs on the gastrointestinal tract: a review. *Hum Pathol.* 2007;38(4):527-536.

A 28-year-old Lebanese man presents to your office with complaints of fatigue and difficulty catching his breath with his normal exercise routine since recently visiting his wife's family. He states he is otherwise healthy. He denies fever/chills/nausea/vomiting/diarrhea. He reports no sick contacts or travel other than to his in-law's house where he ate their famous fava bean soup. Upon further questioning, he reports that his urine has become much more concentrated and dark despite adequate fluid intake. On examination, he is an ill appearing male who appears fatigued/pale. His sclera are icteric and is conjunctiva are pale. His heart rate is slightly tachycardic at 110 beats/minute and his capillary refill is delayed. The remainder of the examination is unremarkable. Urinalysis is collected and revealed very dark urine. His hematocrit is 21% (normal: 40%–49%).

► What is the most likely diagnosis?
► What is the inheritance pattern of this disorder?

# ANSWERS TO CASE 33:
## Glucose 6-Phosphate Dehydrogenase Deficiency

*Summary*: A 28-year-old Lebanese man with new onset fatigue, shortness of breath, jaundice, and anemia following a recent travel to in-law's home where he ate fava bean soup.

- **Likely diagnosis**: Acute hemolytic anemia caused by underlying G6PD deficiency.

- **Inheritance pattern**: X-linked (predominantly seen in males)

## CLINICAL CORRELATION:

Glucose 6-phosphate dehydrogenase (G6PDH) is an X-linked genetic condition that causes instability to the red cell membrane leading to rupture. Fava beans precipitate acute hemolytic anemia in individuals with low levels of G6PDH and, thus, lowered levels of NADPH, reducing equivalents to suppress oxidative damage. Oxidative radical formation damages and compromises the integrity of the red blood cell membrane, leading to hemolysis (hemolytic anemia) and the clinical symptoms described in the case. In addition to Fava bean ingestion, other common causes of glucose-6-dehydrogenase deficiency hemolytic anemia include drugs (primaquine), chemicals (moth balls, aniline dyes, henna compounds), infection (*Escherichia coli*, *Salmonella*), and diabetic ketoacidosis (DKA). Patients confirmed to have this deficiency must be aware of these triggers.

# APPROACH TO:
## Glucose 6-Phosphate Dehydrogenase Deficiency

## OBJECTIVES

1. Describe how NADPH is produced in the red blood cell and its role in maintaining erythrocyte integrity.

2. Explain how dietary challenges can lead to hemolysis in individuals with low G6PDH activity.

3. Recognize the inheritance pattern and population distribution of G6PDH deficiencies.

## DEFINITIONS

**ACUTE HEMOLYTIC ANEMIA:** A pathologic condition in which there is a sudden drop in the number of circulating erythrocytes precipitated by an acute challenge which overwhelms the ability of the erythrocyte to defend against an oxidative attack on the lipids of the erythrocyte membrane resulting in membrane rupture.

**GLUCOSE 6-PHOSPHATE DEHYDROGENASE (G6PDH):** The enzyme catalyzing the rate limiting step of the hexose monophosphate shunt which provides reducing equivalents in the form of NADPH required to inactivate oxygen radicals attacking erythrocyte membrane lipids and protecting the erythrocyte membrane from rupture.

**FAVA BEAN:** *Vicia faba*, a bean of the species *Fabaceae*. It is native to the regions of Southwest Asia and North Africa and is cultivated widely around the world. Evidence indicates that the Fava bean had been cultivated in the Eastern Mediterranean since 6000 BC, if not earlier.

**VICINE, CONVICINE, DIVICINE, AND ISOURAMIL:** Compounds active in precipitating acute hemolytic anemia resulting from ingestion of fava beans by an individual with compromised G6PDH activity. Vicine and convicine are the naturally occurring glycosides while divicine and isouramil are the aglycones resulting from enzymatic removal of the glucoside moiety.

## DISCUSSION

Hemolytic anemia is a condition in which erythrocytes are unable to transport sufficient oxygen to tissues throughout the body to meet the demands for energy generation through metabolism, usually due to premature destruction of red blood cells. The condition may be of either extrinsic or intrinsic origin. Defects in the structural properties of the red blood cell membrane and abnormalities in the proteins (eg, enzymes) within the erythrocyte are intrinsic causes of hemolytic anemia, while abnormalities in erythropoiesis, blood clots in the small vessels, certain infections and the "side effects" of certain therapeutic drugs constitute extrinsic causes of hemolytic anemia. Hemolytic anemias may also be described as chronic (eg, a defect in hemopoiesis) or chronic (eg, an infection or the side effect of a drug or dietary component). Hemolytic anemia arising as a consequence of a deficiency in G6PDH is described as intrinsic (enzyme deficiency) and acute because persons with this condition are free of symptoms until the erythrocytes come into contact with specific toxic drugs or dietary components. In this case, the event prompting the episode of acute hemolytic anemia is the ingestion of fava beans. This sensitivity to fava beans is well known in persons of Mediterranean, Middle Eastern, and African lineages, and it requires a genetic deficiency in G6PDH and a dietary issue, infection, or drug agent for expression of symptoms.

The genetic trait is carried on the X-chromosome at position g28. Because the trait is X-linked and recessive, the condition is more prevalent in males than in females, who would require 2 copies of the altered allele for expression of the condition. More than 400 variant alleles have been identified each leading to reduced G6PDH activity.

### Role of Glucose 6-Phosphate Dehydrogenase in Maintenance of Erythrocyte Membrane Integrity

G6PDH is the first enzyme of 3 and the rate limiting step of the hexose monophosphate shunt (pentose shunt), which oxidizes glucose-6-phosphate to ribulose-5-phosphate, $CO_2$, and 2 molecules of NADPH (shown schematically in Figure 33-1). The product of G6PDH activity is 1 NADPH and gluconolactone-6-P,

**Figure 33-1.** The glutathione reductase and peroxidase system. Glucose 6-phosphate dehydrogenase catalyzes the reaction represented by the first downward arrow in the 3-step conversion of glucose 6-phosphate to ribulose 5-phosphate. This conversion supplies the NADPH that reduces oxidized glutathione (GS-SG). The reduced glutathione (GSH) is used by glutathione peroxidase to reduce organic hydroperoxides to alcohols.

which undergoes hydrolysis by the enzyme gluconolactone-6-P lactonase to form 6-phosphogluconate. A third enzyme, 6-phosphogluconate dehydrogenase, oxidizes 6-phosphogluconate to $CO_2$, ribulose-5-P and the second molecule of NADPH. The $K_m$ values of the dehydrogenases for NADP$^+$ and the $K_i$ values for NADPH are quite close, such that the enzymes are highly regulated, essentially making an NADPH when one is used.

At the opposite end of the scheme shown in Figure 33-1 is illustrated the ultimate use of the NADPH reducing equivalents in the maintenance of red blood cell membrane integrity. Membrane fatty acyl residues present in the phospholipid bilayer can undergo oxidation to form fatty acyl hydroperoxides (R-HCH-CH$_2$-R), which weaken the membrane, making it more susceptible to rupture as the red blood cell squeezes through the narrow diameters of the capillary beds in tissues. Reducing equivalents convert the hydroperoxide to a hydroxyl substituent, making the membrane less susceptible to rupture. This process requires the use of an intermediate carrier of reducing equivalents reduced glutathione and 2 additional enzymes, glutathione reductase, which transfers electrons from NADPH to oxidized glutathione, and glutathione peroxidase, which uses reduced glutathione to reduce the hydroperoxide moiety to the hydroxyl level generating oxidized glutathione as a second product.

If a male has one of the mutations expressing low activity of G6PDH, then he will be at risk for an episode of hemolytic anemia if he eats a meal containing fava beans. The symptoms develop because the deficient G6PDH activity is not able to prevent red blood cell membrane destruction (hemolysis) after eating the fava bean meal. After the fava bean digestion products are eliminated, normal erythropoieses will replace the missing red blood cells and the symptoms will be abated.

### Role of Fava Beans in Prompting a Hemolytic Episode

The active components causing hemolytic episodes in persons with deficient G6PDH activity have been identified as the alkaloid β-glucosides vicine and convicine (Figure 33-2). These 2 compounds give rise by deglycosylation to the 2 aglycones divicine and isouramil, which also cause red blood cell hemolysis. In fact, divicine has been shown to be more toxic to erythrocytes than vicine and seems to be a direct cause of favism—erythrocyte hemolysis following exposure to these compounds. As seen in Figure 33-2, the structures of divicine and isouramil are redox active,

**Figure 33-2.** Structures of the alkaloid glucosides vicine and convicine present in fava beans. Each is metabolized to the corresponding aglycones, divicine, and isouramil.

allowing the reduction of the quinone form to the hydroxyl form and the reverse process as well. These compounds can be reduced with NADPH as the ultimate electron donor, and in individuals with deficient G6PDH activity the capacity to provide reducing equivalents is quickly overwhelmed. This makes possible the formation of superoxide anion ($O_2^{\bullet-}$) and the hydroxyl radical ($OH^{\bullet}$) which can damage lipids in the membrane, predisposing the red blood cell to rupture by the physical pressures exerted on the erythrocyte as it traverses the narrows of the capillary network. The result is acute hemolytic anemia prompted by ingestion of fava beans.

## COMPREHENSION QUESTIONS

33.1  A young otherwise healthy male patient complains of weakness and has a low erythrocyte count. You suspect a recent hemolytic crisis and check his erythrocytes and G6PDH levels. His erythrocyte count is down and his G6PDH is normal. You know that the pathway for protecting the erythrocyte membrane from damage is complex and that glutathione peroxidase is involved. Peroxidases use reducing equivalents produced by metabolism from glucose to reduce organic hydroperoxides to the hydroxyl level. Which of the following statements best describes the action of glutathione peroxidase?

A. Glutathione peroxidase reduces glutathione disulfide back to reduced glutathione.

B. Glutathione peroxidase produces 1 molecule of $CO_2$ in its reaction cycle.

C. Glutathione peroxidase requires a selenium ion cofactor.

D. Glutathione peroxidase reduces organic hydroperoxides to organic hydroxyl compounds.

E. Glutathione peroxidase can use NADPH or NADH directly as a source of reducing equivalents.

33.2 A patient in your care has had a hemolytic crisis event and you have on your differential diagnosis notes that the event may indicate a dysfunction of G6PDH. You know that G6PDH in the red blood cell uses glucose 6-phosphate from the glycolytic pathway to form NADPH through a series of reactions. A person with deficient G6PDH would be expected to have all of the following characteristics except which of the following?

A. Increased proportion of glucose metabolism to pyruvate versus ribulose 5-phosphate than in normal

B. Decreased glutathione reductase activity

C. Decreased glutathione peroxidase activity

D. Increased reduction of organic hydroperoxides to hydroxyl products

E. Decreased production of gluconolactone-6-phosphate

33.3 During your third year, while on your hematology rounds, you are assigned a patient who has had an episode of hemolysis. Based on his recent consumption of fava bean soup and his Middle Eastern heritage you suspect a fava bean induced episode of active oxygen radicals may have caused the hemolysis. You know that fava beans contain divicine, isouramil, and aglycones that are redox active, permitting the transfer of electrons from one compound to another. When oxygen radical species are formed in individuals with deficient G6PDH activity, membrane lipids can undergo hydroperoxide formation. Which of the following statements is least accurate about erythrocytes in your patient?

A. Red blood cell membrane elasticity is reduced.

B. Red blood cells are more easily hemolyzed.

C. Red blood cells are more permeable.

D. Red blood cells easily traverse capillary beds.

E. Red blood cells are less able to reduce fatty acyl hydroperoxides to hydroxyl forms.

33.4 A young male patient with an episodic hemolytic crisis returns to your clinic several months later with another episode. He did not follow your advice to avoid certain foodstuffs. You now have another opportunity to pinpoint the precise cause of the malady. You know that G6PDH, the rate-limiting step of the hexose monophosphate shunt is regulated by the ratio of NADPH/NADP$^+$ and that changes in binding efficiency could change the ability to protect the erythrocyte. Which condition would signal the enzyme to increase its activity?

| Condition | NADPH/NADP$^+$ | Fatty Acyl Peroxide Content | Vicine + Convicine Concentration |
|---|---|---|---|
| A | ↓ | ↓ | ↓ |
| B | ↑ | ↑ | ↑ |
| C | ↓ | ↑ | ↑ |
| D | ↑ | ↓ | ↓ |
| E | ↑ | ↑ | ↓ |

# ANSWERS

33.1 **D.** Glutathione peroxidase is the enzyme active in removing hydroperoxide products, resulting from reactive oxygen species attacks on membrane fatty acid substituents. Glutathione reductase reduces glutathione disulfide to reduced glutathione. 6-phosphogluconate dehydrogenase produces a molecule of $CO_2$, an NADPH and ribulose-5-phosphates. Glutathione reductase requires a selenium cofactor. Glutathione peroxidase can only use reduced glutathione as an electron donor not NADPH and not NADH.

33.2 **D.** If G6PDH is deficient, then the pathway stops there and no reduced glutathione can be produced and, therefore, no removal of hydroperoxides occurs.

33.3 **D.** Erythrocytes with fatty acyl hydroperoxides have "stiff" membranes, which cannot squeeze through the smaller diameters of the capillaries. Membrane permeability is increased and the erythrocytes rupture rather than pass through the capillaries.

33.4 **C.** Elevated NADPH levels would inhibit G6PDH activity because [NADP$^+$], a required substrate for the reaction, is decreased. Thus, choices B, D, and E can be eliminated. Decreased membrane fatty acyl hydroperoxide content would require less peroxidase activity and, therefore, less G6PDH activity, whereas elevated levels would tend to increase G6PDH activity if NADPH levels are reduced. Elevated vicine and convicine levels would increase membrane fatty acid hydroperoxide content, thus an increased need for peroxidase activity, and, therefore, increased G6PDH activity if NADPH levels are low. Choice A can be eliminated because there is a lack of a need for G6PDH activity due to low levels of acyl hydroperoxides and vicine/convicine. Condition C will tend to increase G6PDH activity.

## BIOCHEMISTRY PEARLS

▶ Glucose-6-dehydrogenase deficiency is an X-linked inherited disease.

▶ Glucose-6-dehydrogenase aids in the conversion of glucose-6-phosphate to 6-phosphogluconate with resultant NADPH formation.

▶ NADPH reducing equivalents act to suppress oxidative damage to the red blood cell membrane. Patients with this deficiency do not have the NADPH reducing ability, leading to red blood cell membrane instability and hemolysis.

▶ Consumption of fava beans is only one potential triggering agent of hemolysis in patients with this deficiency. Other etiologies include drugs, chemicals, infection, and DKA.

# REFERENCES

McMillan DC, Bolchoz LJC, Jollous, DS. Favism: effect of divicine on rat erythrocyte sulfhydryl status, hexose monophosphate shunt activity, morphology and membrane skeletal proteins. *Toxicol Sci.* 2001;62:353-359.

Glader B, Schrier S, Mahoney D, Landaw S. Clinical Manifestations of Glucose-6-phosphate Dehydrogenase Deficiency. www.uptodate.com.

A 49-year-old woman presents to your clinic for follow-up after initiating a new medication (lovastatin) for her elevated cholesterol. She is currently without complaints and is feeling well. On repeat serum cholesterol screening, there is noted to be a decrease in the cholesterol level. The patient asks if she needs to continue the medication and what the potential side effects and benefits might be. Her physician explains that this medication inhibits the rate-limiting step and key enzyme in cholesterol biosynthesis.

▶ What is the mechanism of action of this medication?

# ANSWER TO CASE 34:
## Statin Medications

*Summary:* A 49-year-old woman with history of elevated cholesterol on lovastatin that appears to be improving serum cholesterol levels.

- **Mechanism action of lovastatin:** β-Hydroxy-β-methylglutaryl coenzyme A (HMG CoA) reductase inhibitor.

## CLINICAL CORRELATION

Hyperlipidemia is one of the most treatable risk factors of coronary heart disease. Initially, when the fasting low-density lipoprotein (LDL) cholesterol is measured and found to be elevated, lifestyle modification is recommended such as dietary adjustments, exercise, and weight loss. The lipids are measured again after a 3- to 6-month interval. If the LDL cholesterol level is again found to be above threshold, then pharmacologic therapy is entertained. One of the most common medications is a statin agent, acting to inhibit HMG-CoA reductase. The potential side effects include elevated liver function tests, increased muscle creatine phosphokinase (CPK) secondary to myopathy and rarely rhabdomyolysis. Other agents that may be considered include bile acid sequestrants, nicotinic acid, fibric acid, and fish oils.

# APPROACH TO:
## Cholesterol Synthesis

### OBJECTIVES

1. Describe the role of HMG-CoA reductase in cholesterol synthesis.
2. Explain the mechanism of action of statin medications.
3. Describe how cholesterol gives rise to the steroid hormones.
4. Be aware that niacin decreases lipolysis in adipose tissue and very-low-density lipoprotein (VLDL) synthesis in liver.

### DEFINITIONS

**CYTOCHROME P450 ENZYME SYSTEM:** The cytochromes P450 are mixed-function oxidases that require both NADPH and $O_2$. They are involved in a number of reactions in the conversion of lanosterol to cholesterol, as well as important steps in the synthesis of steroid hormones. Cytochromes P450 are very important in the detoxification of xenobiotics and in the metabolism of drugs.

**HMG CoA REDUCTASE:** β-Hydroxy-β-methylglutaryl-CoA reductase; the enzyme that catalyzes the rate limiting and committed step in the synthesis of cholesterol. It converts β-hydroxy-β-methylglutaryl-CoA (HMG-CoA) to mevalonate.

**ISOPRENOID:** Any of a number of hydrophobic compounds derived from the polymerization of isopentenyl pyrophosphate and its isomer, dimethylallyl pyrophosphate. The isoprene unit is a 5-carbon branched hydrocarbon (2-methyl-1, 3-butadiene).

**STATIN:** Any of a number of drugs that competitively inhibit the rate-limiting enzyme in cholesterol biosynthesis, HMG-CoA reductase.

## DISCUSSION

Cholesterol is mainly synthesized in the liver by a 3-stage process. All 27 carbon atoms in the cholesterol molecule are derived from acetyl-CoA. The first stage is the synthesis of the activated 5-carbon isoprene unit, **isopentenyl pyrophosphate.** Six molecules of isopentenyl pyrophosphate then condense to form **squalene** in a sequence of reactions that also synthesize isoprenoid intermediates that are important in protein isoprenylation modifications. The characteristic 4-ring structure of cholesterol is then formed by cyclizing of the linear squalene molecule. Several demethylations, the reduction of a double bond, and the migration of another double bond result in the formation of cholesterol. Figure 34-1 provides an overview of cholesterol biosynthesis.

The key enzyme in the synthesis of cholesterol is β-hydroxy-β-methylglutaryl-CoA reductase **(HMG-CoA reductase), which catalyzes the synthesis of mevalonate from HMG-CoA in an irreversible, rate-limiting reaction.** Mevalonate

**Figure 34-1.** Overview of cholesterol synthesis.

Figure 34-2. General biosynthetic pathway of the steroid hormones.

is the immediate 6-carbon precursor to isopentenyl pyrophosphate. HMG-CoA reductase is localized on the membrane of the endoplasmic reticulum and spans the membrane. The active site for this enzyme is found on the cytosolic side of the membrane. HMG-CoA reductase is inhibited by cholesterol in a feedback mechanism and the levels of mRNA for the enzyme are also regulated by the levels of cholesterol. Low concentrations of cholesterol increase the level of messenger RNA (mRNA) for HMG-CoA reductase, whereas high concentrations of cholesterol decrease the mRNA level. Because the enzyme HMG-CoA reductase is the **rate-limiting step** of cholesterol biosynthesis, this enzyme is the target for many cholesterol-lowering drugs.

The 5 major classes of **steroid hormones** are derived from cholesterol by the pathway illustrated in Figure 34-2. Hydroxylation is important in these conversions. The hydroxylation reactions require NADPH and $O_2$ and are carried out by the **cytochrome P450 enzyme system. The enzyme 21-hydroxylase is required for the synthesis of mineralocorticoids and glucocorticoids.**

Another important hormone derived from cholesterol is **vitamin D.** This steroid-like hormone is involved in regulating calcium and phosphorus metabolism. The complete synthesis of vitamin D requires **ultraviolet light** to convert 7-dehydrocholesterol to previtamin $D_3$. The reaction scheme is shown in Figure 34-3. The active hormone 1,25-dihydroxycholecalciferol (calcitriol) requires reactions that occur in the liver and kidneys and acts in a manner similar to steroid hormones to activate transcription, thereby regulating gene expression.

Lovastatin is a member of a class of drugs (atorvastatin and simvastatin are others in this class) called statins that are used to treat hypercholesterolemia. **The statins act as competitive inhibitors of the enzyme HMG-CoA reductase.** These molecules mimic the structure of the normal substrate of the enzyme (HMG-CoA) and act as transition state analogues. Although the statins are bound to the enzyme, HMG-CoA cannot be converted to mevalonic acid, thus inhibiting the whole cholesterol biosynthetic process. Recent studies indicate that there may be important secondary effects of statin therapy because some of the medical benefits of statins are too rapid to be a result of decreasing atherosclerotic lesions. Statin therapy has been associated with reduced risks of dementia, Alzheimer disease, ischemic cerebral stroke,

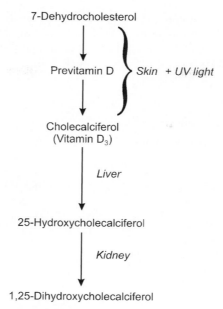

7-Dehydrocholesterol

Previtamin D      } *Skin + UV light*

Cholecalciferol
(Vitamin D$_3$)

*Liver*

25-Hydroxycholecalciferol

*Kidney*

1,25-Dihydroxycholecalciferol

**Figure 34-3.** Biosynthesis of active vitamin D$_3$.

and other diseases that are not correlated with high cholesterol levels. Although this is still an active area of research, it appears that the pleiotropic effects of statins may be a result of a reduction in the synthesis of isoprenoid intermediates that are formed in the pathway of cholesterol biosynthesis.

Niacin is a vitamin that is used in high doses to treat hypercholesterolemia. Niacin acts to decrease VLDL and LDL plasma levels. Its mechanism of action is not clearly understood but probably involves inhibition of VLDL secretion, which in turn decreases the production of LDL. Niacin inhibits the release of free fatty acids from adipose tissue, which leads to a decrease of free fatty acids entering the liver and decreased VLDL synthesis in the liver. This decreases the availability of VLDL for conversion to LDL (containing cholesterol esters). Niacin also increases high-density lipoprotein (HDL; the "good cholesterol") by an unknown mechanism.

## COMPREHENSION QUESTIONS

34.1 Which of the following compounds directly inhibits the expression of the HMG-CoA reductase gene?

A. Squalene

B. HMG-CoA

C. Lanosterol

D. Isopentenyl pyrophosphate

E. Cholesterol

34.2 You decide to treat a patient who has very high levels of serum cholesterol with the statin drug atorvastatin. You know that this drug acts in the metabolic pathway leading to the synthesis of cholesterol. The substrate for the enzyme inhibited by the statin drugs is which of the following?

A. Acetoacetyl-CoA
B. HMG-CoA
C. Farnesol pyrophosphate
D. Isopentenyl pyrophosphate
E. Mevalonate

34.3 Which of the following vitamins can be used in high doses to treat hypercholesterolemia?

A. Niacin
B. Riboflavin
C. Pyridoxine
D. Folic acid
E. Thiamine

## ANSWERS

34.1 **E.** The major regulatory enzyme of cholesterol metabolism, HMG-CoA reductase, is regulated by 3 distinct mechanisms. The first is phosphorylation by a cAMP dependent protein kinase. Phosphorylation of HMG-CoA reductase inactivates the enzyme. The other 2 mechanisms involve the levels of cholesterol. The degradation of the enzyme is controlled by cholesterol levels. The half-life of HMG-CoA reductase is regulated by cholesterol levels with high concentrations of cholesterol leading to a shorter half-life. The final regulatory mechanism involves control of the expression of the HMG-CoA reductase gene. High levels of cholesterol lead to a decrease in the mRNA levels coding for HMG-CoA reductase.

34.2 **B.** The first step in the biosynthesis of cholesterol is the condensation of 2 molecules of acetyl-CoA to form acetoacetyl-CoA. The addition of a third acetyl CoA molecule gives rise to HMG-CoA. HMG-CoA reductase is converted to mevalonate. HMG-CoA reductase is the target of the statin drugs and the substrate used by this enzyme is HMG-CoA.

34.3   **A.** Niacin is the vitamin that can be used, in high doses, to treat hypercholes-terolemia. Niacin acts to decrease VLDL and LDL plasma levels. Its mechanism of action is not clearly understood but probably involves inhibition of VLDL secretion, which, in turn, decreases the production of LDL. Niacin inhibits the release of free fatty acids from adipose tissue, which leads to a decrease of free fatty acids entering the liver and decreased VLDL synthesis in the liver. This decreases the availability of VLDL for conversion to LDL (containing cholesterol esters). Niacin also increases HDL (the "good cholesterol") by an unknown mechanism.

## BIOCHEMISTRY PEARLS

▶ **HMG-CoA reductase** catalyzes the synthesis of mevalonate from HMG-CoA in an irreversible rate-limiting reaction.

▶ The enzyme 21-hydroxylase is required for the synthesis of mineralocorti-coids and glucocorticoids.

▶ The statins act as competitive inhibitors of the enzyme HMG-CoA reductase.

## REFERENCES

Berg JM, Tymoczko JL, Stryer L. *Biochemistry.* 5th ed. New York: Freeman; 2002:722-731.

Devlin TM, ed. *Textbook of Biochemistry with Clinical Correlations.* 7th ed. New York: Wiley-Liss; 2010.

Granner DK. The diversity of the endocrine system. In: Murray RK, Bender DA, Botham KM, et al, eds. *Harper's Illustrated Biochemistry.* 29th ed. New York: Lange Medical Books/McGraw-Hill; 2012.

Liao JK. Isoprenoids as mediators of the biological effects of statins. *J Clin Invest.* 2002;110(3):285-288.

Mayes PA, Botham KM. Cholesterol synthesis, transport, & excretion. In: Murray RK, Bender DA, Botham KM, et al, eds. *Harper's Illustrated Biochemistry.* 29th ed. New York: Lange Medical Books/McGraw-Hill, 2012.

Goldberg AC. *The Merck Manual of Diagnosis and Therapy.* 19th ed. Whitehouse Station, NJ: Merck Sharp & Dohme Corp.; 2013. http://www.merckmanuals.com/professional/endocrine_and_metabolic_disorders/lipid_disorders/overview_of_lipid_metabolism.html.

A 9-year-old boy is brought to the emergency department (ED) by his parents after 2 days of worsening nausea/vomiting and abdominal pain. The abdominal pain is located in the epigastric region and radiates to his back. He has had several episodes of similar pain in the past but none quite as severe as this one. His parents deny fever/chills and change in bowel habits. In the ED, the patient is afebrile and in moderate distress. Both the liver and spleen appear to be enlarged and he has epigastric tenderness. Several small yellow-white papules were noted on his back and buttocks. Laboratory tests reveal elevated amylase and lipase levels. On further questioning, the father reports having high triglyceride levels and several members of the mother's family have had early heart disease. Laboratory tests performed after hospitalization revealed elevated triglyceride levels and reduced lipoprotein lipase (LPL) activity.

▶ What is etiology of the boy's abdominal pain?
▶ What is the likely underlying biochemical disorder?
▶ What is the role of lipoprotein lipase?

# ANSWERS TO CASE 35:

## Hypertriglyceridemia (Lipoprotein Lipase Deficiency)

*Summary:* A 9-year-old boy with acute abdominal pain consistent with pancreatitis, hepatosplenomegaly, eruptive xanthomas, and a family history of hypertriglyceridemia and heart disease.

- **Etiology of abdominal pain:** Acute pancreatitis

- **Underlying biochemical disorder:** Disorder of lipoprotein metabolism

- **Role of lipoprotein lipase:** Hydrolysis of triglycerides from very-low-density lipoprotein (VLDL) and chylomicrons

## CLINICAL CORRELATION

LPL is an enzyme found on the capillary endothelial surface of adipose tissue, heart, and skeletal muscle, and it is required, along with apoC-II, for the hydrolysis of triglycerides. ApoC-II, found on the surface of chylomicrons and VLDL, serves as an activator of LPL. A deficiency in LPL results in elevated levels of triglycerides (VLDL and chylomicrons). The cholesterol level may be normal or slightly elevated. LPL deficiency is inherited in an autosomal recessive pattern. Patients with LPL deficiency often present with recurrent episodes of pancreatitis in their childhood and may have other clinical signs of hypertriglyceridemia, including xanthomas, hepatosplenomegaly, and lipemia retinalis. Reduced serum LPL activity, following an injection of intravenous heparin, confirms the diagnosis of either LPL or apoC-II deficiency. The initial therapeutic intervention consists primarily of dietary modification (reduction of fat intake).

# APPROACH TO:

## Lipid Transport

### OBJECTIVES

1. Describe the metabolism and transport of lipoproteins.

2. Understand the rationale for serum blood test results with the different hypertriglyceridemias.

### DEFINITIONS

**APOLIPOPROTEIN C-II (APOC-II):** The apolipoprotein on the surface of chylomicrons and VLDLs that binds to and activates lipoprotein lipase.

**APOLIPOPROTEIN E (APOE):** The apolipoprotein on the surface of several lipoproteins including chylomicrons, chylomicron remnants, very-low-density lipoprotein (VLDL), VLDL remnants, and intermediate-density lipoprotein (IDL). It mediates the binding of apoE-containing lipoproteins with the LDL receptor and the chylomicron remnant (apoE) receptor.

**LIPOPROTEIN LIPASE (LPL):** An enzyme bound to the surface of the capillary endothelium by heparan sulfate proteoglycans. LPL catalyzes the hydrolysis of triglyceride in chylomicrons and VLDL to free fatty acids and glycerol.

**HEPATIC LIPASE (HL):** An enzyme bound to the surface of sinusoidal endothelial cells of liver. It catalyzes the hydrolysis of mono-, di-, and triglycerides as well as the phospholipids phosphatidyl choline and phosphatidyl ethanolamine.

## DISCUSSION

Triglycerides (TGs) are safely transported in the bloodstream packaged into lipoproteins called chylomicrons or VLDLs. Chylomicrons are formed in the epithelial cells of the intestine and are responsible for the transport of dietary lipids. VLDL is synthesized in the liver and transport endogenously synthesized lipids from the liver to peripheral tissues. Both of these lipoproteins are composed of a core composed primarily of TGs enveloped by a monolayer composed of phospholipids, free cholesterol, and apolipoproteins.

Dietary triglycerides are hydrolyzed by pancreatic lipase in the lumen of the small intestine. Colipase, a protein secreted along with pancreatic lipase, binds to the TG and the pancreatic lipase and improves the hydrolytic process. TG is broken down to free fatty acids and 2-monoacylglycerols, which form micelles along with bile salts and other lipid soluble compounds such as cholesterol and fat-soluble vitamins. The free fatty acids and monoglycerides are absorbed by the microvilli of the intestinal epithelial cells. In the epithelial cell, the fatty acids and monoglycerides are reformed into triglycerides, which are packaged with phospholipids, cholesterol, and apolipoprotein B-48 into chylomicrons.

The newly synthesized chylomicrons are secreted into the lymph and enter the bloodstream via the thoracic duct. In the bloodstream, the chylomicron particles obtain proteins from high-density lipoproteins (HDLs), including apoC II and apoE, which are important for the function of the chylomicron (Figure 35-1).

In the capillary beds in adipose tissue, muscle tissue (especially cardiac muscle) and in lactating mammary glands, apoC II binds to and activates LPL, which is bound to the endothelial surface of the capillaries by heparan sulfate. LPL hydrolyzes the TG in the core of the chylomicron to free fatty acids and glycerol. The fatty acids are taken up by the adipose or muscle cells; glycerol is recycled back to the liver. In muscle, the fatty acids are oxidized to produce ATP and in adipose they are reformed into TG for storage. The TG-depleted chylomicron remnant remains in the blood stream until it binds to the chylomicron remnant receptor located on hepatocytes, a process mediated by apoE. The remnants are taken into the hepatocytes by endocytosis and degraded in the lysosome to fatty acids, amino acids, cholesterol, glycerol, and phosphate.

**Figure 35-1.** Formation and metabolism of chylomicrons. (Abbreviations used are defined in the enclosed box.)

Chylomicrons appear in the blood stream shortly after consumption of a meal containing fat. However, the clearance rate for chylomicrons is fast and blood is usually free of chylomicrons following an overnight fast.

VLDLs are lipoproteins synthesized in the liver from endogenous TG, cholesterol, and phospholipids, along with several apolipoproteins including, apoB-100, apoE, and apoC-II. Following synthesis, the VLDL is secreted into the bloodstream, where it obtains more apoE and apoC II from HDL (Figure 35-2). In a process similar to that of chylomicron degradation, the VLDL apoC-II binds to and activates LPL in the capillary beds of adipose, muscle, and mammary tissue. LPL degrades the VLDL TG core, releasing free fatty acids and glycerol. About one-half of the resulting VLDL remnants bind to receptors in liver cells that recognized apoE and are taken up by endocytosis. The remaining VLDL receptors are further degraded to IDLs, which have their residual TG removed by the action of hepatic lipase to yield low-density lipoproteins (LDLs). HL is synthesized and secreted from liver and is tethered to the external surfaces of liver cells by heparan sulfate. LDL is taken up by receptor-mediated endocytosis upon binding to the LDL receptor in liver and peripheral tissues.

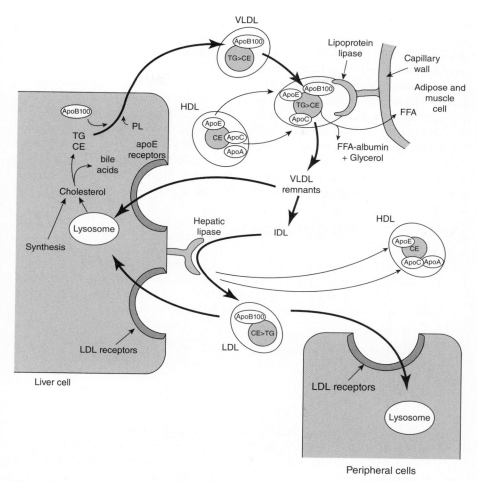

**Figure 35-2.** Formation of very-low-density lipoprotein and metabolism into low-density lipoprotein. (Abbreviations are as used in Figure 35-1.)

Elevated serum TG levels can occur due to a number of factors. Hypertriglyceridemia can be the result of a genetic disorder in one of the proteins involved in lipoprotein metabolism, or it can arise secondarily to a number of other disorders, including diabetes mellitus, obesity, and alcohol abuse, and as an adverse event of some medications such as β-blockers, oral estrogens, and some diuretics. Genetic deficiencies in LPL, apoC-II, or HL can give rise to elevations in circulating TG, as can cause an overproduction of apoB-100 or increased apoE$_2$ levels. ApoE$_2$ has a decreased affinity for hepatic receptors than apoE$_3$ and chylomicron remnants and VLDL remnants containing apoE$_2$ are cleared more slowly from the circulation.

The most common genetic defect leading to hypertriglyceridemia is a deficiency in LPL, which results in increased levels of both chylomicrons and VLDL. Individuals who are homozygous for the defective gene usually present with symptoms of chylomicronemia (TG levels > 2000 mg/dL, abdominal pain, pancreatitis, xanthomas, lipemia retinalis) in childhood. Clinical diagnosis of LPL deficiency requires measurement of LPL activity in plasma following intravenous injection of heparin, which displaces the LPL from its heparan sulfate tether. However, heparin also releases HL into the plasma and the postheparin plasma must be treated with antibodies specific to HL to remove it. Alternatively, LPL can also be measured in adipose tissue, which has no HL activity. A deficiency in apoC II will also show evidence of decreased postheparin plasma LPL activity. An increase in LPL activity when normal apoC II is added to the assay indicates that a defect in apoC-II is the culprit.

A deficiency in HL can also lead to elevated plasma TG levels, however, these increases in TG are usually found in VLDL remnants, LDL, and HDL, which all become more buoyant in their densities. Definitive diagnosis of HL deficiency is made by demonstrating the absence of HL activity in postheparin plasma.

## COMPREHENSION QUESTIONS

35.1   A teenage boy presents with moderate to severe epigastric pain. Physical examination reveals extensive eruptive xanthomas and hepatosplenomegaly. A blood sample reveals milky plasma. Which of the following is the most likely lipoprotein to be elevated in this patient's plasma?

A.   Chylomicrons

B.   Chylomicron remnants

C.   HDL

D.   IDL

E.   LDL

35.2   Laboratory results for a patient with uncontrolled type 1 diabetes mellitus reveal hyperglycemia (634 mg/dL) and hypertriglyceridemia (498 mg/dL). The most likely cause of the hypertriglyceridemia in this patient is which of the following?

A.   Deficiency in apoprotein C-II

B.   Increased hepatic triglyceride synthesis

C.   Decreased lipoprotein lipase activity

D.   Deficiency in LDL receptors

E.   Absence of hormone sensitive lipase

35.3  A 25-year-old woman was referred to a lipid research center for investigation of moderate hypertriglyceridemia because the plasma lipid and lipoprotein profiles showed abnormalities. Both HDL and LDL were more buoyant and showed elevations in TG content with the mass of TG approximately the same as that of cholesterol. A deficiency in which of the following is the most likely cause of this patient's lipid abnormality?

A.  Lecithin-cholesterol acyltransferase

B.  Lipoprotein lipase

C.  Apoprotein C-II

D.  Hepatic lipase

E.  Apoprotein B-100

# ANSWERS

35.1  **A.** This patient presents with classical symptoms of hypertriglyceridemia: milky plasma, eruptive xanthomas, enlarged liver and spleen, and symptoms of pancreatitis. The milky plasma is due to abnormally high chylomicron levels, indicating that TG is not being removed from the transporter of dietary TG and it is accumulating in the plasma. The other lipoproteins listed have low levels of TG are much smaller and would not be expected to lead to milky plasma if elevated.

35.2  **C.** Decreased lipoprotein lipase activity is the result of the failure of the pancreatic β cells to produce and secrete insulin. Insulin stimulates the synthesis of lipoprotein lipase; in the absence of insulin, lipoprotein lipase activity in the capillary beds is low. While a deficiency in apoC-II would also lead to hypertriglyceridemia, this genetic defect is rare. If a patient with type I diabetes mellitus is not given insulin, then the increased glucagon–insulin ratio would stimulate gluconeogenesis and β oxidation in the liver rather than synthesis of triglycerides. Neither a deficiency of LDL receptors nor hormone-sensitive lipase would be expected to increase circulating TG levels.

35.3  **D.** Hepatic lipase. The abnormal buoyancies of the LDL and HDL fractions due to their increased TG content indicate that IDL is not being processed to LDL and HDL is not being remodeled. Both of these processes are accomplished by hepatic lipase. A deficiency in lecithin-cholesterol acyltransferase would lead to elevated serum cholesterol levels, almost all as free cholesterol. Deficiencies in lipoprotein lipase or apoC-II would lead to hypertriglyceridemia as increased chylomicrons and/or VLDL. An apoB-100 deficiency would lead to increased levels of LDL, but they would have the normal TG/cholesterol ratio.

## BIOCHEMISTRY PEARLS

▶ TGs are safely transported in the bloodstream packaged into lipoproteins called chylomicrons or VLDLs.

▶ The most common genetic defect leading to hypertriglyceridemia is a deficiency in lipoprotein lipase, which results in increased levels of both chylomicrons and VLDL.

▶ Individuals who are homozygous for the defective gene for lipoprotein lipase usually present with symptoms of chylomicronemia (TG levels > 2000 mg/dL, abdominal pain, pancreatitis, xanthomas, lipemia retinalis) in childhood.

## REFERENCES

Brunzell JD, Deeb SS. Familial lipoprotein lipase deficiency, apo C-II deficiency, and hepatic lipase deficiency. In: Scriver CR, Beaudet AL, Sly WS, et al, eds. *The Metabolic and Molecular Bases of Inherited Disease*. 8th ed. New York: McGraw Hill; 2001.

Haymore BR, Parks JR, Oliver TG, et al. Hypertriglyceridemia. *Hosp Physician*. 2005;41(3):17-24.

During your medical school training, you spend some time in a pediatric clinic in a third-world country. One of the first patients you encounter is an 8-month-old girl brought to the clinic because of excessive exhaustion and fatigue. On further questioning of the mother, she reports that she was previously breast-feeding but had to stop to return to work. To feed all of her other children, she has had to dilute her formula with water to make the formula last longer for the entire family. After your physical examination is performed, you diagnose the infant with severe malnutrition and aid the mother with resources to increase food intake for their household.

▶ What is this syndrome called (with deficiencies in both calories and protein)?
▶ What is the difference between this syndrome and kwashiorkor syndrome?
▶ What physical findings might differentiate the 2 syndromes?

# ANSWERS TO CASE 36:
## Starvation

*Summary:* An 8-month-old girl presents with exhaustion and excessive starvation secondary to deficient intake of calories and protein.

- **Diagnosis:** Marasmus

- **Differences:** Marasmus has inadequate total caloric intake, whereas kwashiorkor is due to a lack of protein intake.

- **Physical findings of kwashiorkor and not marasmus:** Subcutaneous fat, distended abdomen, hepatomegaly, and fatty liver.

## CLINICAL CORRELATION

Protein-energy malnutrition is caused by inadequate food intake or diseases interfering with food absorption or digestion. The 2 major types of malnutrition are marasmus and kwashiorkor. In marasmus, a child usually between the ages of 1 to 3 years has inadequate caloric intake leading to loss of subcutaneous fat, loose wrinkled skin, and either flat or distended abdomen resulting from atrophic abdominal wall muscles. Often, children are susceptible as they go from breast milk to solid food. The affected child usually has the appearance of an "old person's face." In kwashiorkor, the main issue is lack of protein, leading to edema, sparse hair, enlarged liver, and a distended abdomen. The edema of the face and legs is different from that of marasmus. The therapy for both of these diseases is caloric replacement.

# APPROACH TO:
## Starvation-Related Diseases

## OBJECTIVES

1. Describe the metabolic changes in starvation.
2. Explain the increased formation of ketone bodies in starvation.
3. Describe the oxidation of fatty acids.
4. Contrast the metabolic change in fasting states as compared to starvation.

## DEFINITIONS

**MARASMUS:** Malnutrition resulting from inadequate intake of protein and calories.

**KWASHIORKOR:** Malnutrition resulting from inadequate intake of protein though the intake of total calories is adequate.

**KETONE BODIES:** The short chain fatty acid metabolites acetoacetate, β-hydroxybutyrate, and acetone.

**TRIGLYCERIDE:** A glycerol molecule with each hydroxyl group esterified with a fatty acid moiety.

**DIGLYCERIDE:** A glycerol molecule with 2 hydroxyl groups esterified with a fatty acid moiety.

**MONOGLYCERIDE:** A glycerol molecule with one hydroxyl group esterified with a fatty acid moiety.

## DISCUSSION

Malnutrition and its ultimate form starvation arise from many different causes and are present even in affluent societies. The case description reveals that the child lives in a third-world country, and the physical findings reveal that the child is experiencing protein-calorie-deficient starvation, or marasmus.

Fasting and starvation represent changes from the baseline metabolic interactions between tissues that exist in the fed state. Each of 3 states—fed, fasting, and starvation—must be considered from the standpoint of the whole body primarily because the constituent tissues have different requirements for their nutritional sources. For example, **red blood cells have an absolute requirement for glucose as the exclusive food source from which energy is derived.** Although other tissues use fatty acids and amino acids as well, the red blood cell cannot because it lacks mitochondria and therefore the enzymes required for most of the metabolic steps required in β-oxidation of fatty acids and metabolism of the carbon skeletons of amino acids. **Brain tissue normally has an exclusive preference for glucose,** the exception being in **advanced starvation** when the **brain** can use **ketone bodies** for energy production.

The metabolic interactions of tissues in the fed state are shown in Figure 36-1. Glucose, fatty acids from triglycerides, and amino acids are provided by the diet and used differentially by the tissues. In the **liver, glucose is used for storage as glycogen or converted to fatty acids for formation into triglycerides for storage in adipose tissue.** Amino acid carbon skeletons are used for metabolic intermediates for energy production or fatty acid synthesis. Resting muscle takes up glucose and stores it as glycogen and uses amino acids for protein synthesis. Resting muscle prefers fatty acids and ketone bodies rather than glucose to satisfy its energy demands. In adipose tissue, glucose and fatty acids are taken up. Glucose metabolism provides energy and glycerol 3-phosphate for triglyceride formation and storage using fatty acids transported to adipose cells as triglycerides in lipoprotein particles. The brain and red blood cells take up glucose from blood to meet energy demands.

During circumstances of no food intake for 16 to 20 hours (the postfeeding state), substantial changes occur in the interactions between tissues (Figure 36-2). The liver shifts from consumption of glucose for glycogen storage to mobilization of its glycogen stores to release glucose to the bloodstream to supply the glucose requirements of the brain and red blood cell. Because the hepatic glycogen supply is depleted fairly quickly, metabolic signals increase liver gluconeogenesis, depleting

**Figure 36-1.** The metabolic flow during the fed state. Increased blood glucose triggers release of insulin and a decrease in the release of glucagon and lipolytic hormones.

tricarboxylic acid cycle intermediates and prompting the use of **amino acid carbon skeletons from protein breakdown for new glucose formation.** The energy required for gluconeogenesis is derived by increasing the β-oxidation of fatty acids mobilized from adipose storage sites. Fatty acid synthesis is simultaneously inhibited to prevent a futile cycle. As the tricarboxylic acid cycle's supply of 4-carbon intermediates in liver mitochondria is drained for gluconeogenesis, rapid β-oxidation of fatty acids produces acetyl-CoA faster than the tricarboxylic acid cycle can metabolize the carbon atoms of acetyl-CoA to $CO_2$ and free CoA. The result is a high ratio of acetyl-CoA to free CoA and thus a slowing of β-oxidation and compromise of liver mitochondrial ATP formation. The conversion of the free CoA pool to acetyl-CoA is reversed by the formation of the **ketone body acetoacetate** (and later its reduced product, β-hydroxybutyrate), regenerating free CoA (Figure 36-3). This occurs only in liver mitochondria because of its critical role in gluconeogenesis. The ketone bodies are transported out of the liver mitochondria and the liver into the bloodstream for transport to other tissues where they reenter metabolism by being converted to

## POSTFEEDING FAST (16-20hr)

Figure 36-2. The metabolic flow following a postfeeding fast. Blood glucose levels begin to decrease, triggering homeostatic mechanisms to prevent it from dramatically decreasing.

acetoacetyl-CoA at the expense of succinyl-CoA and then cleaved by β-ketothiolase to produce 2 molecules of acetyl-CoA for metabolism in the TCA cycle.

The β-oxidation of fatty acids that occurs in the mitochondrial matrix provides the energy for gluconeogenesis in the liver. Fatty acids transported from adipose tissues by blood albumin cross the hepatic plasma membrane and are activated by fatty acid thiokinases, producing fatty acid-CoA and requiring ATP (Figure 36-4). The fatty acids are transported across the mitochondrial inner membrane as carnitine derivatives utilizing the carnitine shuttle. All the rest of the reactions occur in the mitochondrial matrix beginning with the oxidation of the fatty acid by flavin adenine dinucleotide (FAD)-linked fatty acyl-CoA dehydrogenase producing

**Figure 36-3.** Mobilization of fatty acids during times in which the liver is synthesizing glucose via the gluconeogenic pathway. The β-oxidation of fatty acids by the liver produces the energy needed for gluconeogenesis; however, because the TCA cycle is slowed because of depletion of $C_4$ acids (used for glucose synthesis), ketone bodies (acetoacetate and β-hydroxybutyrate) are formed from acetyl-CoA to regenerate CoA for continued β-oxidation. The ketone bodies are exported to extrahepatic tissues where they are used as an energy source.

*trans*-$\Delta^2$-enoyl-CoA. This product is hydrated by enoylhydratase producing L-3-hydroxyacyl-CoA. This product undergoes a second oxidation catalyzed by NAD-linked L-3-hydroxy fatty acyl-CoA dehydrogenase, producing 3-ketoacyl-CoA. This product is cleaved by β-ketothiolase, producing one molecule of acetyl-CoA and a new activated fatty acyl-CoA, 2 carbon atoms shorter than at the outset in a reaction that requires another molecule of free CoA. The newly produced fatty acyl-CoA repeats the cycle of steps in β-oxidation releasing another acetyl-CoA and onward until the last cleavage step that hydrolyzes acetoacetyl-CoA to 2 molecules of acetyl-CoA.

Although the postfeeding fast represents a normal state reflective of the alternation of feeding and not feeding, the starvation state shown in Figure 36-5 represents an abnormal state and reflects a dramatic increase in the metabolic changes observed in the postfeeding state, illustrated in Figure 36-3. Thus, starvation represents an

**Figure 36-4.** The activation of fatty acids and transport into the mitochondrion via the carnitine shuttle. (*Reproduced, with permission, from: D.B. Marks, et al,* Basic Medical Biochemistry: A Clinical Approach, *Philadelphia: Lippincott Williams & Wilkins, 1996:361.*)

intensification of the metabolic adjustments of the fasting state with some significant differences seen only in prolonged starvation. Two marked changes in plasma concentrations occur, a decrease in glucose concentration and a dramatic increase in the concentration of ketone bodies, reflecting altered metabolic poise. In the liver the tricarboxylic acid (TCA) cycle is slowed by the drainage of 4-carbon intermediates to gluconeogenesis, fatty acid breakdown continues apace, and body proteins continue to be broken down to replenish the tricarboxylic acid cycle intermediates. In muscle the fuels used for energy generation are fatty acids and ketone bodies. Muscle activity decreases as result of the mobilization of muscle protein, which itself slows as the period of starvation increases. In adipose tissue, the breakdown of triglycerides to fatty acids is accelerated. In the brain and the central nervous system (CNS) an adaptive change occurs, allowing this tissue to use ketone bodies as an energy source relieving both the total body demand for glucose and the use of muscle protein as a carbon source for gluconeogenesis in the liver. Ketone body concentration increases in the blood, reflecting the accelerated breakdown

## PROLONGED STARVATION

**Figure 36-5.** The metabolic flow during prolonged starvation. The brain adapts to use ketone bodies as a source of energy, thus decreasing its utilization of glucose.

of triglycerides in adipose tissue and the slower hepatic TCA cycle. In spite of the utilization of ketone bodies by peripheral tissues and the brain and CNS tissues after 5 to 6 weeks of starvation, ketone body blood levels rise, spill over into the urine and are excreted in significant quantity, wasting material that could be used for energy generation because the tissues capable of using ketone bodies as fuel are already using the maximum possible amount. Thus, the major differences between starvation and the postfeeding fast are the adaptive ability of the brain and central nervous system to use ketone bodies to satisfy some of their energy demand and in the levels of circulating ketone bodies that are high enough to spill over into the urine in significant quantities.

# COMPREHENSION QUESTIONS

36.1 In cases of starvation many metabolic changes take place to meet the metabolic demands of the body. Which of the following illustrates starvation-triggered changes in intermediary metabolism?

A. Increased dependence of liver on glucose for its energy supply

B. Increased synthesis of proteins in muscle tissue

C. Increased use of ketone bodies for energy source in brain

D. Decreased mobilization of triglycerides by adipose tissue

E. Adaptation of red blood cells to use ketone bodies for energy

Use the reactions below for question 36.2:

1. Acetoacetyl-CoA + acetyl-CoA → β-hydroxy-β-methylglutaryl-CoA + CoA

2. Acetoacetate + NADH → β-hydroxybutyrate + $NAD^+$

3. β-hydroxy-β-methylglutaryl-CoA + $H_2O$ → acetoacetate + acetyl-CoA

4. Acetyl-CoA + acetyl-CoA → acetoacetyl-CoA + CoA

5. Acetoacetate + succinyl-CoA → acetoacetyl-CoA + succinate

36.2 Using the above reactions, which of the following correctly describes the pathway of ketone body formation?

A. 3 → 2 → 1 → 4

B. 4 → 1 → 3 → 2

C. 4 → 2 → 3 → 1

D. 5 → 1 → 2 → 3

E. 5 → 2 → 3 → 1

36.3 During starvation muscle activity decreases, and muscle protein is broken down to provide a carbon source for the liver production of glucose via gluconeogenesis. Which of the following amino acids remains in the muscle cell to provide a source of energy for the muscle?

A. Alanine

B. Aspartate

C. Leucine

D. Glutamate

E. Threonine

## ANSWERS

36.1 **C.** In starvation a major metabolic adjustment is that the brain activates the ketone body metabolic pathway and uses ketone bodies for energy, thus sparing somewhat the breakdown of body proteins to generate amino acid carbon skeletons for gluconeogenesis in the liver. In cases of starvation, the liver derives most of its energy from β-oxidation of fatty acids. Muscle proteins are broken down to generate carbon skeletons during starvation. Triglyceride stores in adipose tissue are being used to provide fatty acids for β-oxidation in the liver. Red blood cells are not able to use ketone bodies because they have no mitochondria.

36.2 **B.** The synthesis of ketone bodies begins with the combination of 2 molecules of acetyl-CoA to generate one molecule of free CoA and a molecule of acetoacetyl-CoA, which combines with another molecule of acetyl-CoA to yield another free CoA molecule and β-hydroxy-β-methylglutaryl-CoA (HMG-CoA). HMG-CoA undergoes hydrolysis to produce 1 molecule acetyl-CoA and 1 molecule of acetoacetate, which can be reduced to β-hydroxybutyrate. The reaction of succinyl-CoA and acetoacetate is a reaction in the pathway of ketone body utilization but not in the pathway of ketone body formation.

36.3 **C.** None of the other amino acids listed, except for leucine, is a branched-chain amino acid. The muscle has a very active branched-chain amino acid metabolic pathway and uses that pathway to provide energy for its own use. The products of leucine metabolism are acetyl-CoA and acetoacetate, both of which are used in the TCA cycle. Acetoacetate is activated by succinyl-CoA and cleaved to 2 molecules of acetyl-CoA in the β-ketothiolase reaction. The other branched-chain amino acids, valine, and isoleucine, yield succinyl-CoA and acetyl-CoA as products of their catabolism.

## BIOCHEMISTRY PEARLS

▶ Red blood cells have an absolute requirement for glucose as the exclusive food source from which energy is derived.

▶ **Brain tissue normally has an exclusive preference for glucose,** the exception being in **advanced starvation** when the brain can use **ketone bodies** for energy production.

## REFERENCE

Devlin TM, ed. *Textbook of Biochemistry with Clinical Correlations.* 7th ed. New York: Wiley-Liss; 2010.

A 45-year-old man with history of hepatitis C infection and now cirrhosis of the liver is brought to the emergency department by family members after he experienced acute changes in his mental status. The family reports that the patient has been very disoriented and confused over the last few days and has been nauseated and vomiting blood. The family first noticed disturbances in his sleep pattern followed by alterations in his personality and mood. On examination, he is disoriented with evidence of icteric sclera. His abdomen is distended with a fluid wave appreciated. He has asterixis and hyperreflexia on neurologic exam. His urine drug screen and ethyl alcohol (EtOH) screen are both negative. A blood ammonia level was noted to be elevated, and all other tests have been normal.

▶ What is the most likely cause of the patient's symptoms?
▶ What is asterixis?
▶ What was the likely precipitating factor of the patient's symptoms?

# ANSWERS TO CASE 37:

## Cirrhosis

*Summary:* A 45-year-old man presents with cirrhosis, likely secondary to hepatitis C infection, with acute mental status change coinciding with the recent onset of hematemesis. Patient has an elevated serum ammonia level and otherwise negative workup.

- **Diagnosis:** Hepatic encephalopathy likely secondary to elevated ammonia levels.

- **Asterixis:** Nonspecific to hepatic encephalopathy. Nonrhythmic asymmetric tremor with loss of voluntary control of extremities while in a sustained position. It is also known as "liver flap."

- **Precipitating factor:** Increased nitrogen load from upper gastrointestinal bleed.

## CLINICAL CORRELATION

Cirrhosis is a chronic condition of the liver with diffuse parenchymal injury and regeneration leading to distortion of the liver architecture and increased resistance of blood flow through the liver. The patient usually manifests malaise, lethargy, palmar erythema, ascites, jaundice, and hepatic encephalopathy in the late stages. Toxins accumulating in the blood stream affect the patient's mental status. The most common etiologies of cirrhosis are toxins such as alcohol, viral infections such as hepatitis B or C infection, or metabolic diseases in children (Wilson disease, hemochromatosis, or $\alpha_1$-antitrypsin deficiency). Treatment depends on the exact etiology, although the common therapy includes avoidance of liver toxins, salt restriction, and possibly procedures to reduce the portal pressure.

# APPROACH TO:

## Amino Acid Metabolism and Ammonia

### OBJECTIVES

1. Describe the urea cycle.

2. Describe the strategy in amino acid metabolism.

3. Explain the biochemical means of removing excess ammonia.

### DEFINITIONS

**GLUTAMATE DEHYDROGENASE:** A mitochondrial enzyme present in all tissues that metabolizes amino acids. It catalyzes the oxidative deamination of glutamate to $\alpha$-ketoglutarate using $NAD^+$ as the electron acceptor to also produce nicotinamide adenine dinucleotide (NADH) and ammonia. The enzyme uses the reducing equivalents of nicotinamide adenine dinucleotide phosphate (NADPH) to perform the reverse reaction.

**ORNITHINE:** An α-amino acid similar in structure to lysine but having one methylene group less in the side chain. It is carbamoylated to form citrulline to begin the urea cycle and is regenerated in the final step that releases urea.

**TRANSAMINASE:** An aminotransferase; a pyridoxal phosphate-requiring enzyme that transfers an amino group from an α-amino acid to an α-keto acid.

**UREA CYCLE:** The series of reactions that occur in the liver to synthesize urea for the excretion of nitrogen. The 2 nitrogen atoms present in urea arise from ammonium ion and the α-amino group of aspartate. The cycle also requires $CO_2$ ($HCO_3^-$) and the expenditure of 4 high-energy phosphate bonds and produces fumarate.

## DISCUSSION

Amino acids differ from carbohydrates and fats in that they contain nitrogen as part of their molecular structure. For the carbons in amino acids to enter into the energy generating metabolic pathways, the amino groups must first be removed so that they can be detoxified and excreted. The amino acid nitrogen is excreted predominantly as urea, but some is also excreted as free ammonia in order to buffer the urine.

The **first step** in the **catabolism of most amino acids** is the **transfer of the α-amino group from the amino acid to α-ketoglutarate (α-KG).** This process is catalyzed by transaminase (aminotransferase) enzymes that require pyridoxal phosphate as a cofactor. The products of this reaction are glutamate (Glu) and the α-ketoacid analog of the amino acid destined for catabolic breakdown. For example, aspartate is converted to its α-keto analog, oxaloacetate, by the action of aspartate transaminase (AST), which also produces Glu from α-KG. The transamination process is freely reversible, and the direction in which the reaction proceeds is dependent on the concentrations of the reactants and products. These reactions do not effect a net removal of amino nitrogen; the amino group is only transferred from one amino acid to another.

For net removal of amino nitrogen, a second enzymatic reaction must take place that removes the amino group from Glu for disposal. The net removal of the amino nitrogen is accomplished by the mitochondrial enzyme **glutamate dehydrogenase (GDH),** which catalyzes the oxidative deamination of Glu to α-KG in a reaction that uses NAD⁺ as the electron acceptor. The enzyme can also catalyze the reverse reaction to produce Glu, but in this case it uses the reducing equivalents from NADPH instead of NADH. The oxidative deamination reaction is allosterically activated by adenosine diphosphate (ADP) and guanosine diphosphate (GDP), whereas the reductive amination is activated by GTP and adenosine triphosphate (ATP). The overall process for net removal of the amino group from α-amino acids is summarized in Figure 37-1.

**Ammonia is produced by almost all cells in the body; however, only the liver has the enzymatic machinery to convert it to urea.** Therefore, extrahepatic ammonia must be transported to the liver. However, ammonia in the blood is toxic

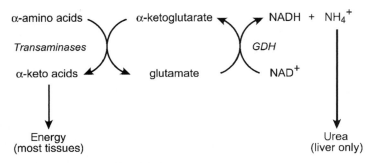

**Figure 37-1.** Summary of amino acid catabolism.

to cells, and therefore the nitrogen from amino acid catabolism is transported in blood either as glutamine or alanine. Glutamine is synthesized from Glu and ammonia in an ATP-requiring reaction catalyzed by glutamine synthetase. Alanine is formed from pyruvate in a transamination reaction catalyzed by alanine transaminase (ALT).

Glutamine and alanine are transported to the liver in the blood where they are taken up by cells in the periportal region. Ammonia is released by the combined action of ALT (in the case of alanine), glutaminase (in the case of glutamine), and GDH. The $\alpha$-amino group of alanine is transferred to $\alpha$-KG to form Glu and pyruvate. Glutaminase catalyzes the hydrolysis of the side-chain amide group releasing ammonia and Glu. Ammonia and Glu enter the mitochondria, where Glu is oxidatively deaminated by GDH. The ammonia that is released by glutaminase and GDH then enters the urea cycle (Figure 37-2), which includes enzymes that are located both in the mitochondria and the cytosol.

Ammonia is condensed with bicarbonate and ATP in the mitochondrion to form carbamoyl phosphate in a reaction catalyzed by carbamoyl phosphate synthetase I. Two molecules of ATP are used in this reaction; one provides the phosphate, and the other is hydrolyzed to ADP and inorganic phosphate ($P_i$) to provide the energy that drives the reaction to products. The activated carbamoyl group is then transferred to the amino acid ornithine by the mitochondrial enzyme ornithine transcarbamoylase to form citrulline. Citrulline then is transported out of the mitochondrion to the cytosol, where the rest of the reactions that are required to synthesize urea take place. The second nitrogen of urea comes directly from the amino acid aspartate. The side chain of citrulline condenses with the $\alpha$-amino group of aspartate to form argininosuccinate in a reaction that is thermodynamically driven by the conversion of ATP to AMP and inorganic pyrophosphate ($PP_i$). The rapid hydrolysis of $PP_i$ by pyrophosphatase releases energy and removes the $PP_i$, thus making the formation of argininosuccinate thermodynamically irreversible. Argininosuccinate is then cleaved to arginine and fumarate by argininosuccinase (argininosuccinate lyase). Arginase then hydrolyzes the guanidino group of arginine, releasing urea and regenerating ornithine, which can then re-enter the mitochondrion and accept another carbamoyl group from carbamoyl phosphate. The urea is transported to the kidney for excretion.

**Figure 37-2.** Urea cycle.

Glutamine is also used by the kidney as a source of ammonia that is used to buffer the urine. Ammonia is released from glutamine by the same enzymes that are active in the liver. The free ammonia accepts a proton to form ammonium ion, thus decreasing the acidity of the urine.

Although most of the ammonia detoxified by the liver arises from the breakdown of amino acids in dietary protein or endogenous protein that is being turned over, ammonia is also produced by bacteria in the gut. This is absorbed into the portal venous blood and directly taken to the liver for conversion into urea.

When liver function is severely impaired or when collateral links between the portal and venous blood vessels arise as occurs in **cirrhosis,** the **ability of the liver to detoxify ammonia to urea is compromised** resulting in **hyperammonemia.** This can be **exacerbated** by an **increase in the ammonia load,** such as can occur from **gastrointestinal bleeding.** When blood ammonia levels rise, ammonia builds up inside the cells and drives the GDH reaction to form Glu, thus depleting $\alpha$-KG stores and slowing the tricarboxylic acid (TCA) cycle. This is particularly devastating to the brain, which must have an active TCA cycle to produce the energy needed for brain function.

## COMPREHENSION QUESTIONS

37.1   An 8.5-month-old infant was admitted to the hospital in a coma and a temperature of 102.9°F (39.4°C). His pulse was elevated, his liver was enlarged, and findings on electroencephalography were grossly abnormal. Because the infant could not retain milk given by gavage feeding, intravenous glucose was administered. He improved rapidly and came out of the coma within 24 hours. Analysis of his urine showed abnormally high amounts of glutamine and uracil, which suggested a high blood ammonium ion concentration. The laboratory confirmed this. Considering the data, which enzyme may be defective in this patient?

A.   Arginase

B.   Carbamoyl phosphate synthetase I

C.   Glutamate dehydrogenase

D.   Glutaminase

E.   Ornithine transcarbamoylase

37.2   A newborn male infant was diagnosed as having phenylketonuria and is immediately placed on diet low in phenylalanine (Phe). Careful compliance with the diet and frequent monitoring of the patient's plasma Phe level resulted in the level being maintained at the lower limit of the normal range. The patient appeared to be developing normally until 4 months of age, when he developed truncal hypotonia and spasticity of the limbs. Despite being on a low-phenylalanine diet, at 5 months the patient had several grand mal (epileptic) seizures. After an abnormal Phe-loading test, the patient's urine was found to have a markedly elevated urinary biopterin concentration. Which of the following enzymes is most likely deficient in this patient?

A.   Dihydropteridine reductase

B.   GTP cyclohydrolase I

C.   Phenylalanine hydroxylase

D.   Tryptophan hydroxylase

E.   Tyrosine hydroxylase

37.3   Which treatment regimen would be most beneficial to this patient in question 37.2?

A.   A low-Phe diet with biopterin supplementation

B.   A low-Phe diet with cobalamin (vitamin $B_{12}$) supplementation

C.   A low-Phe diet + L-dopa (3,4-dihydroxyphenylalanine)

D.   A low-Phe diet + L-dopa and 5-hydroxytryptophan

E.   A diet completely free of Phe

# ANSWERS

37.1  **E.** The patient exhibits signs of a defect in the urea cycle. The presence of elevated uracil in addition to ammonia and glutamine points to an accumulation of carbamoyl phosphate. If ornithine transcarbamoylase is deficient, carbamoyl phosphate will accumulate in the mitochondria and leak into the cytosol, providing the starting compound for the synthesis of uracil.

37.2  **A.** The patient, despite being put on a low-Phe diet, exhibits neurologic problems resulting from an inability to synthesize catecholamine and indoleamine neurotransmitters. This is caused by a deficiency in dihydropteridine reductase (DHPR). DHPR regenerates tetrahydrobiopterin ($BH_4$), which is oxidized to dihydrobiopterin by phenylalanine hydroxylase, as well as tyrosine hydroxylase and tryptophan hydroxylase (tryptophan 5-monooxygenase). If phenylalanine hydroxylase were deficient, then a diet low in Phe would alleviate the effects. Because the urinary biopterin concentration is elevated, a deficiency in GTP cyclohydrolase I is eliminated because that is an enzyme in the biosynthetic pathway of $BH_4$. Phe hydroxylase, Tyr hydroxylase, and Trp hydroxylase activities are low because of a lack of $BH_4$.

37.3  **D.** Because of the DHPR deficiency, the activities of Phe hydroxylase and Tyr hydroxylase are low, hence the synthesis of catecholamine neurotransmitters are depressed. The synthesis of the indoleamine neurotransmitter serotonin is also depressed because $BH_4$ is required for the hydroxylation of tryptophan. The best treatment is to decrease the Phe load by a low-Phe diet and provide the precursors for the catecholamine and indoleamine neurotransmitters that occur after the enzymes affected by the deficiency of $BH_4$, which would be L-dopa and 5-hydroxytryptophan.

## BIOCHEMISTRY PEARLS

► Ammonia is produced by almost all cells in the body; however, only the liver has the enzymatic machinery to convert it to urea.

► Liver disease such as cirrhosis affects the ability of the liver to detoxify ammonia to urea resulting in hyperammonemia.

► Hyperammonemia can be exacerbated by an increase in the ammonia load, such as what can occur from gastrointestinal bleeding.

## REFERENCES

Coomes MW. Amino acid metabolism. In: Devlin TM, ed. *Textbook of Biochemistry with Clinical Correlations*. 7th ed. New York: Wiley-Liss; 2010.

Rodwell VW. Catabolism of proteins & of amino acid nitrogen. In: Murray RK, Bender DA, Botham KM, et al, eds. *Harper's Illustrated Biochemistry*. 29th ed. New York: Lange Medical Books/McGraw-Hill; 2012.

A 1-year-old girl is brought to her pediatrician's office with concerns about her development. She had an uncomplicated birth outside the United States at term. The mother reports that the baby is not achieving the normal milestones for a baby of her age. She also reports an unusual odor to her urine and some areas of hypopigmentation on her skin and hair. On examination, the girl is noted to have some muscle hypotonia and microcephaly. The urine collected is found to have a "mousy" odor.

▶ What is the most likely diagnosis?
▶ What is the biochemical basis of the hypopigmented skin and hair?

## ANSWERS TO CASE 38:

## Phenylketonuria

*Summary:* A 1-year-old girl born outside the United States with developmental delays, hypotonia, hypopigmentation, and foul smelling urine.

- **Likely Diagnosis:** Phenylketonuria (PKU)

- **Biochemical basis of hypopigmentation:** Phenylalanine is competitive inhibitor of tyrosinase (key enzyme in melanin synthesis)

## CLINICAL CORRELATION

Elevated phenylalanine can be caused by a variety of different enzyme deficiencies resulting in impaired conversion of phenylalanine to tyrosine. The most common deficiency is in phenylalanine hydroxylase (autosomal recessive) resulting in the classic picture of PKU. Two other enzyme deficiencies leading to PKU include dihydropteridine reductase and 6-pyruvoyl-tetrahydropterin synthase, an enzyme in the biosynthetic pathway of tetrahydrobiopterin. With PKU, the baby appears normal at birth but then fails to reach normal developmental milestones. If unrecognized, the child will develop profound mental retardation and impairment of cerebral function. A mousy odor of the skin, hair, and urine can often be detected clinically. Areas of hypopigmentation develop secondary to the disruption of melanin synthesis. In the United States, all children are screened for PKU in hopes to prevent the serious life-long complications. Treatment consists of dietary modifications with limitation of phenylalanine intake and supplementation of tyrosine. The diagnosis of PKU and initiation of diet modification must be implemented prior to 3 weeks of age to prevent mental retardation and the other classic signs of PKU.

## APPROACH TO:

## Phenylketonuria

### OBJECTIVES

1. Describe the biochemical conversion of phenylalanine to tyrosine.

2. Describe the biochemical events that occur when conversion of phenylalanine to tyrosine is inhibited.

### DEFINITIONS

**HYPOPIGMENTATION:** Lack of color in skin or hair due to the absence or low quantity of the skin and hair pigment melanin, a product of tyrosine (and phenylalanine) metabolism.

**TETRAHYDROBIOPTERIN:** A 4-electron-reduced form of the reducing agent biopterin required to supply electrons to phenylalanine hydroxylase for conversion of phenylalanine to its hydroxylated product, the amino acid tyrosine.

**PHENYLKETONURIA:** The presence of elevated amounts of phenylketones—primarily phenylpyruvate—in urine; a primary indication of disturbance of phenylalanine metabolism resulting from elevated transamination of phenylalanine due to reduction in phenylalanine hydroxylation to tyrosine.

## DISCUSSION

Phenylketonuria is a disease readily diagnosable in childhood, and it is important for an optimal clinical outcome for it to be diagnosed as early as possible. Laboratory tests can be performed in the neonatal period and now genetic testing can identify the trait before birth.

Phenylketonuria obtains from an elevated level of phenylpyruvate in the urine of the patient. As shown in Figure 38-1, phenylpyruvate is the cognate α-ketoacid of the amino acid phenylalanine. It is formed by transaminating phenylalanine and α-ketoglutarate to yield glutamate and phenylpyruvate. This reaction is freely reversible; therefore, it is driven by elevated concentrations of reactants or products. For large scale conversion of phenylalanine to phenylpyruvate an increase in the concentration of phenylalanine must occur to drive the transamination reaction toward the formation of phenylpyruvate. Such an elevated phenylalanine level will be reflected in the blood as hyperphenylalaninemia, which is defined as a plasma phenylalanine level above 120 μmol/L. The most likely cause is a disturbance in the phenylalanine hydroxylase reaction. Disease states resulting from disturbances of the phenylalanine hydroxylase reaction can be found (1) at the level of the enzymes in the reaction reflected in absent or altered proteins, (2) at the metabolic level reflected in cognate effects on other metabolic processes, and (3) at the cognitive level reflected in changes in brain function and mental retardation.

*Phenylalanine Hydroxylation Reaction and Its Components.* As shown in Figure 38-2, the phenylalanine hydroxylation reaction is the pathway whereby dietary phenylalanine can be converted into tyrosine relieving some of the dietary requirement for tyrosine. It is catalyzed by phenylalanine hydroxylase, a monooxygenase requiring molecular oxygen and a specific 2-electron donor tetrahydrobiopterin. One atom of

**Figure 38-1.** Transamination of phenylalanine to yield phenylpyruvate, a phenylketone.

**Figure 38-2.** Normal conversion of phenylalanine into the amino acid tyrosine catalyzed by phenylalanine hydroxylase.

molecular oxygen appears in the product tyrosine as a hydroxyl group in the para position, the remaining oxygen atom appearing in the product water.

The provision of reducing equivalents to phenylalanine hydroxylase is dependent on reduction of dihydrobiopterin by NADH catalyzed by the enzyme dihydropteridine reductase (Figure 38-2). This reduction is dependent on the availability of biopterin and therefore on the biopterin synthetic pathway. Thus, any genetic or protein folding defect in either dihydropteridine reductase or the biopterin biosynthetic enzymes would compromise the efficacy of phenylalanine hydroxylation to tyrosine resulting in hyperphenylalaninemia and also phenylketonuria resulting from increase transamination of phenylalanine to phenylpyruvate.

The principal enzyme in this pathway is phenylalanine hydroxylase. The gene for phenylalanine hydroxylase is located on chromosome 12 at band region q 23.2 and comprises 100 kb of genomic DNA. Several hundred alleles causing disease states have been recognized for this gene, more than 60% of which are classified as missense alleles. European and Chinese populations show 1 order of magnitude higher incidence than persons of African descent. This population specific expression of disease causing alleles may explain the wide range of incidence reported for this disease entity (5-350 cases/million live births).

## Fates of Tyrosine

Tyrosine can be degraded by oxidative processes to acetoacetate and fumarate which enter the energy generating pathways of the citric acid cycle to produce $CO_2$ and ATP as indicated in Figure 38-2. Tyrosine can be further metabolized to produce various neurotransmitters such as dopamine, epinephrine, and norepinephrine. Hydroxylation of tyrosine by tyrosine hydroxylase produces dihydroxyphenylalanine (DOPA). This enzyme, like phenylalanine hydroxylase, requires molecular oxygen and tetrahydrobiopterin. As is the case for phenylalanine hydroxylase, the tyrosine hydroxylase reaction is sensitive to perturbations in dihydropteridine reductase or the biopterin synthesis pathway, any one of which could lead to interruption of tyrosine hydroxylation, an increase in tyrosine levels, and an increase in transamination of tyrosine to form its cognate α-keto acid, para-hydroxyphenylpyruvate, which also would appear in urine as a contributor to phenylketonuria.

**Figure 38-3.** Conversion of tyrosine to dopaquinone by the enzyme tyrosinase, a $Cu^{+2}$-dependent enzyme in melanocytes.

Tyrosine is also the precursor to melanin formation in melanocytes, the first step of which is catalyzed by tyrosinase as shown in Figure 38-3. This reaction is a 2-step reaction in which DOPA is an intermediate in the formation of dopaquinone. Ring closure of the alanine portion of dopaquinone forms a pyrrole ring and subsequent reactions give rise to the melanins, the primary dark pigment associated with skin color being eumelanin. The absence of tyrosinase gives rise to classic albinism. Phenylalanine is a competitive inhibitor with tyrosine for tyrosinase. Thus in a situation wherein phenylalanine hydroxylase activity is deficient, not only does the α-keto cognate transamination product phenylpyruvate increase but so does the level of phenylalanine. Thus, excess phenylalanine inhibits tyrosinase and melanin formation resulting in hypopigmentation of skin and hair in affected persons.

## COMPREHENSION QUESTIONS

38.1  A 3-month-old boy presents with elevated levels of phenylalanine, para-hydroxyphenylpyruvate, and phenylpyruvate in the serum. His skin color is pale. Your differential diagnosis is PKU. Which of the following would be consistent in such a case?

A.  Elevated levels of homogentisic acid in the serum

B.  Deficiency in vitamin $B_{12}$ (cobalamin)

C.  Elevated levels of pyridoxal phosphate in the serum

D.  Urine in the boy's diaper smells like fresh maple syrup

E.  Phenylalanine hydroxylase activity is only 2% of normal

38.2 A 1-year-old girl presents at your clinic the day after you saw the 3-month-old boy. The symptoms are the same so you order a test on phenylalanine hydroxylase to confirm your diagnosis of phenylketonuria. To your surprise, the phenylalanine hydroxylase activity is well within the normal range. Which of the following might you check next to support your diagnosis?

A. Tyrosine: α-ketoglutarate transaminase

B. Tyrosinase

C. Homogentisic acid oxidase

D. Dihydropteridine reductase

E. Dopamine hydroxylase

38.3 Skin color is the aggregate result of the expression of a number of genes modified by ethnic origin and genetic inheritance. Hypopigmentation may be caused by which of the following?

A. Excess formation of melanin

B. Excess phenylalanine in the serum and tissues

C. Hyposecretion of melatonin

D. Excessive stimulation of tyrosinase

E. Low levels of para-hydroxyphenylpyruvate

## ANSWERS

38.1 **E.** The correct response is very low levels of phenylalanine hydroxylase, a key enzyme in the metabolic sequelae of phenylketonuria—ie, elevated phenylalanine, phenylpyruvate, and para-hydroxyphenylpyruvate in blood. Homogentisic acid is an intermediate in the breakdown of tyrosine to fumarate and acetoacetate. Vitamin $B_{12}$ is required in the metabolism of branched-chain amino acids not phenylalanine. The α-keto acids of the branched chain amino acids produce the maple-syrup odor.

38.2 **D.** The correct response is dihydropteridine reductase. This enzyme reduces dihydrobiopterin to tetrahydrobiopterin the obligate electron donor for phenylalanine hydroxylase. Tyrosinase is the first enzyme on the pathway to melanin. Dopamine hydroxylase and tyrosine transaminase are enzymes on other tyrosine metabolic tracts. Homogentisic acid oxidase is an enzyme on the pathway of tyrosine to fumarate and acetoacetate.

38.3 **B.** Excess phenylalanine inhibits tyrosinase the first step toward melanin production, thus resulting in hypopigmentation. Excess melanin leads to hyperpigmentation. Melatonin is a hormone involved in the sleep cycle. Excessive stimulation of tyrosinase would lead to more melanin and therefore hyperpigmentation. Para-hydroxyphenylpyruvate means less transamination and perhaps more tyrosine converted to melanin and hyperpigmentation.

## BIOCHEMISTRY PEARLS

▶ PKU is an autosomal recessive disorder of amino acid metabolism affecting approximately 1 out of 10,000 of infants in North America.

▶ It is most often due to deficiency of the enzyme phenylalanine hydroxylase, which causes the accumulation of harmful metabolites, including phenylketones.

▶ The gene for phenylalanine hydroxylase is located on chromosome 12 at band region q 23.2.

▶ If untreated, PKU may lead to mental retardation, seizures, psychoses, eczema, and a distinctive "mousy" odor.

▶ PKU is a disease readily diagnosable in childhood and it is important for an optimal clinical outcome for it to be diagnosed as early as possible.

## REFERENCES

Devlin TM, ed. *Textbook of Biochemistry with Clinical Correlations.* 7th ed. New York: Wiley-Liss; 2010.

Scriver CR, Beaudet AL, Sly WS, et al. *The Metabolic and Molecular Basis of Inherited Disease.* 8th ed, New York: McGraw Hill; 2001:1667-1776.

The mother of a 16-year-old girl calls the clinic because of concerns about her daughter's eating habits. The mother states that she will not eat anything and is obsessed with exercise and losing weight. She also states that her daughter has been more withdrawn from friends and family. After discussion with the mother, the patient comes in for a physical examination. The patient is 5 foot 1 inch tall and weighs 85 pounds. She is in no acute distress but appears to have a depressed affect. The patient states she is worried that her friends will think she is fat if she eats more. She denies any binge eating. Her physical examination is normal, other than dry skin and thin fine hair on extremities. Laboratory tests reveal that she is anemic and has a low albumin and magnesium level. She has normal liver and thyroid tests.

- ► What is the most likely diagnosis?
- ► What potential medical problems may develop in a patient with this disorder?
- ► How can this disorder affect her menstrual cycles?

# ANSWERS TO CASE 39:
## Anorexia Nervosa

*Summary:* A thin 16-year-old girl who is obsessed with her body appearance and weight to the point of not wanting to eat and is excessively exercising.

- **Diagnosis:** Anorexia nervosa. This is differentiated from bulimia because she denies binge eating with associated guilty feelings.
- **Medical complications:** Dry skin, lanugo, bradycardia, hypotension, dependent edema, hypothermia, anemia, osteoporosis, infertility, cardiac failure, and death.
- **Menstrual complications:** Amenorrhea secondary to depression of the hypothalamic-pituitary axis. Infertility will result secondary to anovulation.

## CLINICAL CORRELATION

Anorexia nervosa is a disease affecting primarily young women who have distorted body images. Although their weight is less than 30% below ideal body weight, they see themselves as overweight. Anorectics often use diuretic and laxative agents to accomplish their weight loss. Patients with bulimia, who usually induce emesis, may be at normal weight or even above ideal body weight; by contrast, anorectics are almost always under ideal body weight. Often, affected individuals become amenorrheic, have fine lanugo hair, and become hypothermic. Therapy must be multifaceted and include family and individual counseling, behavioral modification, and possibly medication. Severe cases may be fatal.

# APPROACH TO:
## Amino Acid and Negative Protein Balance

### OBJECTIVES

1. Describe protein digestion and amino acid absorption.
2. Explain how nitrogen is added and removed from amino acids.
3. Describe amino acid metabolism in various tissues (muscle, gastrointestinal [GI], kidney).
4. List the special products derived from amino acids.

### DEFINITIONS

**ANOREXIA NERVOSA:** A mental disorder in which the patient has an extreme fear of becoming obese and an aversion to food. The disorder usually occurs in young women and can result in death if the condition is not successfully treated.

**NITROGEN BALANCE:** The condition wherein the amount of nitrogen ingested (via protein) is equal to that excreted. **Negative nitrogen balance** is a condition wherein more nitrogen is excreted than ingested, usually during prolonged periods of calorie restriction. Positive nitrogen balance results when more nitrogen is ingested than excreted, as in growing children.

**PYRIDOXAL PHOSPHATE:** The coenzyme that is required for transaminase (aminotransferase) reactions, as well as other enzymes. It is the active form of pyridoxine (vitamin $B_6$).

## DISCUSSION

Proteins are polymers of $\alpha$-amino acids covalently linked via peptide bonds. $\alpha$-Amino acids consist of a central ($\alpha$) carbon atom to which an amino group, a carboxylic acid group, a hydrogen atom, and a side-chain group are covalently linked. **Twenty different amino acids are used for protein synthesis, each of which is encoded by at least 1 codon (the 3 nucleotide genetic code) and differ only in their side-chain group.** Amino acids can be divided into 2 classes, essential and nonessential amino acids. **Essential amino acids cannot be synthesized by humans** (unlike nonessential amino acids) and, thus, must be ingested to meet the requirements of the organism. Certain nonessential amino acids can become pseudoessential if the starting material from which they are synthesized becomes limiting (eg, methionine-derived cysteine). Amino acids are also used for the synthesis of nonprotein biomolecules (eg, nucleotides, neurotransmitters, antioxidants), as well as participating in critical whole body processes, such as interorgan nitrogen transfer and acid–base balance. Unlike carbohydrate and fatty acids, **no storage form of excess amino acids exists** per se. Instead, dietary amino acids in excess to the body's synthetic needs are used as an energy source and/or **converted to glycogen and lipid.** During periods of **insufficient nutrient ingestion** (eg, starvation, anorexia nervosa), **noncritical skeletal muscle and liver proteins are preferentially degraded** to release utilizable amino acids, to meet both the biosynthetic and energy needs of the body (Figure 39-1).

The **major sites of ingested protein digestion are the stomach and the small intestine.** Gastric, pancreatic, and intestinal peptidases hydrolytically cleave peptide bonds. The released amino acids, dipeptides, and tripeptides are transported into small intestinal epithelial cells, wherein dipeptides and tripeptides are further degraded to free amino acids. The latter are subsequently released into the circulation. A healthy, well-fed adult is generally in nitrogen balance. This means that the amount of nitrogen ingested (as protein) is equal to that excreted (primarily as urea). When rates of dietary amino acid incorporation into new protein exceed rates of amino acid degradation and nitrogen excretion, the individual is said to be in positive nitrogen balance. Growing children are normally in positive nitrogen balance. By contrast, an individual is said to be in **negative nitrogen balance when more nitrogen is excreted than ingested.** This occurs during prolonged periods of calorie restriction (eg, starvation, anorexia nervosa), when protein is degraded to release amino acids as an utilizable energy source.

A general tactic employed during catabolism of amino acids is the removal of the $\alpha$-amino group, followed by conversion of the remaining carbon skeleton into a

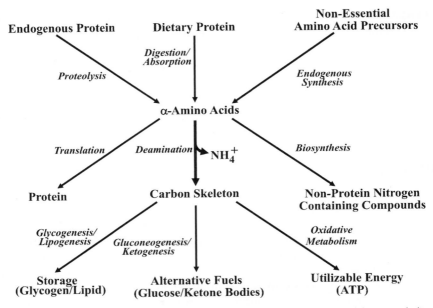

**Figure 39-1.** Schematic diagram showing the source and utilization of α-amino acids in metabolic processes.

major metabolic intermediate. The **main way in which α-amino groups are removed** is through **transamination,** the transfer of an amino group from an α-amino acid to an α-keto acid. This transamination reaction is catalyzed by a class of enzymes called transaminases (or aminotransferases). These enzymes use pyridoxal phosphate, a vitamin $B_6$ derivative, during the catalytic process. Pyridoxal phosphate acts as an initial acceptor of the α-amino group, forming a Schiff base ($-CH = N-$) intermediate. The pyridoxamine phosphate intermediate subsequently donates the amino group to an acceptor α-keto acid, forming a new α-amino acid. The acceptor α-keto acid is most often α-ketoglutarate, thus resulting in glutamate generation. Not all amino acids are substrates for transaminases. Certain amino acids are initially converted into an intermediate that is subsequently transaminated (eg, asparagine is hydrolyzed to aspartate, the latter of which is transaminated by aspartate aminotransferase, forming oxaloacetate). Given that the majority of amino acids use transaminases in their pathways of degradation (although a select few amino acids can also be directly deaminated, eg, threonine), glutamate formation increases markedly during periods of increased amino acid catabolism. Ultimately, the majority of this glutamate is oxidatively deaminated in the liver, where the released ammonium is incorporated into urea, via the urea cycle, and subsequently excreted in urine (Figure 39-2).

The carbon skeleton released during amino acid catabolism can undergo multiple fates, depending on the metabolic situation during which it was formed, the cell type within which it was generated, and the amino acid from which it is derived. For example, during periods of **excess amino acid ingestion, the amino acid–derived**

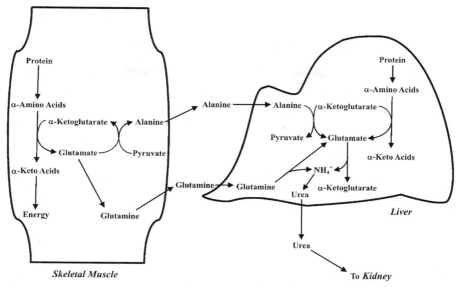

Figure 39-2. General pathway for the degradation of amino acids showing the relationship between extrahepatic tissues and the liver, which is the site of the formation of urea.

carbon skeleton is either used as a metabolic fuel or converted to glycogen or lipid. By contrast, when rates of amino acid catabolism are increased as a result of prolonged caloric insufficiency, a large portion of the carbon skeleton is used by the liver for the synthesis of either glucose or ketone bodies, depending on the specific amino acid. Indeed, glucogenic amino acids (those amino acids whose carbon skeleton can generate net glucose through gluconeogenesis) are essential for maintenance of blood glucose levels during prolonged caloric insufficiency. Maintenance of blood glucose is also made possible by increased reliance of skeletal muscle on amino acids as a fuel source, thereby decreasing glucose utilization.

Certain amino acids are preferentially used in a tissue-specific manner. For example, skeletal muscle has a relatively high capacity for branched-chain amino acid (leucine, isoleucine, and valine) utilization. Following transamination, the carbon skeleton is oxidatively metabolized as an energy source during situations such as sustained exercise and caloric insufficiency. The amino group is transported in the circulation to the liver as either glutamine (formed by the enzymatic addition of an amino group to the side-chain group of glutamate) or alanine (formed by enzymatic transfer of the α-amino group from glutamate to pyruvate). Once at the liver, the transferred amino groups are ultimately used in urea synthesis, as described above (see Figure 39-2).

By contrast to skeletal muscle, which is the primary site of endogenous glutamine synthesis, rapidly dividing cells (eg, lymphocytes, enterocytes) preferentially use glutamine. The reason for this is that rapidly dividing cells require both energy as well as precursors for biosynthetic reactions. The carbon skeleton of glutamine enters intermediary metabolism via α-ketoglutarate, a Krebs cycle intermediate, providing the required energy for cellular processes. In addition, the amino groups of glutamine are used in **purine and pyrimidine biosynthesis,** which in turn are required for the synthesis of both RNA and DNA. Indeed, lymphocyte proliferation is greatly accelerated when glutamine is used as a metabolic substrate (as opposed to glucose), leading to suggestions that glutamine deficiency may result in immunosuppression and therefore increased susceptibility to infection. An additional reason for high rates of glutamine utilization in enterocytes appears to be for the synthesis of citrulline. The latter is transported to the kidney, where it is converted to arginine. Arginine is not only important in protein synthesis but also essential in cellular signaling (via nitric oxide production) and in maintaining adequate levels of urea cycle intermediates (Figure 39-3).

Glutamine also plays an important role in maintenance of whole body acid–base balance. High rates of catabolism of positively charged and sulfur-containing amino acids result in the net formation of hydrogen ions. To maintain an acid–base balance, the kidney uses glutamine as a gluconeogenic precursor, resulting in the formation of glucose, bicarbonate ion, and ammonium ($NH_4^+$) ion formation. The bicarbonate is released into the circulation, where it associates with a proton (forming $CO_2$ and $H_2O$), thereby increasing blood pH. By contrast, the ammonium ion is excreted (see Figure 39-3).

As noted above, amino acids are not only used for protein synthesis but are also essential for the biosynthesis of other biomolecules. These include carnitine (a derivative of lysine), creatine (a derivative of glycine and arginine), glutathione

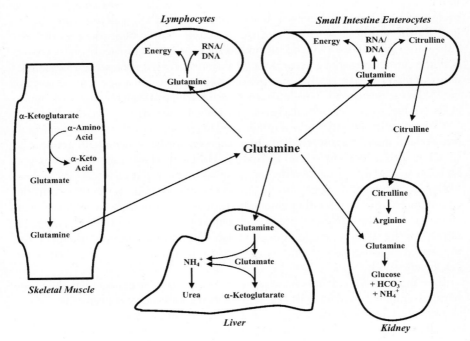

**Figure 39-3.** Schematic diagram showing the central role of glutamine as a transporter of amino acid nitrogen to various tissues.

(a derivative of glutamate, cysteine, and glycine), serotonin and melatonin (derivatives of tryptophan), dopamine, norepinephrine, and epinephrine (derivatives of tyrosine), as well as purines and pyrimidines (requiring aspartate and glutamine for biosynthesis). Alterations in dietary intake of amino acids can influence the rates at which these macromolecules are synthesized. For example, ingestion of a tryptophan-rich meal elevates neuronal serotonin synthesis, resulting in lethargy. Tryptophan crosses the blood–brain barrier via a transporter that is also specific for the branched-chain amino acids. Conditions that influence the tryptophan-to-branched-chain amino acid ratio in the circulation have been shown to affect serotonin levels in the brain because of competition for this transporter. For example, increased skeletal muscle branched-chain amino acid catabolism during starvation is associated with an increase in the blood tryptophan-to-branched-chain amino acid ratio, increased tryptophan uptake in the brain, and increased serotonin synthesis. The latter then influences wakefulness.

Amino acids also play an important role in cellular signaling. The guanidino group from arginine is used in the synthesis of nitric oxide, a ubiquitous, highly reactive signaling molecule that regulates multiple physiologic processes, including blood pressure, immune response, learning, and metabolism. Much less understood is the mechanism by which leucine affects cellular signaling. This amino acid has been termed a "pseudohormone" following the observations that one or more of its early metabolites (eg, α-ketoisocaproate) are among the strongest regulators of protein turnover identified to date.

## COMPREHENSION QUESTIONS

For questions 39.1 to 39.3 refer to the following case: A 12-year-old girl is presented at the clinic with reports of frequent fainting and lethargy. The girl is 5 foot tall and weighs 80 pounds. Skin fold tests show an abnormally low percentage of body fat mass.

39.1  Which of the following is *least likely* to be consistent with the patient's symptoms?

    A.  Anorexia nervosa

    B.  Bulimia

    C.  Type 1 diabetes

    D.  Type 2 diabetes

39.2  Which of the following hormones is likely to be severely diminished in the patient described above?

    A.  Cortisol

    B.  Epinephrine

    C.  Glucagon

    D.  Insulin

39.3 Which of the following metabolic fluxes would be most consistent in this patient?

    A. Protein → amino acids

    B. Glucose → fatty acids

    C. Glucose → glycogen

    D. Fatty acids → triacylglycerol

## ANSWERS

39.1 **D.** Individuals with type 2 diabetes tend to be either overweight (a body mass index [BMI] between 25 and 30 kg/m$^2$) or obese (BMI > 30 kg/m$^2$). This may be due in part to chronic hyperinsulinemia. By contrast, decreased insulin levels associated with type 1 diabetes, anorexia, and bulimia will promote lipolysis and, thus, decreased adipose mass.

39.2 **D.** The low body weight and fat mass observed in the patient are consistent with a metabolically "fasted" state. During such a condition, circulating insulin levels will be low, whereas counter-regulatory hormones (eg, glucagon, epinephrine, and cortisol) will be elevated.

39.3 **A.** Consistent with a metabolically fasted state, decreased circulating insulin levels will signal attenuation of biosynthetic reaction and augmentation of catabolic reactions. The latter will provide necessary fuels to sustain the energetic needs of the body. Elevation of counter-regulator hormones (eg, glucagon, epinephrine, and cortisol) will synergistically stimulate catabolic processes. Increased proteolysis (protein → amino acids) in tissues such as skeletal muscle and the liver provide amino acids as a direct fuel source, as well as ketogenic and gluconeogenic precursors (depending on the individual amino acid).

## BIOCHEMISTRY PEARLS

▶ Twenty different amino acids are used for protein synthesis, each of which is encoded by at least 1 codon (the 3-nucleotide genetic code) and differ only in their side-chain group.

▶ Amino acids can be divided into one of 2 classes, essential and nonessential amino acids. Humans cannot synthesize essential amino acids.

▶ Nitrogen balance refers to whether there is more or less nitrogen (protein) ingested than excreted.

▶ With prolonged caloric insufficiency, a large portion of the carbon skeleton is used by the liver for the synthesis of either glucose or ketone bodies, depending on the specific amino acid.

▶ Rapidly dividing cells (eg, lymphocytes, enterocytes) preferentially use glutamine for energy and biosynthetic purposes.

## REFERENCE

Newsholme EA, Leech AR. *Biochemistry for the Medical Sciences.* New York: Wiley; 1983.

A 20-year-old woman was brought to the emergency department after being found on the dormitory room floor nauseated, vomiting, and complaining of abdominal pain. Her friends were concerned when she did not show up for a biochemistry final at the local university. The patient had been under a lot of stress with finals, a recent breakup with a boyfriend, and trying to find a job. In the dormitory room, one of her friends noticed an empty bottle of acetaminophen near the bed with numerous pills lying on the ground near their friend. On arrival to the emergency department, the patient was found to be in moderate distress and vomiting. The patient was quickly assessed, and laboratory work was obtained. Patient had a hypokalemia noted on electrolytes and elevated liver enzymes. Her white blood cell count was normal. Her urine drug screen was negative, and her acetaminophen blood level was above 200 µg/mL. The emergency department physician prescribes oral N-acetylcysteine to help prevent toxicity from the acetaminophen.

▶ What is the pathophysiology of the liver toxicity?
▶ What is the biochemical mechanism whereby the N-acetylcysteine helps in this condition?

# ANSWERS TO CASE 40:

## Acetaminophen Overdose

*Summary:* A 20-year-old college student under increasing stress was found in moderate distress with nausea, vomiting, and abdominal pain with empty bottle of acetaminophen at her bedside. Oral N-acetylcysteine is prescribed.

- **Pathophysiology:** Acetaminophen is metabolized via the cytochrome P450 enzymes into a deleterious product N-acetyl benzoquinoneimine, an unstable intermediate, which causes arylated derivatives of protein, lipid, RNA, and DNA, causing destruction of these compounds. Because the liver has high levels of cytochrome P450 enzymes, it is the major organ affected by acetaminophen overdose.

- **Biochemical mechanism of N-acetylcysteine:** As glutathione is used to conjugate the acetaminophen toxic metabolite, the antidote N-acetylcysteine helps to facilitate glutathione synthesis by increasing the concentrations of one of the reactants of the first synthetic step.

## CLINICAL CORRELATION

The patient described has all the initial signs of a deliberate overdose of acetaminophen. Normally acetaminophen is cleared by conjugation with either glucuronic acid or sulfate followed by excretion. Metabolism also takes place, producing an active intermediate capable of binding tissue macromolecules. These conjugative and metabolic pathways involve a number of enzymes that may themselves be compromised to such an extent that the threshold for the concentration that constitutes an overdose is substantially lowered. More typically, overdose concentrations are the result of deliberate ingestion, as in this clinical case, or accidental ingestion, often involving either a child who finds a bottle of acetaminophen and consumes its contents or a disoriented elderly person who loses track of how many tablets have been consumed. Usually, the acetaminophen serum level is drawn and plotted on a nomogram to determine the possibility of hepatic damage. Hepatocyte necrosis with clinical manifestations of nausea and vomiting, diarrhea, abdominal pain, and shock may ensue. Few survivors of an overdose have long-term hepatic disease. The initial therapy is gastric lavage, activated charcoal, supportive care, and administration of N-acetylcysteine.

## APPROACH TO:
## Glutathione and Acetaminophen

### OBJECTIVES

1. Describe the role of glutathione in protection of acetaminophen overdose.

2. Explain how an acetaminophen overdose can lead to liver toxicity.

3. Describe the effect of glutathione.

4. Describe the mechanism of action of N-acetylcysteine in treating acetaminophen toxicity.

### DEFINITIONS

**PHASE 1 DRUG METABOLISM:** Oxidative metabolism of drugs usually mediated by cytochrome P450 leading to hydroxylation or epoxidation of substrate compounds.

**PHASE 2 DRUG METABOLISM:** Conjugative metabolism of oxidized drugs usually involving hydration of epoxides by epoxide hydrase producing phenolic derivatives, conjugation by uridine diphosphate (UDP)-glucuronyl transferase to produce glucuronide adducts or S-alkylated adducts, or sulfation by sulfotransferase producing sulfated derivatives.

**DRUG TOXICITY:** Aberrant reaction to a therapeutic agent often depending on individual variations in either the quantity or activity level of specific drug metabolizing enzymes toward the drugs or on individual genetic polymorphisms of drug metabolism enzymes giving higher or lower activities or product profile produced by the genetic variant versus the normally expressed enzyme.

### DISCUSSION

The **major pathway of removal of acetaminophen is by formation of a glucuronide conjugate.** The reactions required for formation of acetaminophen glucuronide are shown in Figure 40-1 and depend on the generation of activated glucuronic acid. The first phase is the formation of activated glucuronic acid from glucose. Glucose is phosphorylated to glucose 6-phosphate by hexokinase in an adenosine triphosphate (ATP)-requiring reaction, which constitutes the first step of glycolysis, the basal pathway for cellular energy generation. Phosphoglucomutase, which plays a critical role in glycogen formation, converts glucose 6-phosphate to glucose 1-phosphate. Glucose 1-phosphate is activated to UDP-glucose by UDP-glucose pyrophosphorylase using UTP and producing pyrophosphate as an additional product. Pyrophosphate is rapidly hydrolyzed to 2 mol of phosphate by pyrophosphatase; this pulls the reaction toward the formation of UDP-glucose. This reaction is also on the pathway to the formation of glycogen. The last step in this activation phase is the oxidation of the sixth carbon of glucose in UDP-glucose to the acid level forming

**Figure 40-1.** Formation of uridine diphosphate (UDP)-glucuronate and acetaminophen glucuronide.

UDP-glucuronic acid. This reaction is catalyzed by UDP-glucose dehydrogenase, which also produces 2 mol of nicotinamide adenine dinucleotide (NADH) as an additional product. UDP-glucuronyl transferase, in the next phase of the reaction, catalyzes the transfer of the glucuronide group to the hydroxyl group of acetaminophen forming acetaminophen glucuronide, which is eliminated without toxic effects to the organism.

Alternatively, acetaminophen can be conjugated with organic sulfate for elimination. This alternative pathway shown in Figure 40-2 also consists of 2 phases. The first phase consists of preparing activated sulfate for transfer as 5′-phosphoadenosine 3′-phosphosulfate (PAPS), and the second consists of transfer of the sulfate moiety to acetaminophen. In the first step of the first phase, ATP-sulfurylase catalyzes the formation of pyrophosphate and adenosine-5′-phosphosulfate (APS) from ATP and

**Figure 40-2.** Formation of 5'-phosphoadenosine 3'-phosphosulfate (PAPS) and sulfated acetaminophen.

sulfate. In the second step, APS-kinase catalyzes the formation of PAPS and adenosine diphosphate (ADP) from ATP and APS. The structure for PAPS is shown in Figure 40-2. In the second phase, phenolsulfotransferase, one of a group of sulfotransferases, transfers the sulfate group from PAPS to acetaminophen to yield adenosine-3', 5'-bisphosphate and acetaminophen sulfate, which is eliminated. In the event that this pathway and the glucuronide-forming pathway are both overwhelmed by overdose, more acetaminophen is metabolized by the cytochrome P450 pathway.

Oxidative metabolism of acetaminophen by the cytochrome P450 system, shown in Figure 40-3, is **catalyzed by various cytochromes P450 such as CYP2E1** and others. The **deleterious product is N-acetyl benzoquinoneimine, an unstable intermediate,** shown in Figure 40-3, which can react with cellular macromolecules, damaging them and the integrity of the cells wherein the metabolic alteration occurs. The tissue with the **highest concentration of cytochromes P450 is the liver,** and it is there (along with kidney) that acetaminophen causes the most damage. In the liver, N-acetyl benzoquinoneimine can form **arylated derivatives of protein, lipid, RNA, and DNA, causing destruction of these compounds as well as any larger structure** with which they are associated, for example, cellular and subcellular membranes, leading to hepatocyte lysis and loss of cellular contents, such as enzymes, to the circulation. However, N-acetyl benzoquinoneimine may also disrupt $Ca^{2+}$

Figure 40-3. Metabolism of acetaminophen.

balance, leading to dramatically increased intracellular $Ca^{2+}$ concentrations, that is, 20 compared with 0.1 μM, which is the normal concentration. $Ca^{2+}$ is a potent and, thus, well-regulated signal. Thus, dramatic increases in $Ca^{2+}$ concentration would have deleterious effects on the balance of many cellular processes, especially energy generation. The low serum calcium and elevated liver enzyme serum levels seen in the patient reflect hepatocyte lysis.

What mechanisms protect against this metabolite-induced destruction of cellular integrity? The primary defense against radical metabolite intermediate-mediated damage is the glutathione (GSH) system. Glutathione is a tripeptide with an active sulfhydryl group that plays a role in protection of cellular macromolecules from attack by radicals such as organic hydroperoxides or active metabolic intermediates such as N-acetyl benzoquinoneimine. The formation of glutathione is summarized in Figure 40-4. γ-Glutamylcysteine synthetase catalyzes the formation of the dipeptide γ-glutamylcysteine from the amino acids glutamate and cysteine using energy provided by the hydrolysis of ATP to ADP and phosphate. Glutathione synthetase

Figure 40-4. Glutathione formation.

catalyzes the addition of glycine to γ-glutamylcysteine to form the tripeptide gluta-thione, again using 1 mol of ATP.

The role of the glutathione in detoxifying N-acetyl benzoquinoneimine is shown in Figure 40-3. The adduct acetaminophen glutathionate is no longer toxic to cells and can be excreted without further damage. **Any process depleting glutathione levels would compromise the ability of the cell to protect itself against N-acetyl benzoquinoneimine.** This includes deficiencies of any of the enzymes involved in the synthesis of glutathione or that keep glutathione in its reduced state as well as any other radical generating process that consumes glutathione. In the case of acetaminophen overdose, in addition to giving activated charcoal to absorb excess stomach and intestinal acetaminophen or its conjugates, a strategy to replenish glu-tathione concentration is important. The most frequently administered compound is **N-acetylcysteine.** Easily obtainable and readily soluble, it serves to **facilitate glu-tathione synthesis by increasing the concentrations of one of the reactants of the first synthetic step.** The committed dipeptide product being made, glutathione is synthesized to replenish depleted supplies. N-acetylcysteine seems most effective when given less than 10 hours after ingestion of acetaminophen but is recommended within the first 35 hours after ingestion.

## COMPREHENSION QUESTIONS

40.1  A patient admitted to the emergency room with nausea and vomiting showed low serum potassium, elevated blood enzymes, and acetaminophen blood level above 200 µg/mL. The patient was diagnosed with acetaminophen overdose. Acetaminophen is a widely used analgesic. What is the most probable explana-tion of how a high dose of acetaminophen might have led to a toxic condition?

A.  Acetaminophen itself is toxic.

B.  Acetaminophen is metabolized to a potential toxic product.

C.  Acetaminophen is metabolized to a potential toxic product that is fully conjugated.

D.  Acetaminophen is metabolized to a potential toxic product that is par-tially conjugated.

E.  None of the above is correct.

40.2  In acetaminophen toxicity, which of the following compounds is a potential toxic intermediate?

A.  Acetaminophen glucuronide

B.  Acetaminophen sulfate

C.  N-Acetyl benzoquinoneimine

D.  Acetaminophen glutathionate

E.  N-Acetyl-p-aminophenol

40.3 Glutathione is a critical tripeptide involved in conjugation reactions and in reactions that protect cells from reactive oxygen species. Which of the following components compose glutathione?

A. Glutamic acid, alanine, methionine

B. Glutamine, alanine, cysteine

C. Glutamate, glycine, cysteine

D. Alanine, glycine, cysteine

E. Methionine, glycine, cysteine

## ANSWERS

40.1 **D.** Acetaminophen is not itself toxic, but its intermediate metabolite N-acetyl benzoquinoneimine can be toxic unless it is adequately conjugated. In the case presented, a high dose of acetaminophen overwhelmed the conjugative processes, allowing the toxic intermediate to interact with body components and thus causing the nausea, vomiting, and elevated blood enzymes observed.

40.2 **C.** N-acetyl benzoquinoneimine is toxic whereas acetaminophen glucuronide, acetaminophen sulfate, and acetaminophen glutathionate are nontoxic acetaminophen conjugates. N-acetyl-p-aminophenol is another name for acetaminophen.

40.3 **C.** Glutathione ($\gamma$-glutamylcysteinylglycine) is a tripeptide of glutamic acid, cysteine, and glycine in which the amino terminal glutamate residue is in a peptide linkage through its side-chain carboxyl group to the cysteine residue.

## BIOCHEMISTRY PEARLS

► The major pathway of removal of acetaminophen is by formation of a glucuronide conjugate.

► Acetaminophen is oxidized by the cytochrome P450 system, yielding the deleterious product N-acetyl benzoquinoneimine, an unstable intermediate that can react with cellular macromolecules and thus damage them.

► The liver has a high concentration of cytochrome P450 and is particularly susceptible to acetaminophen toxicity.

► N-acetylcysteine is the antidote to acetaminophen toxicity and facilitates glutathione synthesis by increasing the concentrations of one of the reactants of the first synthetic step.

## REFERENCE

Brunton L, Chabner B, Bjorn Knollman, eds. *Goodman and Gilman's The Pharmacological Basis of Therapeutics*. 12th ed. New York: McGraw-Hill; 2010.

A 37-year-old woman presents to your clinic to discuss her plans for a new vegetarian diet. The patient heard from a friend about a new vegetarian diet that promised rapid weight loss. The diet consists of many leafy vegetables with no pork, chicken, beef, eggs, or milk. She is also planning on working out regularly with the goal of running a marathon within the year. After listening to the patient, you refer her to a nutritionist for further assistance and guidance.

▶ What is an essential amino acid, and how many are there?
▶ List the essential amino acids.

## ANSWERS TO CASE 41:

# Vegetarian Diet (Essential Amino Acids)

*Summary:* A 37-year-old woman who is planning to undertake a radical new vegetarian diet is in your office for counseling.

- **Essential amino acids:** The amino acids that cannot be synthesized by the body. There are a total of nine essential amino acids.

- **List of essential amino acids:** Histidine, isoleucine, leucine, lysine, methionine, phenylalanine, threonine, tryptophan, and valine.

## CLINICAL CORRELATION

The vegetarian should be careful to ensure a balanced ingestion of proteins, fats, carbohydrates, and vitamins. Most animal proteins contain all the essential amino acids; however, vegetable proteins often lack one or more of them. Often, plant amino acids are of low biologic value and incompletely digested. Vegans often benefit from nutritional consultation, which would allow the patient to make sure that she ate foods that complemented each other in providing the essential amino acids.

## APPROACH TO:

# Essential Amino Acids

## OBJECTIVES

1. Explain the importance of essential amino acids.

2. Outline the synthesis of other amino acids.

3. Describe some of the problems that arise with inadequate essential amino acid intake.

## DEFINITIONS

**ESSENTIAL AMINO ACIDS:** Amino acids that the human body cannot synthesize (or cannot synthesize in sufficient quantities to meet cellular needs) and must be taken in the diet. If essential amino acids are deficient, the result is a condition of negative nitrogen balance.

**NONESSENTIAL AMINO ACIDS:** Those amino acids that are synthesized by the human body in sufficient quantities to meet cellular needs.

**PHENYLALANINE HYDROXYLASE:** The enzyme that converts the essential amino acid phenylalanine to the amino acid tyrosine using tetrahydrobiopterin and molecular oxygen. A genetic deficiency in this enzyme gives rise to the disease phenylketonuria.

**PHENYLKETONES:** Normally minor metabolites of phenylalanine that result from the transamination of phenylalanine and further reduction. These include phenylpyruvate and phenylacetate. These metabolites are elevated when the conversion of phenylalanine to tyrosine is impaired.

**PKU:** Phenylketonuria (PKU); the pathologic condition of increased excretion of phenylketones in the urine because of impaired conversion of phenylalanine to tyrosine. Classical PKU is because of a genetic deficiency of phenylalanine hydroxylase; however, other causes are deficiencies in dihydropteridine reductase or in the biosynthesis of tetrahydrobiopterin.

## DISCUSSION

All 20 amino acids are needed for normal cellular growth and function. Amino acids are the basic building blocks for all proteins synthesized in the cell. In addition, the metabolism of amino acids provides carbon and nitrogen units used in the synthesis of numerous important biomolecules including neurotransmitters, heme, purines, pyrimidines, polyamines, and various cellular-signaling molecules. The carbon skeletons of amino acids can also be used as an energy source. After removal of the amino group, amino acids can either be directly oxidized or converted to glucose in the liver, providing carbon units to other tissues for the production of adenosine triphosphate (ATP) through glycolysis and the tricarboxylic acid (TCA) cycle. Certain amino acids can be directly interconverted to intermediates of the TCA cycle to provide a rapid source of carbon units. Finally, catabolism of amino acids provides a means of nitrogen and carbon removal from the body through their metabolism to urea and $CO_2$. Thus, all amino acids are necessary for life.

Apart from their biologic importance, amino acids are classified as essential or nonessential based on their ability to be synthesized in the body. **The term *essential* amino acid is used to identify those amino acids that must be taken in through the diet** (Table 41-1). There are 10 such amino acids for which biosynthetic pathways do not exist in cells of the human body. By contrast, there are 11 amino acids that are termed *nonessential*, for which the human body has biosynthetic pathways for their generation. One of these amino acids, **tyrosine,** is **synthesized from the essential amino acid phenylalanine** (Figure 38-2). In addition, it should be noted that arginine is listed as both an essential and nonessential amino acid. Arginine is considered nonessential because biosynthetic pathways for its generation do exist in certain cells of the body. Arginine can be synthesized from the amino acid glutamate. **Glutamate** is first converted to **ornithine,** which is then converted to **arginine** by enzymes of the urea cycle. The urea cycle is found only in the liver, and thus the production of arginine through this pathway is limited. The production of arginine through this pathway is likely sufficient for healthy adults but may not be sufficient in times of growth when increased protein synthesis augments the need for amino acids. Thus, in growing children and in adults following surgery or trauma, arginine becomes an essential amino acid.

There is a **continuous need for amino acids for protein synthesis, energy utilization, and the production of biologic mediators.** The most readily available source of all amino acids, but particularly the essential amino acids, is the diet. Protein is taken

| Table 41-1 • ESSENTIAL AND NONESSENTIAL AMINO ACIDS | | |
|---|---|---|
| | Nonessential Amino Acids | |
| Essential Amino Acids | Synthesized From Glucose | Synthesized From an Essential Amino Acid(s) |
| Histidine | Alanine | Tyrosine |
| Isoleucine | Arginine | |
| Leucine | Asparagine | |
| Lysine | Aspartate | |
| Methionine | Cysteine | |
| Phenylalanine | Glutamate | |
| Threonine | Glutamine | |
| Tryptophan | Glycine | |
| Valine | Proline | |
| Arginine[a] | Serine | |

[a]Required for growth

in through the diet and digested to smaller peptides and amino acids in the stomach and small intestine by specific proteolytic enzymes known as proteases. Because of their different specificities, enzymes work to cleave specific peptide bonds within proteins. Individual digestive enzymes are not capable of completely digesting proteins themselves, but in concert with many different enzymes, most proteins can be efficiently digested. Once released by the digestive enzymes, amino acids are absorbed by epithelial cells of the small intestine for distribution and utilization throughout the body.

Composition of the diet is an important consideration when trying to understand and plan for the uptake of essential amino acids. Not all dietary constituents are equal with regard to the type and amounts of proteins present or the amino acids that can be derived from these proteins by the human digestive tract. Proteins derived from vegetable matter may not contain all the essential amino acids needed and digestion of certain plant proteins can be insufficient to produce certain individual amino acids. By contrast, proteins found in animal products are readily digestible and contain all essential amino acids. Therefore, careful consideration should be given to the dietary intake of individuals who may have or will be undergoing an increased level of exertion.

**Regulation of the dietary intake of amino acids** can also be important when considering the treatment of certain defects in amino acid biosynthesis. **Phenylalanine** is an essential amino acid that is also used to generate the nonessential amino acid tyrosine. The enzyme that carries out this reaction is the mixed function oxidase **phenylalanine hydroxylase** (PAH). **Inherited deficiencies in PAH are associated with a condition known as phenylketonuria (PKU; see case 38).** The absence of PAH results in elevations of phenylalanine and various phenylketones, the accumulation of which is associated with the neurologic defects seen in this disorder. PKU can be treated by controlling the dietary intake of phenylalanine. Diets low in phenylalanine will help prevent excessive elevations in phenylalanine. Phenylalanine cannot be completely eliminated from the diet because it is an essential amino acid needed for protein synthesis. In the absence of PAH activity, tyrosine becomes an essential amino acid because it cannot be generated from phenylalanine.

## COMPREHENSION QUESTIONS

41.1   All amino acids are needed for the production of proteins in cells and for the synthesis of important biomolecules. Which of the following amino acids, all of which can be synthesized by the human body, must be taken in the diet because it is not synthesized in sufficient quantities to meet the body's needs?

    A.  Asparagine

    B.  Glutamine

    C.  Methionine

    D.  Proline

    E.  Tyrosine

41.2   A young child is in an automobile accident that requires surgical intervention and substantial recovery time in the hospital. A consultation with a nutritionist results in a specific dietary plan. The plan included the supplementation of an amino acid that is typically considered a nonessential amino acid. Which of the following amino acids is an essential amino acid under conditions of enhanced growth or surgical recovery?

    A.  Alanine

    B.  Arginine

    C.  Glycine

    D.  Serine

    E.  Tyrosine

41.3   As part of a standard neonatal screen, an infant is diagnosed with a loss of function genetic defect in the enzyme phenylalanine hydroxylase. Defects in this enzyme can result in a condition known as PKU, which results from the toxic effects of phenylalanine-derived phenylketones. Fortunately, this condition can be managed by regulating the amount of phenylalanine provided in the diet. Which of the following nonessential amino acids will need to be supplied in the diet of this infant?

    A.  Alanine

    B.  Aspartate

    C.  Glycine

    D.  Serine

    E.  Tyrosine

## ANSWERS

41.1 **C.** Methionine can be synthesized by the methylation of homocysteine by the enzyme methionine synthase, which requires the participation of vitamin $B_{12}$ and 5-methyltetrahydrofolate. It is actually the homocysteine component of methionine that is required, since this reaction has the capacity to synthesize enough methionine. However, there is no good dietary source of homocysteine. This conversion of homocysteine to methionine also serves the purpose of making tetrahydrofolate (THF) available for other biosynthetic reactions.

41.2 **B.** Arginine is considered nonessential because biosynthetic pathways for its generation do exist in certain cells of the body. Arginine is synthesized from the amino acid glutamate. Glutamate is first converted to ornithine, which is then converted to arginine by enzymes of the urea cycle. The urea cycle is found only in the liver; therefore, the production of arginine through this pathway is limiting. The production of arginine through this pathway is likely sufficient for healthy adults, but it may not be sufficient in times of growth where increased protein synthesis augments the need for amino acids. Thus, in growing children and in adults following surgery, arginine becomes an essential amino acid.

41.3 **E.** Phenylalanine is an essential amino acid that is also used to generate the nonessential amino acid tyrosine. Because tyrosine is made from phenylalanine, it becomes an essential amino acid when phenylalanine levels are limited because of the absence of phenylalanine hydroxylase activity.

## BIOCHEMISTRY PEARLS

▶ The term *essential* amino acid is used to identify those amino acids that must be taken in through the diet and cannot be manufactured.

▶ There are 10 such essential amino acids for which biosynthetic pathways do not exist in cells of the human body.

▶ Phenylalanine is an essential amino acid that is also used to generate the nonessential amino acid tyrosine.

## REFERENCE

Marks DB, Marks AD, Smith CM. *Basic Medical Biochemistry: A Clinical Approach.* Baltimore, MD: Lippincott Williams & Wilkins; 1996:569-646.

A 38-year-old vegetarian (vegan) Caucasian woman presents to her primary care doctor with fatigue and tingling/numbness in her extremities (bilateral). The symptoms have been gradually getting worse over the last year. Upon further questioning she reports frequent episodes of diarrhea and weight loss. On examination, she is pale and tachycardic. Her tongue is beefy red and a neurologic examination reveals numbness in all extremities with decreased vibration senses. A complete blood count demonstrates megaloblastic anemia.

▶ What is the most likely diagnosis?
▶ What is the most likely underlying problem for this patient?
▶ What are the 2 most common causes of megaloblastic anemia and how would this patient's history and examination differentiate these 2 causes?

# ANSWERS TO CASE 42:
## Cobalamin Deficiency (Vitamin B$_{12}$)

*Summary:* A 38-year-old vegetarian woman with gradually worsening fatigue, neurologic and gastrointestinal (GI) symptoms, and megaloblastic anemia.

- **Diagnosis:** Cobalamin (vitamin B$_{12}$) deficiency.

- **Underlying problem:** Lack of cobalamin intake with complete vegetarian diet (vegan).

- **Causes of megaloblastic anemia:** Folate and cobalamin deficiency. Patients with folate deficiency have similar hematologic and GI findings but do *not* have the neurologic symptoms as with cobalamin deficiency.

## CLINICAL CORRELATION

The 2 most common etiologies of megaloblastic anemia are deficiencies in folate or cobalamin. Cobalamin deficiency can occur from a lack of intake (such as with complete vegetarians), absence of intrinsic factor (either inherited or from removal/damage to gastric mucosa), intestinal organisms, or ileal abnormalities (tropical sprue). Patients present with anemic symptoms, including fatigue, weakness, palpitations, vertigo, and tachycardia. GI symptoms include sore, beefy-red tongue, weight loss, and diarrhea. Both folate and cobalamin deficiencies have similar anemic and GI symptoms. However, cobalamin deficiency also can present with numerous neurologic manifestations including: numbness, paresthesia, weakness, ataxia, abnormal reflexes, diminished vibratory sensation, and disturbances in mentation (from irritability to psychosis). Treatment consists of identifying/treating the underlying cause of deficiency and replacement of cobalamin or folate.

## OBJECTIVES

1. Describe the role of cobalamin in red blood cell formation.

2. Explain why cobalamin deficiency leads to megaloblastic anemia.

3. Develop a comprehension of the role of cobalamin in metabolism.

## DEFINITIONS

**COBALAMIN (VITAMIN B$_{12}$) DEFICIENCY:** Inadequate uptake of cobalamin from the diet; often due to lack of intrinsic factor an intestinal transport protein or less often due to unaugmented vegetarian diet that strictly avoids meat or meat products, the source of dietary cobalamin.

**MEGALOBLASTIC ANEMIA:** A disturbance in erythroid cell synthesis due to an impaired DNA synthesis. This results in cells with small nuclei and normal cytoplasm, and a high RNA to DNA ratio. Impaired DNA synthesis is due to decreased thymidylate synthetase conversion ($C_1$ transfer) of deoxyuridine monophosphate (dUMP) to deoxythymidine monophosphate (dTMP) as a result of insufficient cobalamin or folate pool impairment.

**ONE-CARBON POOL:** Folate derivatives that carry a single carbon in various oxidation states (formyl, methenyl, methylene, and methyl) for transfer to acceptor molecules; that is, transfer to deoxyuridine monophosphate to form deoxythymidine monophosphate; transfer to homocysteine to form methionine.

## DISCUSSION

The structure of cobalamin (vitamin $B_{12}$) is shown in Figure 42-1. Cobalamin is somewhat analogous to heme in its structure having as its base a tetrapyrrole ring. Instead of iron as a metal cofactor for heme, cobalamin has cobalt in a coordination state of 6 with a benzimidazole group nitrogen coordinated to one axial position, the 4 equatorial positions coordinated by the nitrogens of the 4 pyrrole groups and the sixth position occupied by either a deoxyadenosine group, a methyl group or a CN⁻ group in the commercially available form in vitamin tablets. Dietary cobalamin is absorbed in the $Co^{3+}$ oxidation state and must be reduced by intracellular reductases to the $Co^+$ form for use.

**Figure 42-1.** The structure of cobalamin, vitamin $B_{12}$. X = deoxyadenosine in deoxyadenyosylcobalamin; X = $CH_3$ in methylcobalamin; X = CN⁻ in cyanocobalamin, the commercial form found in vitamin tablets.

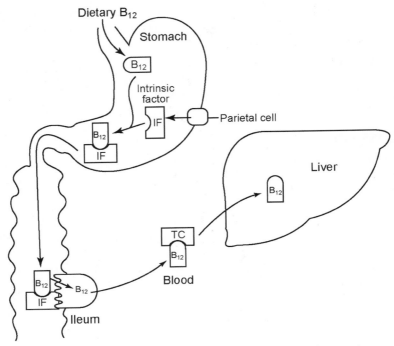

**Figure 42-2.** Absorption, transport, and storage of vitamin B$_{12}$. IF = intrinsic factor, a glycoprotein secreted by gastric parietal cells; TC = transcobalamins, blood proteins that carry cobalamin to the liver. *(Reproduced, with permission, from D.B. Marks, et al.* Basic Medical Biochemistry: A Clinical Approach. *Philadelphia: Lippincott Williams & Wilkins; 1996:619.)*

Dietary cobalamin is absorbed from animal food sources by a multistage process shown in Figure 42-2. Cobalamin absorption requires the presence of a protein (the intrinsic factor) secreted from the parietal cells of the stomach to bind cobalamin and aid in its absorption in the ileum. The protein is released into the ileum while the cobalamin is transported to the blood stream where it binds specialized serum proteins, the transcobalamins, which transport it to other tissues such as liver where cobalamin can be stored (usually several milligrams are present in liver). In the absence of the intrinsic factor inadequate amounts of cobalamin are absorbed (the dietary requirement is approximately 200 ng/day) resulting in megaloblastic anemia. When the root cause of the resultant megaloblastic anemia is absence of or inadequate amounts of intrinsic factor the condition is called pernicious anemia. Other conditions or choices may also eventuate in cobalamin deficiency–induced megaloblastic anemia. This condition is also observed in vegetarians who strictly avoid meat and meat products.

The cause of megaloblastic anemia seen in strict nonsupplemented vegetarians is attributed to the effects of cobalamin deficiency on DNA synthesis, specifically the thymidylate synthetase reaction, which converts dUMP to dTMP. Inadequate dTMP restricts DNA but not RNA synthesis, leading to the appearance of large erythroid cells with small nuclei containing a high ratio of RNA to DNA. These cells

**Figure 42-3.** The role of cobalamin as a cofactor in the methylation of homocysteine to methionine.

are removed from the circulation, thus stimulating erythrogenesis and giving rise to anemia with an elevated presence of megaloblasts.

This process focuses on the role of cobalamin in folate metabolism. As shown in Figure 42-3, cobalamin is required for the conversion of homocysteine into methionine. Cobalamin must first undergo methyl transfer to form methyl cobalamin. It receives the methyl group from $N^5$-methyltetrahydrofolate thus regenerating tetrahydrofolate to participate in other one-carbon transfers in purine metabolism or pyrimidine remodeling. If there is a cobalamin deficiency, then the methionine synthase reaction cannot occur, $N^5$-methyltetrahydrofolate accumulates and the other C-1 donor forms of tetrahydrofolate cannot be formed. If $N^5$, $N^{10}$-methylenetetrahydrofolate, which is required for the methylation of dUMP to dTMP, cannot be formed, then the thymidylate synthase reaction will be slowed and dTMP levels will drop. An added complication is that the thymidylate synthase reaction produces dihydrofolate unlike all the other C-1 pool reactions, which produce tetrahydrofolate. The dihydro-form must be reduced to the tetrahydro-form by dihydrofolate reductase, which can be inhibited by many drugs. Thus, in the absence of cobalamin, methionine synthesis from homocysteine ceases, allowing the "trapping" of the folate pool as $N^5$-methyltetrahydrofolate, diminishing levels of $N^5$, $N^{10}$-methylenetetrahydrofolate, and impairing dTMP formation and, thus, DNA synthesis. Cells requiring regeneration due to turnover feel the brunt of this situation early and thus megaloblastic anemia is a result.

### Role of Cobalamin in Metabolism

Cobalamin plays a vital role in the catabolism of odd-chain fatty acids, threonine, methionine, and the branched-chain amino acids (leucine, isoleucine, and valine), as shown in Figure 42-4. The degradation of each of the compounds named above produces the same metabolite, propionyl-CoA. This activated 3-carbon fatty acid enters the energy generating metabolic pathway at the level of the citric acid cycle as succinyl-CoA. The process requires 3 specialized enzymes. Propionyl-CoA carboxylase adds another carbon to propionyl-CoA to form D-methylmalonyl-CoA in a reaction that requires ATP and the $CO_2$-binding cofactor biotin. A racemase converts the D isomer of methylmalonyl-CoA to the L isomer. The last step is catalyzed by methylmalonyl-CoA mutase, a deoxyadenosylcobalamin-requiring enzyme that moves the acyl-CoA group from the methylene carbon to the methyl carbon to form succinyl-CoA. In cases of cobalamin deficiency this reaction is compromised and leads to an accumulation of methylmalonyl-CoA in serum, which has been suggested as a possible source of neurologic defects seen in cobalamin deficiency by decreasing lipid synthesis. Alternatively, impaired biosynthesis of phosphatidyl

**Figure 42-4.** The role of vitamin $B_{12}$ in the conversion of propionyl-CoA to succinyl-CoA.

choline due to decreased levels of methionine and S-adenosylmethionine may play a role for the neurologic symptoms of cobalamin deficiency by compromising the repair of demyelination.

## COMPREHENSION QUESTIONS

42.1 A patient with a tentative diagnosis of cobalamin deficiency is awaiting a comprehensive blood analysis. Which of the following perturbations would NOT fit with the putative diagnosis?

A. Elevated levels of methylmalonic acid

B. Elevated levels of propionic acid

C. Elevated levels of para-hydroxyphenylpyruvate

D. Decreased levels of erythrocytes

E. Elevated levels of megaloblasts

42.2 In evaluating the case presented above your resident asks questions of the role of cobalamin in metabolism. Which of the following statements is true?

A. Cyanocobalamin is the principal form of cobalamin physiologically used.

B. Cobalamin is equally active with an iron cofactor.

C. Enterocytes produce an intrinsic factor required for uptake of cobalamin in the gut.

D. Cobalamin is transported in the blood to tissues by proteins named trans-cobalamins.

E. Cobalamin is active in its 3+ oxidation state.

42.3  Megaloblastic anemia has 2 most likely causes, deficiency of folate and deficiency of cobalamin. Often treatment of patients with cobalamin deficiency improves in terms of their hematologic features with treatment with folate but not in their neurologic symptoms. What is the most likely explanation for this explanation?

A.  Cobalamin deficiencies are not serious.

B.  Excess folate blunts the trapping of folate as $N^5$-methyltetrahydrofolate.

C.  Folate in high concentrations can serve as cofactor for the conversion of homocysteine to methionine.

D.  Excess folate directly inhibits the destruction of red blood cells.

E.  Excess folate stimulates erythropoietic tissues to synthesize cobalamin in situ.

## ANSWERS

42.1  **C.** Para-hydroxyphenylpyruvate is the $\alpha$-keto acid cognate of tyrosine and is not affected by cobalamin levels. All others result from cobalamin deficiency.

42.2  **D.** Cobalamin is transported in the blood by transcobalamins. Cyanocobalamin, the pharmacologic preparation of cobalamin available in vitamin pills, is a active as is. Cobalamin is not active with an iron cofactor. The intrinsic factor is produced by parietal cells in the stomach. Cobalamin must be reduced to the $Co^+$ state for activity.

42.3  **B.** Excess folate, by overwhelming the folate pool trapped as $N^5$-methyltetrahydrofolate, can allow for formation of $N^5$, $N^{10}$-methylenetetrahydrofolate, which is required for the thymidylate synthase reaction for DNA synthesis and red blood cell formation. Folate is not recognized as a methyl donor by methionine synthase. Folate does not inhibit destruction of erythrocytes. Cobalamin is an important critical vitamin not synthesized by humans.

## BIOCHEMISTRY PEARLS

▶ Vitamin $B_{12}$ (cobalamin) plays a critical role in DNA synthesis and neurologic function.

▶ Cobalamin deficiency can lead to a wide spectrum of hematologic, neuropsychiatric, and cardiovascular disorders that can often be reversed by early diagnosis and prompt treatment.

▶ Cobalamin absorption from the GI tract requires the presence of a protein (the intrinsic factor) secreted from the parietal cells of the stomach to bind cobalamin and aid in its absorption in the ileum.

## REFERENCES

Devlin TM, ed. *Textbook of Biochemistry with Clinical Correlations*. 7th ed. New York: Wiley-Liss; 2010.

Longo D, Fauci AS, Kaspar D, et al, eds. *Harrison's Principles of Internal Medicine*. 18th ed. New York: McGraw-Hill; 2011.

Scriver CR, Beaudet AL, Sly WS, et al. *The Metabolic and Molecular Basis of Inherited Disease*. 8th ed, New York: McGraw Hill; 2001:2165-2193.

A 46-year-old man presents to the emergency department with severe right toe pain. The patient was in usual state of health until early in the morning when he woke up with severe pain in his right big toe. The patient denies any trauma to the toe and no previous history of such pain in other joints. He did say that he had a "few too many" beers with the guys last night. On examination, he was found to have a temperature of 100.8°F (38.2°C) and in moderate distress secondary to the pain in his right toe. The right big toe was swollen, warm, red, and exquisitely tender. The remainder of the examination was normal. Synovial fluid was obtained and revealed rod- or needle-shaped crystals that were negatively birefringent under polarizing microscopy, consistent with gout.

▶ What is the likely diagnosis?
▶ How would you make a definite diagnosis?
▶ What is the pathophysiology of this disorder?

# ANSWERS TO CASE 43:
## Gout

*Summary:* A 47-year-old man presents with an acute onset of right toe pain in the middle of night after drinking alcohol and no history of trauma or any other joint pain.

- **Diagnosis:** Gouty arthritis.

- **Confirming diagnosis:** Demonstration of the presence of the monosodium urate crystals within the synovial leukocytes or in material derived from tophi under polarizing microscopy.

- **Pathophysiology:** Increased conversion of purine bases to uric acid or a decreased excretion of uric acid by the kidney. Elevated levels of the insoluble uric acid result in precipitation of urate crystals in the joints.

## CLINICAL CORRELATION

Gout is a disorder that occurs when uric acid crystallizes in the joints of the body, usually the great toe or large joints. Hyperuricemia is a clinical condition characterized by elevated levels of uric acid. This leads to the formation of sodium urate crystals, which are found primarily in the joints of the extremities and in the renal interstitium. The presence of urate crystals is associated with extreme swelling and tenderness in the joints of the extremities. This condition is often referred to as gout or gouty arthritis. In this condition, elevated levels of uric acid are detectable in the blood and urine, and definitive diagnosis can be made by observing the presence of urate crystals in synovial fluid removed from affected joints. The preference of urate crystal formation in the joints of the extremities, such as the big toe, is thought to be associated with the decreased temperature of the extremities that aids in urate crystal formation when levels exceed solubility.

# APPROACH TO:
## Uric Acid Crystallization

## OBJECTIVES

1. Describe the uric acid pathway.

2. Outline purine base metabolism.

3. Explain the rationale for treating gout with allopurinol and colchicine.

# DEFINITIONS

**ALLOPURINOL:** An inhibitor of the enzyme xanthine oxidase used to treat gout to decrease the amount of sodium urate in the blood and thus prevent its crystallization in the joints.

**COLCHICINE:** A tricyclic, water-soluble alkaloid isolated from the autumn crocus. Colchicine will inhibit microtubule formation and inhibit phagocytosis of urate crystals, thus preventing the inflammatory events associated with a gouty attack.

**GOUT:** An inflammatory event triggered by the crystallization of sodium urate crystals in the joints as a result of increased levels of sodium urate in the blood.

**HGPRT:** Hypoxanthine-guanine phosphoribosyltransferase; the enzyme that catalyzes the synthesis of inosine monophosphate (IMP) and guanosine monophosphate (GMP) from hypoxanthine and guanine, respectively. It makes up part of the purine salvage pathway, a way of recycling purine bases back to the nucleotides.

**LESCH-NYHAN SYNDROME:** A genetic disease caused by a deficiency in hypoxanthine-guanine phosphoribosyltransferase (HGPRT) that is characterized by mental retardation and self-destructive behavior. Lesch-Nyhan patients have increased levels of uric acid and sodium urate that lead to gout and kidney stones.

**PURINE SALVAGE PATHWAY:** The synthesis of purine nucleotides by the condensation of the purine bases with phosphoribosyl pyrophosphate. As the name suggests, it is a way in which purine bases can be recycled back to nucleotides. The purine salvage pathway consists of 2 enzymes, HGPRT and adenine phosphoribosyltransferase (APRT).

**URIC ACID:** The final product in the degradation of purine nucleotides in human metabolism. The salt form of uric acid, sodium urate, is present at about saturation levels in the bloodstream. When sodium urate levels increase above this point, it can crystallize into sharp crystals, usually in the joints where the temperature is lower.

**XANTHINE OXIDASE:** The enzyme that catalyzes the final steps in purine degradation to produce urate. This enzyme is inhibited by compounds such as allopurinol in treatment regimens designed to decrease sodium urate concentrations in the blood.

# DISCUSSION

**Purine bases are used in many important biologic processes including the formation of nucleic acids** (RNA and DNA), **energy currency** (adenosine triphosphate [ATP]), **cofactors** (nicotinamide adenine dinucleotide, flavin adenine dinucleotide), and **cellular signaling** (guanosine triphosphate [GTP], ATP, adenosine). Purines are both synthesized de novo and taken in through the diet. Their degradation is a ubiquitous process; however, increased levels of the enzymes that carry out the metabolism of purine bases suggest that purine catabolism is higher in the liver and the gastrointestinal tract. Abnormalities in purine biosynthesis and degradation are associated with numerous disorders suggesting that the regulation of purine levels is essential.

Degradation of purine nucleotides, nucleosides and bases follow a common pathway (Figure 43-1). During purine catabolism, the purine nucleotides adenosine monophosphate (AMP) and GMP are generated from the dephosphorylation of ATP and GTP, respectively. AMP is then deaminated to IMP by AMP deaminase. Subsequently, GMP and IMP are dephosphorylated by specific nucleotidases to produce the nucleosides inosine and guanosine. Alternatively, AMP can be dephosphorylated to form adenosine, which is then deaminated by adenosine deaminase to form inosine. Inosine and guanosine are further broken down by the cleavage of the purine base from the ribose sugar to yield ribose 1-phosphate and hypoxanthine and guanine, respectively. Similar reactions are carried out for the degradation of purine deoxyribonucleotides and deoxyribonucleosides. Guanine is deaminated to form xanthine, whereas hypoxanthine is oxidized to form xanthine by the enzyme xanthine oxidase. Xanthine is further oxidized, again by xanthine oxidase, to form uric acid, which is excreted in the urine. Uric acid has a $pK_a$ of 5.4 and is in the ionized urate form at physiologic pH. Urate is not very soluble in an aqueous environment and the concentration of urate in human blood is very close to saturation. Therefore, conditions that lead to excessive degradation of purine bases can lead to the formation of urate crystals.

Metabolic abnormalities that lead to the overproduction of purine nucleotides through the de novo pathway lead to increased purine degradation and subsequent hyperuricemia. An example of this is an increase in the activity of 5-phosphoribosyl-1-pyrophosphate (PRPP) synthetase. This enzyme is responsible for the production of PRPP, which is an important precursor of both purine and pyrimidine de novo biosynthesis. Elevations in PRPP lead to increased purine nucleotide production that can in turn increase the rate of degradation and hence increased uric acid production. Hyperuricemia can also result from defects in the purine salvage pathway. The enzyme HGPRT is responsible for reforming IMP and GMP from hypoxanthine and guanine, respectively. In this manner purine bases are salvaged back into the purine nucleotide pool. Lesch-Nyhan syndrome results from an inherited deficiency in HGPRT. This syndrome is associated with mental retardation and self-destructive behavior, which may be associated with inadequate production of purine nucleotides through the salvage pathway in certain neuronal cells. In addition, patients with Lesch-Nyhan syndrome have gout resulting from the inability to salvage purine bases, which leads to increased levels of uric acid. Hyperuricemia and gout can also arise from numerous undefined mechanisms that include dietary issues.

One approach for the treatment of gout is to decrease the production of uric acid to prevent the development of urate crystals. **Allopurinol is an inhibitor of xanthine oxidase enzymatic activity** (see Figure 43-1). The administration of allopurinol is an effective treatment of gout because it decreases the amount of uric acid produced, which, in turn, alleviates the amount of sodium urate crystals that are formed. Additional drugs used for the treatment of gout include alloxanthine, another inhibitor of xanthine oxidase, and **colchicine, which inhibits microtubule formation and prevents phagocytic cells from engulfing the urate crystals.** This prevents the urate crystals from rupturing the phagocytes and causing inflammation in the joints.

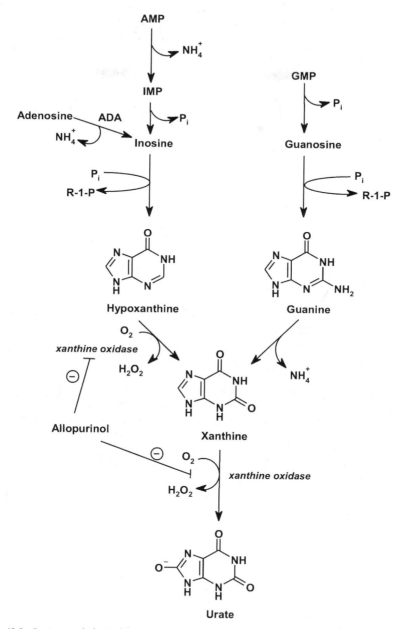

**Figure 43-1.** Purine catabolic pathway. The enzyme steps inhibited by allopurinol are indicated.

## COMPREHENSION QUESTIONS

43.1 A patient presents with extreme swelling and tenderness in the joints of the extremities. Examination of synovial fluid extracted from the big toe reveals the presence of urate crystals and confirms the diagnosis of gouty arthritis. The drug allopurinol is prescribed to inhibit which of the following enzymes?

A. Adenosine deaminase

B. AMP deaminase

C. Nucleoside phosphorylase

D. Uricase

E. Xanthine oxidase

43.2 Hyperuricemia (gout) is a clinical condition characterized by elevated levels of uric acid that lead to the formation of sodium urate crystals that are found primarily in the joints of the extremities. Which of the following factors contributes most to the formation of urate crystals in the extremities?

A. Decreased blood flow

B. Decreased temperature

C. Exposure to sunlight

D. Increased blood flow

E. Increased mobility

43.3 Inherited defects in components of purine catabolism and salvage are associated with various conditions and syndromes. The enzyme HGPRT is a key enzyme in the purine salvage pathway. It is responsible for reforming IMP and GMP from hypoxanthine and guanine, respectively. In this manner purine bases are salvaged back into the purine nucleotide pool. Genetic defects that lead to the loss of HGPRT activity are the primary cause for which of the following conditions?

A. Gout

B. Lesch-Nyhan syndrome

C. Orotic aciduria

D. Severe combined immunodeficiency syndrome

E. Tay-Sachs disease

# ANSWERS

43.1  **E.** One approach for the treatment of gout is to decrease the levels of uric acid production to prevent the development of urate crystals. Allopurinol is an inhibitor of xanthine oxidase enzymatic activity. The administration of allopurinol is an effective treatment of gout because it decreases the amount of uric acid produced, which in turn alleviates the formation of sodium urate crystals.

43.2  **B.** Uric acid has a pKa of 5.4 and is ionized in the body to form urate. Urate is not very soluble in an aqueous environment, and the quantity of urate in human blood is very close to the solubility range. Therefore, situations that lead to excessive degradation of purine bases can increase the urate concentration past the solubility point and lead to the formation of urate crystals. The decreased body temperature found in the joints contributes to the formation of urate crystals under these conditions.

43.3  **B.** Lesch-Nyhan syndrome results from an inherited deficiency in HGPRT. This syndrome is associated with mental retardation and self-destructive behavior, which may be associated with inadequate production of purine nucleotides through the salvage pathway in certain neuronal cells. In addition, Lesch-Nyhan patients have gout resulting from the inability to salvage purine bases, which leads to increased levels of uric acid. However, most patients with gout do not have a defect in HGPRT but have hyperuricemia resulting from a number of factors, including diet.

## BIOCHEMISTRY PEARLS

▶ Purine bases are used in many important biologic processes, including the formation of nucleic acids.

▶ Because urate is not very soluble in an aqueous environment and the concentration of urate in human blood is very close to saturation, conditions that lead to excessive degradation of purine bases can lead to the formation of urate crystals.

▶ Allopurinol is an inhibitor of xanthine oxidase enzymatic activity.

▶ Colchicine inhibits microtubule formation and prevents phagocytic cells from engulfing the urate crystals.

## REFERENCES

Becker MA. Hyperuricemia and gout. In: Scriver CR, Beaudet AL, Sly WS, et al, eds. *The Metabolic and Molecular Basis of Inherited Disease.* 8th ed. New York: McGraw-Hill; 2001:2513-2535.

Marks DB, Marks AD, Smith CM, eds. *Basic Medical Biochemistry.* Baltimore, MD: Lippincott Williams & Wilkins; 1996:633-635.

A 21-year-old healthy male college student went to celebrate his birthday with some friends at a bar. His friends convinced him to have his first beer since he just turned 21 years of age. After consuming the beer, he began to experience intense, worsening abdominal pain that was nonspecific in location and described as cramping. Nausea and vomiting then ensued and he was taken to the emergency department. Upon arrival to the emergency department, he was found to be very anxious with hallucinations. He was noted to be hypertensive, tachycardic, and diaphoretic. Peripheral neuropathy was also noticed on examination. Initial laboratory test revealed a normal complete blood count, drug screen, and EtOH level. Serum and urine aminolevulinic acid (ALA) and porphobilinogen (PBG) levels were both found to be elevated.

► What is the likely diagnosis?
► What is the underlying biochemical problem?

# ANSWERS TO CASE 44:

## Porphyria (Acute Intermittent Porphyria)

*Summary:* A 21-year-old healthy male patient with sudden onset abdominal pain, nausea and vomiting, hypertension, tachycardia, and peripheral neuropathy after consumption of his first alcoholic beverage. Further testing revealed elevated levels of both serum and urine ALA and PBG.

- **Diagnosis:** Porphyria (likely acute intermittent porphyria, ie, variegate)
- **Biochemical problem:** Enzymatic deficiency in heme biosynthetic pathway

## CLINICAL CORRELATION

Porphyrias are inherited disorders in the heme biosynthetic pathway. Porphyrias are classified as either hepatic or erythropoietic depending on primary site of accumulation. Inheritance is usually autosomal dominant. Patients often are asymptomatic unless exposed to factors that increase production of porphyrias (drugs, alcohol, sunlight). Erythropoietic etiologies primarily present with photosensitivity. Hepatic porphyrias can present with primarily neurovisceral symptoms, which may include abdominal pain, nausea and vomiting, tachycardia and hypertension, peripheral neuropathy, and mental symptoms (hallucinations, anxiety, seizures). Diagnosis is confirmed with elevated levels of ALA and PBG in the urine and serum. Specific tests can be performed to detect which enzyme is deficient (ie, variegate porphyria is caused by deficiency in the protoporphyrinogen oxidase [PPO] enzyme). Treatment is supportive with avoidance of triggers in the future.

## OBJECTIVES

1. Describe the biosynthesis of heme.
2. Explain why certain triggers (such as EtOH) cause increases in ALA and PBG levels.
3. Explain why treatment with intravenous heme or hematin is effective.

## DEFINITIONS

**AMINOLEVULINIC ACID SYNTHASE (ALAS):** Mitochondrial matrix enzyme that catalyzes the rate-limiting synthesis of ALA via condensation of succinyl-CoA and glycine.

**ALA DEHYDRATASE (ALAD):** Cytosolic enzyme that catalyzes the asymmetric condensation of 2 molecules of ALA to form PBG.

**AUTONOMIC NEUROPATHY:** Autonomic nervous disruption or deregulation affecting the cardiovascular, urogenital, gastrointestinal systems. Symptoms include abdominal pain, nausea and vomiting, tachycardia, and hypertension (also known as visceral neuropathy).

**COPROPORPHYRINOGEN OXIDASE (CPO):** Mitochondrial enzyme that catalyzes specifically the conversion of coproporphyrinogen III to protoporphyrinogen IX.

**FERROCHELATASE:** Assists in the insertion of the ferrous iron into the protoporphyrin IX; the final step in heme synthesis.

**HEMATIN:** Compound similar in structure to heme, except that the iron is in the ferric state (tetracoordinated with the pyrrole nitrogens and a hydroxyl group); can restore negative regulation of ALAS.

**HEME:** An essential metalorganic cofactor, consisting of 1 ferrous iron atom coordinated within a tetrapyrrole ring, protoporphyrin IX.

**PORPHOBILINOGEN DEAMINASE (PBGD):** Cytosolic enzyme that processes 6 PBG molecules through a hexapyrrole adduct to catalyze the formation of a free linear tetrapyrrole, hydroxymethylbilane (also known as **uroporphyrinogen I synthase**).

**PORPHYRIA:** Any of a number of diseases characterized by derangement in porphyrin metabolism; many are caused by genetic defects in the biosynthetic enzymes.

**PROTOPORPHYRINOGEN OXIDASE (PPO):** Catalyzes the oxidation of protoporphyrinogen IX to produce protoporphyrin IX.

**PYRIDOXAL PHOSPHATE:** Coenzyme active derivative of vitamin $B_6$.

**UROPORPHYRINOGEN (URO) III COSYNTHASE:** Cytosolic enzyme that catalyzes formation of the URO III isomer from hydroxymethylbilane.

**URO DECARBOXYLASE (UROD):** Cytosolic enzyme that catalyzes the removal of the carboxyl groups from the side chains of both URO isoforms converting them to their respective coproporphyrinogens (ie, COPRO I and COPRO III).

## DISCUSSION

The cofactor heme is required for numerous processes throughout the body. Most importantly, the heme iron facilitates systemic oxygen transfer via hemoglobin, participates in mitochondrial electron transport, and mediates oxidative drug metabolism in the liver through various cytochromes P450. All cellular tissues are capable of synthesizing heme, but expression of the pathway enzymes and levels of intermediates are greatest in erythropoietic and hepatic tissues due to high demand for heme incorporation into hemoglobin and cytochromes, respectively. Heme is a metalorganic compound, consisting of 1 ferrous iron atom coordinated within a tetrapyrrole ring, protoporphyrin IX. Protoporphyrin IX is derived from 8 molecules each of succinyl-CoA and glycine. Heme is a relatively planar molecule and highly stabilized by strong resonance throughout the tetrapyrrole ring system. The structure of heme is shown in Figure 44-1.

The biosynthetic pathway includes eight steps, shown in Figure 44-2. The first step is the rate-limiting condensation reaction between succinyl-CoA and glycine to form δ-ALA. This reaction is catalyzed by a mitochondrial matrix enzyme,

**Figure 44-1.** Structure of heme.

**ALA synthase** (ALAS), and requires the cofactor **pyridoxal phosphate.** The ALAS protein is produced in the cytosol but remains unfolded or inactive until it is directed to the mitochondrial matrix where its N-terminal signaling sequence is cleaved. In addition, this enzyme catalyzes the primary regulatory step in heme biosynthesis and is negatively regulated by any accumulation of free heme in the mitochondrial matrix. In the next step of the pathway, **ALA dehydratase** catalyzes the asymmetric condensation of 2 molecules of ALA to form PBG. Through the addition of water and the removal of 4 amino groups, **PBG deaminase** produces the linear tetrapyrrole intermediate, hydroxymethylbilane (HMB) from 4 molecules of PBG. At this point, HMB can close either in an enzyme-independent manner to form uroporphyrinogen (URO) I, or in an enzyme-dependent manner through **uroporphyrinogen III cosynthase** to form uroporphyrinogen III, the intermediate that will ultimately lead to heme formation. URO I and URO III differ in the order of the carboxymethyl and carboxyethyl substituents around the tetrapyrrole ring. In the last cytosolic steps, **URO decarboxylase** (UROD) recognizes either isomer URO I or III and removes specific carboxyl groups leaving coproporphyrinogen I or III, respectively. **Coproporphyrinogen oxidase** (CPO) acts exclusively on the type III isomer of coproporphyrinogen; after its substrate enters the mitochondrion CPO catalyzes the conversion of COPRO III to protoporphyrinogen III. This intermediate is oxidized by PPO to form protoporphyrin IX. In the final step of heme synthesis, the enzyme **ferrochelatase** inserts a ferrous iron into water-insoluble protoporphyrin IX. The excess protoporphyrin IX not converted to heme is removed via biliary excretion into the intestine.

The porphyrias are a group of inherited disorders resulting from specific enzymatic defects of the heme biosynthetic pathway. Figure 44-3 shows the heme biosynthetic

**Figure 44-2.** Heme biosynthetic pathway involving (1) ALAS, (2) ALAD, (3) PBGD, (4) UROS, (5) UROD, (6) CPO, (7) PPO, and (8) ferrochelatase. CE = carboxyethyl, CM = carboxymethyl, HMB = hydroxymethylbilane, M = methyl, V = vinyl.

pathway and characteristics of porphyrias associated with each step. A derangement in any of the involved enzymes can result in an overproduction or backlog of heme precursors prior to the deficient enzymatic step. All of the intermediate compounds in this pathway are potentially toxic. The disorders are divided into 2 broad groups, erythropoietic and hepatic porphyrias, based on the primary source of precursor accumulation. Furthermore, the porphyrias are also categorized based on the appearance of distinctive acute or chronic symptoms. Pressure to overcome the metabolic "roadblock" contributes to the rapid accumulation of precursors in acute attacks. Early pathway intermediates—that is, ALA and PBG are associated with acute neurovisceral symptoms—whereas later intermediates (which undergo porphyrinogen-porphyrin conversions upon exposure to light) cause skin photosensitivity through free-radial damage. The porphyrins can be detected and identified by spectrofluorometry based on characteristic excitation and emission wavelengths for each porphyrin. For example, serum uroporphyrin levels can be determined by

Succinyl-CoA + Glycine

↓

Aminolevulinic Acid

↓

Porphobilinogen

↓

Hydroxymethylbilane

↓

Uroporphyrinogen III

↓

Coproporphyrinogen III

↓

Protoporphyrinogen IX

↓

Protoporphyrin IX

↓

Heme

| Disease | Inheritance | Enzyme | Type | Manifestation | Symptoms |
|---|---|---|---|---|---|
| ADP | Autosomal Recessive | 2. ALA Dehydrase | Hepatic | Urinary ALA | Neurovisceral |
| AIP | Autosomal Dominant | 3. PBG Deaminase | Hepatic | Urinary ALA & PBG | Neurovisceral |
| CEP | Autosomal Recessive | 4. URO III Synthase | Erythropoietic | Urinary & RBC URO I and COPRO I | Photosensitivity |
| PCT, HEP | Variable, Autosomal Recessive | 5. URO Decarboxylase | Hepatic/ Erythropoietic | Urinary URO- and Heptaporphyrin; Fecal isocoproporphyrin | Photosensitivity, Hemolytic anemia |
| HCP | Autosomal Dominant | 6. COPRO Oxidase | Hepatic | Urinary ALA, PBG, coproporphyrin | Neurovisceral, Photosensitivity |
| VP | Autosomal Dominant | 7. PROTO Oxidase | Hepatic | Urinary ALA & PBG; Fecal protoporphyrin | Neurovisceral, Photosensitivity |
| EPP | Autosomal Dominant | 8. Ferrochelatase | Erythropoietic | RBC protoporphyrin; Fecal protoporphyrin | Photosensitivity |

**Figure 44-3.** Heme biosynthetic pathway and characteristics associated with specific enzyme-deficiency porphyrias. ADP = ALA dehydratase deficiency porphyria, AIP = acute intermittent porphyria, CEP = congenital erythropoietic porphyria, EPP = erythropoietic protoporphyria, HCP = hereditary coproporphyria, HEP = hepatoerythropoietic porphyria, PCT = porphyria cutanea tarda, VP = variegate porphyria.

detection at 615 nm after excitation at 395 to 398 nm, while protoporphyrin is detected at 626 nm. The excretion pathway of the porphyrins is determined by their water solubility. The first possible porphyrin byproduct of the heme biosynthetic pathway, uroporphyrin is by far the most water-soluble, while protoporphyrin the least soluble. Accordingly, uroporphyrin is excreted predominantly in urine, copro-porphyrin in urine and in bile, and protoporphyrin exclusively in bile.

In most cases, these disorders are inherited in an autosomal dominant manner where the individual carries one normal allele and one loss-of-function allele. Under normal circumstances, the wild type allele allows for expression of enough functional enzymes to meet the individual's requirement for heme (symptom-free carriers). However, certain environmental triggers, for example, drugs, alcohol, steroids, fasting, trauma, and/or high stress can increase this demand beyond a level that can be compensated by the single functional allele. Upon exposure to the trigger(s), patients with acute hepatic porphyrias can shift from a compensated phase to a decompensated latent phase (increased precursor production and excretion without symptoms) or to a clinically manifest stage (marked by abdominal, peripheral neurologic, cardiovascular, and psychiatric symptoms).

Alcohol ingestion induces increased activity of ALAS significantly in the liver and moderately in peripheral tissues. This effect is mediated by alleviating the negative regulation of ALAS by free heme. Mitochondrial concentrations of free heme are diminished by increased heme utilization and/or reduced activity of downstream pathway enzymes. In the liver, the demand for heme is exacerbated by requirement for heme incorporation into alcohol-eliminating cytochromes P450. Upon increased activity of ALAS, a genetic defect in either ALAD or PBGD would cause the rapid accumulation of ALA or both ALA and PBG, resulting in **ALAD deficiency porphyria** (very rare) or **acute intermittent porphyria**, respectively. During an attack, excess ALA and PBG produced in the liver are secreted into systemic circulation and are later excreted in the urine. In circulation, these neurotoxic compounds have the greatest effect on the autonomic and peripheral nervous systems resulting in the peripheral neuropathy and neurovisceral symptoms, that is, abdominal pain, nausea and vomiting, tachycardia, and hypertension.

Alternatively, patients with cutaneous porphyrias, for example, **porphyria cutanea tarda** or **hereditary coproporphyria,** chronic symptoms develop as a result of sun exposure (400 nm radiation). The excess porphyrins accumulated in the skin can absorb light energy and transfer it to damaging chemical reactions, such as peroxidation of membrane lipids. This manifests as thickening of the dermal vessel walls leading to damage of the epidermal basement membrane, excessive fragility, blistering, and scarring. In **variegate porphyria,** patients can present with neurovisceral symptoms (acute symptoms are identical but often milder than those of acute intermittent porphyria [AIP]) and/or cutaneous symptoms.

Porphyrias are diagnosed after demonstration and biochemical identification of the increased porphyrin precursor(s). Acute porphyrias are often misdiagnosed, and attacks can be fatal. The intravenous administration of heme or hematin can aid in reestablishing the negative regulation of ALAS during acute attacks. With ALAS activity attenuated, the precursor backlog at the enzymatic deficient step can begin to return to manageable levels, and the patient's condition can shift back to the compensated, symptom-free phase. After diagnosis of acute porphyria is confirmed, strict avoidance of environmental triggers can prevent acute attacks. Most patients with acute porphyrias can lead a normal life; however, complications such as hypertension, chronic renal failure, and hepatoma can become problematic.

## COMPREHENSION QUESTIONS

For questions 44-1 and 44-2 refer to the following case:

A 30-year-old white woman enters the emergency department complaining of nausea, severe abdominal pain, and prolonged constipation. She appeared distraught and was sweating. She described beginning an extremely low calorie diet within the past 2 months in an attempt to lose weight. Physical examination determined rapid heart rate, moderate hypertension, and weakness in the extremities. In addition, mild dermatitis/blistering is noted on her hands as well as scarring on her face.

44.1 You suspect porphyria. Which biochemical laboratory test(s) would be sufficient to determine the type of porphyria?

    A. Urinary ALA and PBG

    B. Urinary and fecal PBG and porphyrins

    C. Porphyrin spectrofluorometry (plasma scan)

    D. None of the above is sufficient alone

44.2 Laboratory tests revealed elevated levels of urinary PBG and coproporphyrin and plasma fluorescence emission at 626 nm. Which type of porphyria does the patient have and what is the most likely biochemical explanation?

A. Acute intermittent porphyria; PBGD heterozygous enzyme deficiency causing PBG backlog

B. Porphyria cutanea tarda; UROD homozygous enzyme deficiency causing uroporphyrin backlog

C. Variegate porphyria; PPO heterozygous deficiency causing protoporphyrin IX backlog

D. Variegate porphyria; PPO homozygous deficiency causing protoporphyrin IX backlog

44.3 The second enzyme in the heme pathway, ALAD, is very sensitive to inhibition by heavy metals (eg, lead). Which of the following test results would distinguish lead-based poisoning from acute intermittent porphyria?

A. Decreased serum and urinary ALA and PBG levels

B. Increased serum and urinary ALA and PBG levels

C. Increased serum and urinary ALA levels, decreased serum and urinary PBG levels

D. Decreased serum and urinary ALA levels, increased serum and urinary PBG levels

## ANSWERS

44.1 **C.** Given the patient's symptoms (neurologic *and* cutaneous), the main porphyrias to consider are hereditary coproporphyria and variegate porphyria. Both hereditary coproporphyria and variegate porphyria show elevated ALA and PBG levels during acute attacks; therefore, urine and serum tests for these molecules would not distinguish between these two possiblities. Similarly, both disorders show coproporphyrin in stool. In this case, spectrofluorometric assay alone to distinguish between coproporphyrin and protoporphyrin in plasma would be sufficient.

44.2 **C.** Variegate porphyria patients present with the same, but generally milder, symptoms as AIP. The emission wavelength at 626 nm is characteristic of protoporphyrin IX; the compound is responsible for the skin sensitivity not observed in AIP. Porphyria cutanea tarda can also be ruled out because the characteristic fluorescence emission for uroporphyrin is 615 nm. Homozygous deletion of PPO is unlikely because the patient's symptoms were triggered by stress in the form of caloric restriction. Patients with homozygous deficiency in the heme synthesis enzymes show early onset and more severe symptoms.

44.3 **C.** An increase in urine/serum ALA levels without concomitant increase in PBG indicates disrupted activity of ALAD. ALA alone can cause the same neurovisceral symptoms as ALA and PBG together cause in AIP. ALAD-deficiency porphyria is an extremely rare autosomal recessive disorder.

## BIOCHEMISTRY PEARLS

▶ The porphyrias are a group of inherited disorders resulting from specific enzymatic defects of the heme biosynthetic pathway.

▶ The major types of porphyria are each caused by mutations in one of the genes required for heme production.

▶ The first step in heme formation is the rate-limiting condensation reaction between succinyl-CoA and glycine to form δ-ALA. This reaction is catalyzed by the mitochondrial matrix enzyme ALAS.

▶ Forms of porphyria include ALAS-deficiency porphyria, acute intermittent porphyria, congenital erythropoietic porphyria, erythropoietic protoporphyria, hepatoerythropoietic porphyria, hereditary coproporphyria, porphyria cutanea tarda, and variegate porphyria.

## REFERENCES

Awad W. Iron and heme metabolism. In: Devlin TM, ed. *Textbook of Biochemistry with Clinical Correlations*. 7th ed. New York: Wiley-Liss; 2010.

Doss MO, Kuhnel A, Gross U. Alcohol and porphyrin metabolism. *Alcohol.* 2000;35(2):109-125.

Kauppinen R. Porphyrias. *Lancet.* 2005;365(9455):241-252.

Sassa S. Modern diagnosis and management of the porphyrias. *Br J Haematol.* 2006;135(3):281-292.

A 65-year-old woman presents to the clinic feeling tired and fatigued all the time. She has also noticed an increasing problem with constipation despite adequate fiber intake. She is frequently cold when others are hot. Her skin has become dry, and she has noticed a swelling sensation in her neck area. On examination she is afebrile with a pulse of 60 beats/minute. She is in no acute distress and appears in good health. She has an enlarged, nontender thyroid noted on her neck. Her reflexes are diminished, and her skin is dry to the touch.

▶ What is the most likely diagnosis?
▶ What laboratory test would you need to confirm the diagnosis?
▶ What is the treatment of choice?

## ANSWERS TO CASE 45:

## Hypothyroidism

*Summary:* A 65-year-old woman presents with weakness, fatigue, cold intolerance, constipation, dry skin, and goiter.

- **Diagnosis:** Hypothyroidism
- **Laboratory tests:** Thyroid-stimulating hormone (TSH) and free thyroxine ($T_4$)
- **Treatment:** Thyroid hormone replacement with levothyroxine

### CLINICAL CORRELATION

Hypothyroidism is quite common in older adults and may present with an indolent course, or it may induce dramatic mental changes such as coma or pericardial effusion with tamponade. The most common etiology is primary hypothyroidism, or failure of the thyroid gland to manufacture and release sufficient thyroid hormone. The diagnosis is established by an elevated TSH. The treatment is by thyroxine replacement.

## APPROACH TO:

## Thyroid Gland

### OBJECTIVES

1. Describe thyroid hormone metabolism.
2. Explain the regulation of thyroid hormones.
3. Explain the role of iodine on synthesis of thyroid hormone.

### DEFINITIONS

**GRAVES DISEASE:** An autoimmune disorder in which antibodies overstimulate the production of thyroid hormones leading to a condition of hyperthyroidism, or elevated thyroid hormone synthesis and secretion.

**HASHIMOTO THYROIDITIS:** An autoimmune disorder in which the thyroid gland is destroyed by the action of antibodies leading to a condition of hypothyroidism, or decreased thyroid hormone synthesis and secretion.

**THYROID RESPONSE ELEMENTS (TREs):** A domain on DNA that will bind the complex formed by thyroid hormone binding to the thyroid hormone receptor. When the complex binds to the TRE, which are located in the promoter region of the DNA, it activates transcription of the gene. When thyroid hormone is not bound to the receptor the receptor acts as a transcription repressor.

**THYROXINE:** $T_4$; a thyroid hormone derived from the amino acid tyrosine that contains 4 iodine atoms per molecule.

**TRH:** Thyrotropin-releasing hormone; a tripeptide hormone that is released by the hypothalamus and that acts on the anterior pituitary to stimulate the release of thyroid-stimulating hormone.

**TRIIODOTHYRONINE:** $T_3$; a thyroid hormone derived from the amino acid tyrosine that contains 3 iodine atoms per molecule.

**TSH:** Thyroid-stimulating hormone or thyrotropin; a glycoprotein hormone released from the anterior pituitary in response to increased levels of TRH. TSH binds to TSH receptors on the basal membrane of epithelial cells of the thyroid gland to stimulate the release of the thyroid hormones, $T_3$ and $T_4$.

## DISCUSSION

The major circulating forms of thyroid hormone are thyroxine ($T_4$), containing 4 iodine atoms per molecule, and triiodothyronine ($T_3$), with 3 iodine atoms per molecule (Figure 45-1). Of these, $T_3$ is eightfold more active. These are synthesized

**Figure 45-1.** Structures of the thyroid hormones thyroxine ($T_4$) and triiodothyronine ($T_3$). Also shown are the intermediates monoiodotyrosine (MIT) and di-iodotyrosine (DIT) that are also formed on thyroglobulin.

in the thyroid gland following TSH stimulation. **TSH binds a G protein–coupled receptor to activate adenylate cyclase and trigger a signaling cascade leading to thyroid hormone biosynthesis.** TSH is released from the pituitary in response to negative feedback by circulating levels of thyroid hormone as well as regulation by circulating levels of TRH, a tripeptide synthesized in the hypothalamus.

**Thyroid hormones are the only major biochemical species known to incorporate iodine.** In fact, **in third-world countries, iodine deficiency is the major cause of hypothyroidism** (deficiency of thyroid hormones). Iodine deficiency is characterized by the development of a goiter, representing enlargement of the thyroid gland. In the **developed world, where iodine deficiency is rare because of the use of iodized salt, autoimmune disorders are a leading cause of thyroid disease.** These are characterized by the presence of antibodies in the blood that either stimulate or damage the thyroid gland. The most common examples are Graves disease, characterized by antibody overstimulation of thyroid hormone production, and Hashimoto thyroiditis, leading to autoimmune destruction of the thyroid gland. In addition, inherited human disorders resulting in mutations in the thyroid hormone receptor, which may abolish hormone binding, have been reported. These individuals exhibit symptoms of hypothyroidism as well as a high incidence of attention-deficit disorder. This trait is genetically dominant, indicating that the mutant receptors act in a dominant negative manner.

Thyroid hormone biosynthesis (Figure 45-2) involves the concentrative uptake of iodide into thyroid cells where it is converted into iodine by **thyroid peroxidase** in the colloid space of the follicular lumen. Iodine is incorporated into tyrosine residues of thyroglobulin contained within the colloid space at the basal surface of the thyroid follicular cell. Tyrosine residues are iodinated at either one or 2 sites, and then these residues are coupled to generate either $T_3$ or $T_4$ residues within thyroglobulin. The iodinated thyroglobulin is then taken up from the extracellular matrix into the cytoplasm of the thyroid cell where lysosomal proteases cleave $T_3$ and $T_4$ from thyroglobulin. The hormones are then carried in the blood bound primarily to thyroid-binding globulin. $T_4$ is converted to $T_3$ **in the liver** and to a lesser extent other tissues, accounting for 80% of circulating $T_3$.

**Thyroid hormones stimulate protein synthesis in most cells of the body.** They also **stimulate oxygen consumption by increasing the levels of the $Na^+$, $K^+$-ATPase ion transporter.** The generation of plasma membrane $Na^+$ and $K^+$ gradients by the $Na^+$, $K^+$-ATPase is a major consumer of cellular adenosine triphosphate (ATP), leading to stimulation of ATP synthesis in the mitochondria thus directly increasing mitochondrial energy metabolism. By this means, **thyroid hormones aid the conversion of food into energy and heat.** In all of its known actions, thyroid hormone exerts its effects by interaction with its receptor in the cell nucleus and activation of transcription of the target genes.

Thyroid hormone receptors are members of a large nuclear receptor super-family that includes receptors for steroid hormones, vitamin $D_3$, and retinoic acid. Members of this receptor superfamily contain a **DNA-binding domain** responsible for binding to hormone response elements contained within the **promoters of target genes.** In addition, members of this superfamily contain a region responsible for specific binding to the hormone or biologically active agent. DNA-binding specificity is

**Figure 45-2.** Biosynthesis of the thyroid hormones T₃ and T₄ in the thyroid follicular cell and release into the bloodstream. DIT = diiodotyrosine, MIT = monoiodotyrosine, $T_3$ = triiodothyronine, $T_4$ = thyroxine, TG = thyroglobulin.

mediated by receptor sequence motifs known as *zinc fingers*, owing to their chelation of one zinc ion per loop, or *finger*. In the case of thyroid hormone, receptors bind thyroid response elements (TREs). Thyroid hormone receptors can bind TREs as monomers, as homodimers, or as heterodimers with the retinoid X receptor, another member of this superfamily. The latter exhibits the highest DNA-binding affinity and is the major functional form of the receptor.

In essence, these **receptors serve as hormone-activated transcription factors that directly regulate transcription of messenger RNA (mRNA) from target genes.** By contrast to other members of this superfamily, thyroid hormone receptors bind their sites on the promoter regions of DNA in the absence of bound hormone, usually resulting in transcriptional repression. **Binding of thyroid hormone triggers a conformational change in the receptor, converting it to a transcriptional activator.** In this state, it is competent to bind a group of coactivator proteins including histone transacetylase, an activity that serves to create a more open configuration on adjacent chromatin. Mammalian thyroid receptors are encoded by 2 different genes, each of which can be alternatively spliced, and, thus, yield 4 different receptor isoforms. These isoforms differ in their functional characteristics as well as their tissue-specific and developmental stage–dependent expression, underscoring the complexity of the multiple physiologic effects of thyroid hormones.

## COMPREHENSION QUESTIONS

45.1 A 25-year-old woman sought treatment for her constant fatigue, lethargy, and depression. She was small in stature and had previously been diagnosed with attention-deficit/hyperactivity disorder. On physical examination she was found to have an enlarged thyroid gland (goiter). Blood tests revealed elevated levels of $T_3$, $T_4$, and TSH, yet she did not exhibit typical symptoms of hyperthyroidism. Which one of the following possibilities offers the most likely explanation of her symptoms?

A. Thyroid hormone overproduction because of a thyroid gland tumor

B. Hypersecretion of TSH because of a pituitary tumor

C. Genetic alteration in the thyroid receptor reducing its ability to bind thyroid hormone

D. Mutation in the TSH receptor in the thyroid gland reducing its ability to bind TSH

E. Iodide deficiency in the diet

45.2 In individuals with iodide deficiency, which one of the following is most likely?

A. TSH levels are elevated and directly stimulate growth of the thyroid gland to a very large size.

B. Mono- and diiodinated thyroid hormone molecules are produced, and elevated levels of these derivatives compensate for the deficiency.

C. TSH levels are decreased, relieving their inhibitory effects on thyroid cell proliferation.

D. Synthesis of the $Na^+$, $K^+$-ATPase is increased.

E. Tissue utilization of oxygen is increased.

45.3  In women taking thyroid hormone replacement pills, the dosage must be adjusted if they start taking birth control pills. Which one of the following best explains this situation?

A.  Thyroid hormones block the action of estrogens, so the estrogen dose must be increased.

B.  Estrogens block the action of thyroid hormones, so the dose of thyroid hormone must be increased.

C.  Progestins block the action of thyroid hormone, so the dose of thyroid hormone must be increased.

D.  Thyroid hormones stimulate the action of estrogens, so the estrogen dose must be decreased.

E.  Estrogens stimulate the action of thyroid hormone, so the dose of thyroid hormone must be decreased.

## ANSWERS

45.1  **C.** The patient exhibits symptoms of hypothyroidism including goiter, yet thyroid hormone levels are elevated. This pattern can only be explained by resistance of target cells to thyroid hormone, for example, a mutation of the receptor decreasing its binding affinity for hormone. Iodide deficiency would lead to goiter but not increased hormone levels.

45.2  **A.** Elevation of TSH is the mechanism for goiter formation. Decreased thyroid hormone levels reduce feedback inhibition of TSH secretion by the pituitary. Therefore, TSH secretion is increased. TSH acts as a growth factor for the thyroid gland, increasing its mass and, thus, its capacity to synthesize thyroid hormones.

45.3  **B.** Estrogens partially block the action of thyroid hormones, making them less effective.

## BIOCHEMISTRY PEARLS

▶ The major circulating forms of thyroid hormone are $T_4$, containing 4 iodine atoms per molecule, and tri-iodothyronine $(T_3)$, with 3 iodine atoms per molecule.

▶ TSH binds a G protein–coupled receptor to activate adenylate cyclase and trigger a signaling cascade leading to thyroid hormone biosynthesis.

▶ In developed countries, where iodine deficiency is rare because of the use of iodized salt, **autoimmune disorders are a leading cause of thyroid disease.**

▶ Thyroid hormone receptors bind their sites on the promoter regions of DNA in the absence of bound hormone, usually resulting in transcriptional repression.

▶ **Binding of thyroid hormone triggers a conformational change in the receptor, converting it to a transcriptional activator.**

## REFERENCES

Barrett EJ. The thyroid gland. In: Boron WF, Boulpaep EL, eds. *Medical Physiology: A Cellular and Molecular Approach.* 2nd ed. Philadelphia, PA: W.B. Saunders; 2011.

Bowen RA, Austgen L, Rouge M. *Pathophysiology of the Endocrine System.* Colorado State University, 2006. http://arbl.cvmbs.colostate.edu/hbooks/pathphys/endocrine/.

Litwack G, Schmidt TJ. Biochemistry of hormones I: polypeptide hormones. In: Devlin TM, ed. *Textbook of Biochemistry with Clinical Correlations.* 7th ed. New York: Wiley-Liss; 2010.

A 32-year-old man was seen in the emergency department yesterday after experiencing a concussion and head trauma from a motor vehicle accident. The patient was stabilized in the emergency department and transferred to the intensive care unit (ICU) for observation. The patient had computed tomography (CT) scan of the head that revealed a small amount of cerebral edema but was otherwise normal. During the second day in the ICU, the nurse informs you that the patient has had a large amount of urine output in the last 24 hours. The nursing records report his urine output during the last 24 hours was 6400 cc. He has been given no diuretic medications. A urine osmolality was ordered and was found to be low. His physician remarks that the kidneys are not concentrating urine normally.

▶ What is the most likely diagnosis for the increasing dilute urine output?
▶ What is the biochemical mediator that is responsible for this disorder?

# ANSWERS TO CASE 46:

## Diabetes Insipidus

*Summary:* A 32-year-old man with head trauma is in stable condition in the ICU with increasing dilute urine output.

- **Diagnosis:** Diabetes insipidus (DI).

- **Biochemical mechanism:** Absence of vasopressin leading to inability to retain free water.

## CLINICAL CORRELATION

Vasopressin is a hormone produced in the hypothalamus and stored in the posterior pituitary gland. It is also called antidiuretic hormone, because its presence stimulates water resorption in the distal renal tubule. Excess antidiuretic hormone can lead to "water intoxication" and hyponatremia. By contrast, lack of vasopressin leads to excess loss of free water and hypernatremia. The clinical presentation is that of a patient who is excessively thirsty, having to drink large amounts of water, and urinating large amounts of dilute urine. Head trauma is one of the most common causes, particularly if the posterior pituitary stalk is disrupted. Excessive water (psychogenic water drinking) may present similarly, but these individuals will have normal decreased urine response to water restriction, and during sleep. By contrast, patients with DI will have excessive urinary loss even with water restriction and even during the night. The treatment is administration of desmopressin acetate (DDAVP), a synthetic analogue of arginine vasopressin (AVP).

# APPROACH TO:

## Vasopressin and Water Balance

### OBJECTIVES

1. Explain the role of vasopressin in the control of water metabolism.

2. Describe the role of aldosterone in regulating salt and water balance.

3. Describe the role of the hormones renin and angiotensins I, II, and III in the regulation of salt and water balance.

### DEFINITIONS

**ALDOSTERONE:** A mineralocorticoid hormone that is synthesized from cholesterol in the adrenal cortex and released in response to angiotensin II or III. It increases the ability of the kidney to absorb $Na^+$, $Cl^-$, and water from the glomerular filtrate.

**ANGIOTENSIN-CONVERTING ENZYME:** An enzyme found primarily in the lung (as well as the vascular epithelium and other tissues) that removes 2 amino acids from angiotensin I to form angiotensin II.

**ANGIOTENSINOGEN:** $\alpha_2$-Globulin; a 14-amino acid peptide that circulates in the plasma. It is cleaved by the protease renin to give the inactive decapeptide **angiotensin I.** Angiotensin converting enzyme hydrolyzes 2 amino acids from the C-terminus of angiotensin I to give the active **angiotensin II,** which gives rise to **angiotensin III** by the action of an aminopeptidase.

**DIABETES INSIPIDUS (DI):** The chronic excretion of large quantities of very pale urine of low specific gravity resulting in dehydration and extreme thirst.

**NEUROPHYSIN:** A protein that is secreted with oxytocin and vasopressin from the posterior pituitary gland. Neurophysin binds to these 2 hormones and stabilizes them.

**RENIN:** A protease that is synthesized by the juxtaglomerular cells of the kidney and secreted into the bloodstream in response to conditions of hypovolemia and hyponatremia. It hydrolyzes circulating angiotensinogen to angiotensin I.

**VASOPRESSIN:** Antidiuretic hormone; a nine-amino acid peptide that is synthesized by the hypothalamus and controls resorption of water by distal tubules of the kidney. It stimulates the insertion of water channels (aquaporins) into the apical membranes of kidney tubules.

## DISCUSSION

**Vasopressin (antidiuretic hormone) is a nonapeptide that controls resorption of water** by distal tubules of the kidney to regulate the osmotic pressure of blood. It functions to conserve body water by reducing the output of urine, and thus it is known as an **antidiuretic. Vasopressin is synthesized in the supraoptic nucleus of the hypothalamus** where it is bound to a neurophysin protein carrier, packaged in granules, and delivered by intracellular transport to nerve terminals in the **posterior pituitary.** Vasopressin bound to neurophysin is released from the granules in response to increased extracellular osmolarity sensed by hypothalamic osmoreceptors, signaling by atrial stretch receptors or after a rise in angiotensin II levels. **Its secretion is increased by dehydration or stress and decreased after alcohol consumption.**

**Vasopressin promotes increased resorption of water in the renal distal tubule by stimulating insertion of water channels or aquaporins into the apical membranes of kidney tubules.** Water is resorbed across the renal epithelium into the blood leading to a decrease in plasma osmolarity and an increase in the osmolarity of urine. In DI, this process is impaired, leading to excessive urine production. In the absence of vasopressin, the kidney cannot resorb water and it flows out as urine. This condition can arise from a deficiency in vasopressin secretion from the posterior pituitary as a result of hypothalamic tumors, injury (as in the case of this patient) or infection. Alternately, the condition may result from mutations in the vasopressin receptor or aquaporin genes or other diseases impairing renal response to vasopressin. When injected in pharmacologic doses, vasopressin acts as a vasoconstrictor.

There are 2 major types of vasopressin receptors, V1 and V2. The V1 receptor occurs in vascular smooth muscle and is coupled via $G_q$ to activation of the phosphoinositide cascade-signaling system and generation of the second messenger inositol trisphosphate ($IP_3$) and diacylglycerol. V2 receptors are found in kidney and are coupled via $G_s$ to activation of adenylate cyclase and production of the second messenger cyclic AMP.

The steroid hormone aldosterone, synthesized in the zona glomerulosa of the adrenal cortex, also plays an important role in maintaining blood osmolarity. It binds its receptors in the cytoplasm of epithelial cells of the distal colon and the renal nephron, followed by translocation of the hormone-receptor complex to the nucleus and activation of transcription of ion transport genes to increase $Na^+$ reabsorption and $K^+$ secretion. Water follows $Na^+$ movement by osmosis. These transporters include the luminal amiloride-sensitive epithelial $Na^+$ channel, the luminal $K^+$ channel, the serosal $Na^+$, $K^+$-ATPase, the $Na^+/H^+$ exchanger, and the $Na^+/Cl^-$ cotransporter.

Vasopressin and aldosterone each act on the kidney to increase fluid retention and both are in turn regulated by angiotensin II. Renin is a proteolytic enzyme that is released from the kidney in response to sympathetic neuron stimulation, renal artery hypotension, or decreased $Na^+$ delivery to renal distal tubules. Renin cleaves circulating angiotensinogen to form the decapeptide angiotensin I. Then angiotensin-converting enzyme found primarily in lung removes 2 amino acids from angiotensin I to form the octapeptide angiotensin II. In addition to other important targets in regulating blood volume, arterial pressure and cardiac and vascular function, angiotensin II stimulates aldosterone release from the adrenal cortex and vasopressin release from the posterior pituitary. The actions of angiotensin II are mediated by plasma membrane seven-helix receptors coupled via $G_q$ signaling by the phosphoinositide pathway.

## COMPREHENSION QUESTIONS

For questions 46.1 to 46.3 refer to the following case scenario:

Following brain surgery involving trans-sphenoidal removal of a pituitary adenoma, a patient experienced polyuria, polydipsia, and nocturia. These symptoms appeared shortly after the surgery and had never been previously observed. Osmolarity of the urine was below normal, even if liquid consumption was restricted. Administration of desmopressin alleviated these symptoms.

46.1 Which of the following possibilities is the most likely hypothesis to explain these symptoms?

A. Damage to the thirst mechanism from surgical trauma, leading to excessive consumption of liquids

B. Damage to the pituitary or hypothalamus from surgical trauma, leading to decreased secretion of vasopressin

C. Onset of diabetes mellitus following surgery

D. Renal injury

E. Oversecretion of angiotensin II following surgery

46.2 Desmopressin acts mainly by which of the following mechanisms?
   A.  Stimulating aldosterone secretion by the adrenal gland
   B.  Increasing synthesis of $Na^+$ transporters in kidney distal tubule
   C.  Increasing aquaporin insertion into renal distal tubule apical membranes
   D.  Acting as an insulin sensitizer
   E.  Stimulation of angiotensin II release

46.3 Which of the following would be least likely to stimulate vasopressin release from the posterior pituitary?
   A.  Dehydration
   B.  Stress
   C.  Angiotensin II
   D.  Atrial stretch receptors
   E.  Aldosterone

## ANSWERS

46.1 **B.** Desmopressin is a vasopressin analog. Symptoms are consistent with DI arising from surgical trauma to the pituitary or hypothalamus and impairment of vasopressin release. The other possibilities would not be alleviated by desmopressin.

46.2 **C.** Vasopressin, and its analog desmopressin, acts by increasing insertion of aquaporin (water channels) into the renal distal tubule membrane, permitting increased resorption of water from the urinary filtrate.

46.3 **E.** Aldosterone acts independent of vasopressin to increase water resorption by the kidney, by stimulating the insertion of ion transporters into the membrane of distal colon and kidney distal tubule.

## BIOCHEMISTRY PEARLS

▶ Vasopressin (antidiuretic hormone) is a nonapeptide that controls resorption of water by distal tubules of the kidney to regulate the osmotic pressure of blood.

▶ **Vasopressin is synthesized in the hypothalamus and stored in the posterior pituitary.**

▶ Vasopressin is released in response to increased extracellular osmolarity sensed by hypothalamic osmoreceptors, signaling by atrial stretch receptors or after a rise in angiotensin II levels. **Its secretion is increased by dehydration or stress.**

▶ Vasopressin promotes increased resorption of water in the renal distal tubule by stimulating insertion of water channels or aquaporins into the apical membranes of kidney tubules.

## REFERENCES

Booth RE, Johnson JP, Stockand JD. Aldosterone. *Adv Physiol Educ*. 2002;26(1-4):8-20.

de Gasparo M, Catt KJ, Inagami T, et al. International union of pharmacology. XXIII. The angiotensin II receptors. *Pharmacol Rev*. 2000;52(3):415-472.

Litwack G, Schmidt TJ. Biochemistry of hormones I: polypeptide hormones. In: Devlin TM, ed. *Textbook of Biochemistry with Clinical Correlations*. 7th ed. New York: Wiley-Liss; 2010.

Colorado State University. *Pathophysiology of the Endocrine System*. http://www.vivo.colostate.edu/hbooks/pathphys/endocrine/.

A 3-year-old girl was brought to the emergency department (ED) after collapsing while she was playing. Her parents report that she had gone out to play in the back yard with her new dog while her mother prepared breakfast. She began to feel ill after chasing the dog and collapsed in the kitchen. Her parents immediately transported her by car to the ED, which was close by. On arrival at the ED, the child was unconscious, apneic, with sinus bradycardia (52 beats/minute). Cardiopulmonary resuscitation was begun, the girl was intubated and an intravenous line was inserted. Parents denied any recent fever, head trauma, or vomiting. The girl was born full-term without complications and reached developmental milestones. The parents report that their first child died due to sudden infant death syndrome. A bedside glucometer test revealed a blood glucose level of less than 20 mg/dL, which was later confirmed by laboratory analysis. In response, the child was infused with 10% glucose in quarter-normal saline. Laboratory analysis also reported minimal ketones in urine and serum and an elevated blood urea nitrogen level. A urinary organic acid analysis revealed elevated levels of hexanoylglycine and suberylglycine. After spending the night in the intensive care unit, the girl was successfully extubated. There were no neurologic sequelae.

▶ What is the most likely cause for the child's hypoglycemia with low ketone bodies?
▶ What is the most likely molecular mechanism for this disease?
▶ How is this condition treated and managed to prevent further episodes?

# ANSWERS TO CASE 47:

## Medium Chain Acyl-CoA Dehydrogenase Deficiency

*Summary:* A 3-year-old girl with bradycardia, apnea, severe hypoglycemia with low ketone production, and laboratory evidence of a defect in fatty acid oxidation.

- **Most likely cause for hypoglycemia with low ketone bodies:** A defect in fatty acid oxidation

- **Most likely molecular mechanism:** The presence of hexanoylglycine and suberylglycine (medium chain fatty acyl derivatives) suggest that there is a defect in the medium chain fatty acyl CoA dehydrogenase (MCAD), thus preventing the catabolism of fatty acyl-CoA that have fatty acyl groups of 6 to 10 carbons.

- **Treatment and management:** Severe episodes of hypoglycemia are resolved by intravenous administration of glucose. Long-term management of MCAD deficiency involves prevention of long-term fasting via dietary management and adequate caloric intake.

## CLINICAL CORRELATION

A defect in fatty acid oxidation prevents the formation of ketone bodies, resulting in sequestering of CoA into acyl-CoA intermediates in the mitochondria. These intermediates inhibit gluconeogenesis in times of fasting, resulting in low concentrations of blood glucose. Severe episodes of hypoglycemia are resolved by intravenous administration of glucose while long-term management of MCAD deficiency involves prevention of long-term fasting via dietary management and adequate caloric intake. Infections leading to anorexia need to be aggressively managed to prevent hypoglycemia and buildup of toxic metabolites of fatty acid oxidation.

# APPROACH TO:

## Medium Chain Acyl-CoA Dehydrogenase Deficiency

### OBJECTIVES

1. Describe how fatty acids are catabolized to yield energy for cellular processes.

2. Explain how disruption of fatty acid oxidation can lead to decreased biosynthesis of glucose and hypoglycemia.

3. Identify laboratory analyses that can be used to differentiate between mitochondrial fatty acid oxidation disorders.

4. Formulate a treatment and management plan for patients with MCAD deficiency.

## DEFINITIONS

**β-OXIDATION:** The metabolic process by which activated fatty acids (fatty acyl-CoA derivatives) are oxidized to remove acetyl-CoA leaving a fatty acyl-CoA that is 2 carbons shorter.

**ω-OXIDATION:** The sequential oxidation of the terminal methyl group of a fatty acid to a carboxyl group. This oxidation occurs in the endoplasmic reticulum and results in dicarboxylic acids.

**SHORT-CHAIN FATTY ACIDS:** Fatty acids having 4 to 8 carbons.

**MEDIUM-CHAIN FATTY ACIDS:** Fatty acids having 6 to 12 carbons.

**LONG-CHAIN FATTY ACIDS:** Fatty acids having 10 to 16 carbons.

**VERY-LONG-CHAIN FATTY ACIDS:** Fatty acids having 17 to 26 carbons.

**FATTY-ACYL-CoA DEHYDROGENASES:** A family of mitochondrial enzymes that catalyze the first step in the β-oxidation of fatty acids; the enzymes have specificities that preferentially oxidize fatty acyl-CoA derivatives based on their chain length. Short-chain acyl-CoA dehydrogenase (SCAD) will only oxidize fatty acyl groups of 4 to 6 carbons; MCAD prefers those with 4 to 12 carbons; and long-chain acyl-CoA dehydrogenase (LCAD) prefers those with 12 to 18 carbons. Although very-long-chain fatty acids are preferentially oxidized in peroxisomes, mitochondria have a very-long-chain acyl-CoA dehydrogenase (VLCAD) that will oxidize fatty acyl CoA derivatives that have 14 to 20 carbons.

## DISCUSSION

As seen in this case, severe hypoglycemia in pediatric patients can result in cardio-pulmonary deficiencies and even cardiac arrest. When the hypoglycemia is accompanied by low blood ketones, it is an indication that there may be a defect in the catabolism of fatty acids that prevents the biosynthesis of glucose (gluconeogenesis) when blood glucose levels decrease.

To synthesize glucose, the gluconeogenic pathway requires a source of carbons, energy in the form of ATP and reducing equivalents in the form of NADH (see cases 21 and 22 for a discussion of gluconeogenesis and accompanying figures). The sources of carbon are lactate produced by glycolysis in muscle and red blood cells, and glycerol is released from the hydrolysis of triglycerides and the carbon skeletons of glucogenic amino acids. The end product of fatty acid oxidation, acetyl-CoA, cannot be used as a carbon source to synthesize glucose in a net fashion, but the β-oxidation of fatty acids provides the reducing equivalents in the form of $FADH_2$ and NADH that will be used to form ATP through oxidative phosphorylation as well as the NADH that is required for the reduction step in gluconeogenesis.

Fatty acid β-oxidation is a mitochondrial process occurring in most tissues except the brain (fatty acids cannot cross the blood-brain barrier) and red blood cells (which do not have mitochondria). After being taken up by the cell, long-chain fatty acids are activated to the fatty acyl-CoA derivatives by acyl-CoA synthetase in a reaction that converts ATP to AMP and inorganic pyrophosphate. The fatty acyl-CoA can be utilized for synthesis of triglycerides, phospholipids, or cholesteryl esters; however, under conditions of low energy and low blood glucose levels, they are directed to the mitochondria for oxidation. Long-chain fatty acyl-CoA cannot cross the mitochondrial matrix, but must first be converted to carnitine derivatives by a process known as the carnitine shuttle (see Figure 36-4).

After the fatty acyl carnitine moieties enter the mitochondria and are converted back to the CoA derivatives, the CoA-activated fatty acids enter a repeating four-step oxidation process that results in the release of acetyl-CoA, which can be further oxidized to $CO_2$ in the tricarboxylic acid (TCA) cycle or be converted to ketone bodies. This repeating 4-step process known as β-oxidation is presented in Figure 47-1.

The first step in the β-oxidation process is the oxidation of the fatty acyl-CoA to introduce a transdouble bond between the α- and β-carbons (carbons 2 and 3) to produce an enoyl-CoA. This reaction is catalyzed by fatty acyl-CoA dehydrogenases, a family of enzymes that have specificities based on the number of carbons in the fatty acyl chain. The electrons released by the double bond insertion are transferred to flavin adenine dinucleotide (FAD) to form $FADH_2$. The reducing equivalents are then transferred to electron transfer flavoprotein (ETF), which feeds them into the electron transfer chain via ETF:ubiquinone oxidoreductase.

Enoyl-CoA hydratase adds a molecule of water across the *trans*-double bond in the second step of the β-oxidative reaction scheme. This β-hydroxyacyl-CoA product

**Figure 47-1.** β-Oxidation pathway of fatty acyl-CoA.

is then further oxidized by the $NAD^+$-requiring β-hydroxyacyl-CoA dehydrogenase to produce β-ketoacyl-CoA and NADH. The final step is the cleavage of acetyl-CoA from the β-ketoacyl-CoA by β-ketothiolase. This enzymatic cleavage requires free CoA (CoASH) and results in a fatty acyl-CoA moiety that is 2 carbon units shorter than the original. This fatty acyl-CoA derivative can be further cleaved by β-oxidation until acetoacetyl-CoA is cleaved to 2 molecules of acetyl-CoA.

The fatty acyl-CoA dehydrogenases (AD) are a family of 4 enzymes that have different specificities based on the number of carbons in the fatty acyl chain. VLCAD is bound to the inner mitochondrial membrane and will oxidize fatty acyl-CoAs with chain lengths of 14-20 carbons, with its highest activity on palmitoyl-CoA ($C_{16}$). The other AD enzymes are found in the mitochondrial matrix. LCAD prefers fatty acyl-CoAs with 12 to 18 carbons, which overlaps with the specificity of VLCAD. MCAD acts on CoA-activated fatty acids between 4 to 12 carbons, with SCAD only acting on those of 4 to 6 carbons. Thus, a long-chain fatty acyl-CoA such as stearoyl-CoA ($C_{18}$) could be acted upon by as many as 4 fatty acyl-CoA dehydrogenases as it is degraded to 9 acetyl-CoA.

The most common genetic deficiency in the β-oxidative pathway is MCAD deficiency. MCAD deficiency is an autosomal recessive disease that mainly affects those of northwestern European heritage. More than 80% of patients diagnosed with MCAD deficiency have a missense mutation of a guanine residue for an adenine residue (c.985 A > G) that results in the substitution of a glutamate residue for a lysine in an alpha helical portion of the carboxy-terminal half of the molecule. This leads to impairment of the assembly of the tetrameric structure of the enzyme and instability.

A deficiency in MCAD results in a build-up of medium-chain fatty acyl-CoA in the mitochondria and a depletion of both free CoA and acetyl-CoA. Since CoA is tied up as medium-chain fatty-acyl CoA, this inhibits all metabolic processes that require free CoA. Thus, β-oxidation, ketone body formation, the TCA cycle, oxidative phosphorylation, and gluconeogenesis are all compromised. When blood glucose levels drop, after glycogen levels are depleted the liver is unable to make new glucose, and severe hypoglycemia can result. This explains why the affected individuals usually first present following a period of fasting.

Medium-chain fatty acyl moieties can exit the mitochondria as carnitine derivatives and can be exported to the blood. They also can be converted to dicarboxylic acids by Ω-oxidation by cytochromes P450 in the endoplasmic reticulum. These are usually excreted in the urine after N-acylation to glycine, such as suberylglycine. The presence of acylglycines in urine is suggestive of defects in β-oxidation. Specific diagnosis of MCAD deficiency can be definitively confirmed by determining the profile of medium-chain fatty acylcarnitines present in the blood by tandem mass spectrometry.

MCAD deficiency is manageable by means of careful dietary control. The goal of management is to avoid periods of fasting for 10 to 12 hours, which can lead to hypoglycemia and accumulation of toxic fatty acyl intermediates. A high-fat diet should be avoided, and meals high in carbohydrate should be given to children who are ill. L-Carnitine supplementation has been utilized by some physicians as a means of decreasing toxic medium-chain fatty acyl intermediates that accumulate during fasting or infections.

## COMPREHENSION QUESTIONS

47.1 On the third day of life, a female neonate born of nonconsanguineous parents began to vomit and became lethargic and hypotonic. Laboratory analysis indicated that she was hypoglycemic, acidotic (pH 7.3), and hyperammonemic. The patient remained lethargic, hypotonic, and became unresponsive despite administration of intravenous glucose. Further laboratory analyses revealed lactic acidosis, elevated ketones, and increased levels of the organic acids butyrate, adipate, and ethylmalonate in the urine. The neonate most likely is deficient in which of the following?

A. Carnitine palmitoyltransferase I

B. Carnitine acylcarnitine translocase

C. MCAD

D. SCAD

E. Succinate dehydrogenase

47.2 A 5-year-old boy had several unexplained episodes of lethargy and coma associated with fasting, hypoglycemia with low ketones, and dicarboxylic aciduria beginning at about 18 months of age. Hospitalization following a recurrence at 5 years led to the diagnosis of a deficiency of VLCAD. Which of the following would be contraindicated in the management of this patient?

A. Diet high in carbohydrates

B. Carnitine supplementation

C. High fat, ketogenic diet

D. Frequent feeding

E. Medium-chain triglyceride supplementation

47.3 The first step in the β-oxidation of fatty acyl-CoA is catalyzed by a family of enzymes, each of which are specific for different chain length fatty acyl groups. The activity of this family of enzymes would be most negatively affected by a dietary deficiency in which of the following vitamins?

A. Ascorbic acid

B. Biotin

C. Niacin

D. Riboflavin

E. Thiamine

## ANSWERS

47.1 **D.** The presence of the urinary organic acids butyrate, adipate, and ethylmalonate suggest a defect in the catabolism of short-chain fatty acyl groups. Patients deficient in carnitine palmitoyltransferase I usually present with hypoketotic hypoglycemia with elevated levels of plasma carnitine. Blood analysis of patients with a carnitine/acylcarnitine translocase defect would reveal elevated long-chain fatty acyl carnitines. MCAD deficiency would lead to elevations of medium-chain fatty acyl derivatives such as hexanoyl-glycine or suberyl-glycine. Succinate dehydrogenase deficiency would lead to a buildup of succinate and its derivatives. The patient most likely has a defect in SCAD.

47.2 **C.** With a deficiency in VLCAD, patients should avoid intake of large quantities of long-chain triglycerides, which would preclude a high fat, ketogenic diet. Patients are encouraged to eat frequent small meals high in carbohydrates to avoid hypoglycemia. Some also recommend supplementing the diet with carnitine and medium-chain triglycerides to bypass VLCAD.

47.3 **D.** The first step in the β-oxidation pathway of degradation of fatty acyl-CoA is catalyzed by acyl-CoA dehydrogenases. Each of these enzymes requires the participation of flavin adenine dinucleotide, which is a derivative of riboflavin. A deficiency in this enzyme would negatively affect the activity of the fatty acyl CoA dehydrogenases.

---

### BIOCHEMISTRY PEARLS

▶ MCAD results in a build-up of medium-chain fatty acyl-CoA in the mitochondria and a depletion of both free CoA and acetyl-CoA.

▶ Because CoA is tied up as medium-chain fatty-acyl CoA, it inhibits all metabolic processes that require free CoA. Thus, β-oxidation, ketone body formation, the TCA cycle, oxidative phosphorylation, and gluconeogenesis are all compromised.

▶ MCAD deficiency is manageable by means of careful dietary control. The goal of management is to avoid periods of fasting for 10 to 12 hours, which can lead to hypoglycemia and accumulation of toxic fatty acyl intermediates. A high-fat diet should be avoided, and meals high in carbohydrates should be given to children who are ill.

## REFERENCES

Roe CR, Ding J. Mitochondrial fatty acid oxidation disorders. In: Valle D, et al, eds. *The Online Metabolic & Molecular Basis of Inherited Disease.* New York: McGraw-Hill, 2005. http://dx.doi.org/10.1036/ommbid.129.

Salter N, Quin G, Tracy E. Cardiac arrest in infancy: don't forget glucose! *Emerg Med J*.2010;27(9): 720-721.

Sunehag A, Haymond M, Wolfsdorf J, Hoppin A. Etiology of hypoglycemia in infants and children. Accessed March 14, 2013.

A 52-year-old woman presents to your office with complaints of hot flushes, mood swings, irritability, and vaginal dryness and itching. Her last menstrual period was a little over a year ago. She denies any vaginal discharge. The patient is concerned about having thyroid problems because her friend has similar symptoms and was diagnosed with hyperthyroidism. On examination, the patient is in no acute distress with normal vital signs. Her physical is normal other than thin, atrophic vaginal mucosa. A thyroid-stimulating hormone (TSH) level is drawn and is normal. The follicle-stimulating hormone (FSH) level is drawn and is markedly elevated.

▶ What is the organ that secretes FSH?
▶ What is the signal that stimulates the release of FSH?

# ANSWERS TO CASE 48:
## Menopause

*Summary:* A 52-year-old woman presents with hot flushes, mood swings, irritability, vaginal dryness and atrophy, and last menstrual period over 1 year ago.

- **Organ secreting FSH**: Anterior pituitary gland.

- **Signal stimulates FSH release:** Gonadotropin-releasing hormone (GnRH) from the hypothalamus binds to membrane receptors of the anterior pituitary cells, triggered phosphatidylinositol signaling to stimulate FSH production and release.

## CLINICAL CORRELATION

This 52-year-old woman has symptoms of estrogen insufficiency, such as hot flushes, mood swings, and vaginal dryness. Her last menstrual period was 1 year ago, consistent with the menopause. The etiology of the hypoestrogenic state is follicular atresia of the ovaries. Once in puberty, a woman usually has fairly regular menstrual cycles as dictated by the estrogen and progesterone secretion of the ovaries until about the age of 40 to 50 years. During a period of 2 to 4 years, some women may experience irregular menses because of irregular ovulation until finally there are no further menses. The diagnosis of menopause is made by clinical criteria, although gonadotropin, FSH, and luteinizing hormone (LH) levels are usually elevated.

# APPROACH TO:
## Menstrual Cycle

## OBJECTIVES

1. Identify the hormones that control reproduction.

2. Describe about the regulation of the normal menstrual cycle.

3. Explain the hormone changes that occur during menopause.

## DEFINITIONS

**APOPTOSIS:** Programmed cell death that leads to the destruction of cells leaving membrane-bound particles that are shed or taken up by phagocytosis.

**ESTRADIOL:** 17-$\beta$-Estradiol; an estrogen steroid hormone that is synthesized in the granulose cells of the ovary and secreted in response to binding of FSH released from the anterior pituitary.

**FSH:** Follicle-stimulating hormone; a polypeptide hormone that contains $\alpha$ and $\beta$ subunits that is synthesized in and released from the anterior pituitary in response to binding of GnRH. When bound to receptors on the plasma membrane of the granulose cells of the ovarian follicle, it stimulates the synthesis and secretion of estradiol.

**GNRH:** Gonadotropin-releasing hormone; a decapeptide containing an N-terminal pyroglutaminyl residue and a C-terminal glycinamide residue. GnRH is synthesized and secreted from the hypothalamus and binds receptors on the anterior pituitary.

**LH:** Luteinizing hormone; a polypeptide hormone similar in structure to FSH and, like FSH, is synthesized and secreted from the anterior pituitary in response to binding of GnRH. It binds to receptors on the thecal cells of the ovarian follicle to increase synthesis of androgens. When bound to receptors on the corpus luteum, it increases the synthesis of progesterone.

**PROGESTERONE:** A steroid hormone synthesized from cholesterol secreted from the corpus luteum in the luteal phase of the menstrual cycle.

## DISCUSSION

With the onset of **puberty,** the normal menstrual (ovarian) cycle, as shown in Figure 48-1, is initiated by the pulsatile **release of GnRH** from the hypothalamus. **GnRH binds to plasma membrane receptors** in its target cells in the **anterior pituitary** and triggers activation of the **phosphatidylinositol signaling** pathway. This in turn signals the pituitary to release both FSH and LH from the same cell. **FSH binds its plasma membrane receptor in the ovarian follicle to stimulate, via adenylate cyclase activation, cyclic AMP production and protein kinase A activation,** increased ovarian synthesis and secretion of 17-β-estradiol, the female sex hormone. This leads to maturation of the follicle and ovum. **Estradiol also induces progesterone receptors.** Estrogens circulate in the bloodstream to maintain female primary and secondary sex characteristics. The steroid hormones estradiol and progesterone act by activating their intracellular receptors ($E_2R$ and PR, respectively) to bind their response elements in promoter regions of target genes. Together they promote the thickening and vascularization of the uterine endometrium in preparation for implantation of the fertilized ovum. Ovarian synthesis of inhibin, a negative feedback regulator of FSH (but not LH) production, is also stimulated. As **17-β-estradiol levels reach a maximum,** around **day 13** of the cycle, they stimulate a **massive release of LH** and, to a lesser extent FSH, from the pituitary, known as the LH spike. The **LH spike,** together with other factors such as prostaglandin $F_2\alpha$, **triggers ovulation.**

After ovulation, estrogen biosynthesis by the follicle declines, leading to a drop in blood levels of estrogen. The Graafian follicle now differentiates into the corpus luteum, under the mediation of LH. LH binds plasma membrane receptors in the corpus luteum, acting by the adenylate cyclase/protein kinase A signaling pathway, to stimulate progesterone biosynthesis. The uterine endometrial wall becomes secretory in preparation for implantation of the fertilized egg. In the absence of fertilization, the corpus luteum dies, because of decreased levels of LH. This leads to decreased production of progesterone and estradiol, culminating with apoptosis of the uterine endometrial cells, and their shedding at day 28 in menstruation. A new follicle then begins to develop. The decline in blood levels of estradiol and

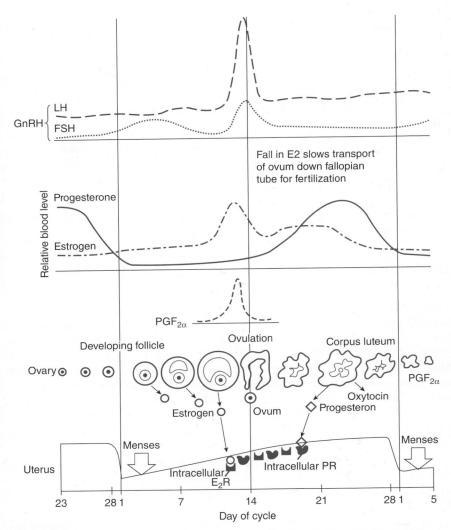

**Figure 48-1.** The ovarian cycle. (*Reproduced, with permission, from Devlin* TM, *ed.* Textbook of Biochemistry with Clinical Correlations. *5th ed. New York: Wiley-Liss, Copyright © 2002:935. This material is used by permission of John Wiley & Sons, Inc.)*

progesterone relieves feedback inhibition of the gonadotropes and the hypothalamus, leading to GnRH release and the initiation of another ovarian cycle.

If fertilization occurs, the corpus luteum remains viable and begins secretion of human chorionic gonadotropin, a function eventually taken over by the placenta. This hormone **is necessary for the maintenance of the endometrium during the first trimester of pregnancy.**

At menopause, beginning, on average, at the age of 51 years, ovarian production of estrogen and progesterone gradually declines. The **resulting release of feedback inhibition on the pituitary leads to its greatly increased release of FSH and LH.**

The adrenal glands continue to produce a minor amount of estrogen. Ovulation stops, and menstruation becomes less frequent and eventually ceases. The postmenopausal ovary and the adrenal gland continue to secrete androgens. The conversion of these androgens to estrogens mainly in fat cells and skin via the enzyme aromatase provides most of circulating estrogen in postmenopausal women.

## COMPREHENSION QUESTIONS

48.1 A 57-year-old woman who is obese did not yet exhibit symptoms of menopause but was diagnosed with polycystic ovary syndrome and insulin resistance. Her plasma levels of testosterone were above normal. Which one of the following is most likely in this case?

A. Hyperinsulinemia leading to androgen overproduction by the ovary and its conversion to estrogen in fat cells

B. Androgen overproduction by the adrenal gland and its conversion to estrogen in fat cells

C. Progesterone overproduction by the polycystic ovary leading to its conversion to estrogen

D. LH/FSH ratio = 1

E. Estrogen overproduction by the ovary and conversion to testosterone

48.2 Which one of the following changes is most likely to be observed in a postmenopausal woman who is not taking hormone supplementation?

A. Cessation of androgen secretion

B. Increased levels of FSH and LH

C. Increased osteoblast activity

D. Decreased levels of gonadotropin-releasing hormone

E. Increased progesterone levels

48.3 In a normal premenopausal woman, which one of the following is stimulated by progesterone?

A. Release of gonadotropin-releasing hormone by the pituitary

B. Ovulation

C. Development of the endometrium in preparation for possible pregnancy

D. Uterine contraction

E. Follicle development

# ANSWERS

48.1  **A.** Hyperandrogenism is primarily ovarian in origin in women with polycystic ovary syndrome, although a minor contribution from the adrenal gland may occur. Hyperinsulinemia is the primary stimulus. Fat cells convert androgens to estrogens. This may explain the late menopause in this case. In normal postmenopausal women, ovarian production of testosterone continues and this provides the main source of circulating estrogen. Typically, an LH/FSH ratio of at least 2.5 is associated with polycystic ovary syndrome.

48.2  **B.** Increased levels of FSH and LH result from decreased estrogen levels and release of feedback inhibition. Androgen secretion continues although diminished. Osteoblast activity decreases, eventually leading to risk of osteoporosis. Progesterone levels decrease and GnRH levels increase.

48.3  **C.** Progesterone is secreted by the corpus luteum under the influence of LH. Together with estrogen, it promotes the thickening and maintenance of the endometrium. Progesterone inhibits GnRH release, uterine contraction, and follicle development.

## BIOCHEMISTRY PEARLS

▶ Puberty is initiated by the pulsatile release of GnRH from the hypothalamus.

▶ GnRH binds to plasma membrane receptors in its target cells in the anterior pituitary and triggers activation of the phosphatidylinositol-signaling pathway, stimulating the release of both FSH and LH from the same cell.

▶ FSH binds its plasma membrane receptor in the ovarian follicle to stimulate, via adenylate cyclase activation, cyclic AMP production, and protein kinase, increasing the ovarian synthesis and secretion of 17-β-estradiol, the female sex hormone.

▶ Follicular atresia is the cause of hypoestrogenemia in the menopause, which is associated with elevated gonadotropin levels (FSH and LH).

## REFERENCES

Bown RA, Austagen L, Rouge M. *Pathophysiology of the Endocrine System.* Colorado State University, 2006. http://arbl.cvmbs.colostate.edu/hbooks/pathphys/endocrine/.

Litwack G, Schmidt TJ. Biochemistry of hormones I: polypeptide hormones. In: Devlin TM, ed. *Textbook of Biochemistry with Clinical Correlations.* 7th ed. New York: Wiley-Liss; 2010.

A 36-year-old man presents to the clinic with concerns about increasing weakness and fatigue. He reports that his symptoms are present at all times, but at times of stress, the weakness is much worse. He has had some nausea, vomiting, and non-specific abdominal pain, resulting in involuntary weight loss. His skin coloration has changed similar to a tan and is all over his body. On exam, he is in no distress with normal vitals other than a slightly low blood pressure. His skin is bronze in color with darkening in elbows and creases of the hand, although he states that he avoids the sun. The remainder of the examination is normal.

► What is the likely diagnosis?
► What is the underlying molecular disorder?

# ANSWERS TO CASE 49:

## Addison Disease

*Summary:* A 36-year-old man presents with fatigue, weakness, nonspecific gastrointestinal symptoms, hypotension, and darkening skin coloration despite being away from sunlight.

- **Diagnosis:** Addison disease

- **Underlying problem:** Adrenal insufficiency with lack of mineralocorticoids and cortisol

## CLINICAL CORRELATION

This 36-year-old man has the clinical stigmata of Addison disease, or adrenocorticoid deficiency. Symptoms of weakness, fatigue, and hypotension are caused by decreased levels of cortisol as well as mineralocorticoids. The darkening of the skin is a result of increased melanocyte-stimulating hormone, metabolized from adrenocorticotropin hormone (ACTH), which is elevated because of the low levels of the adrenal hormones. This is a potentially fatal disorder and requires prompt clinical recognition. Serum electrolytes give a clue to the disorder, because the patient would likely have hyponatremia and hyperkalemia. An ACTH stimulation test revealing low levels of adrenal corticoid response is confirmatory. The treatment includes hydrocortisone (cortisol) to replace glucocorticoid deficiency and a mineralocorticoid supplementation. The most common cause of adrenal insufficiency on a chronic basis is autoimmune destruction of the adrenal gland. Other autoimmune diseases should be sought and tested for, such as diabetes mellitus and systemic lupus erythematosus. Adrenal insufficiency may occur acutely when the adrenal gland is not able to generate high levels of steroids in times of stress, such as surgery or infection; the most common reason in these cases is chronic corticosteroid therapy leading to relative adrenal suppression. These situations can be avoided by the administration of a "stress dose" hydrocortisone intravenously around the time of anticipated physiologic stress.

# APPROACH TO:

## Adrenal Hormones

## OBJECTIVES

1. Describe the clinical manifestations of mineralocorticoid deficiency.

2. Describe the regulation of ACTH and cortisol.

## DEFINITIONS

**α-MELANOCYTE-STIMULATING HORMONE (α-MSH):** A polypeptide hormone derived from the breakdown of ACTH (the N-terminal 13-amino acid residues). Released from the anterior pituitary, it acts on skin cells to cause skin darkening by the dispersion of melanin.

**ACTH:** Adrenocorticotropin, adrenocorticotropic hormone; a polypeptide hormone released from the anterior pituitary into the bloodstream in response to the binding of corticotropin-releasing hormone (CRH). ACTH binds to receptors in the adrenal cortex, causing the synthesis and release of cortisol.

**CRH:** Corticotropin-releasing hormone; a polypeptide hormone consisting of 41 amino acids that is released from the hypothalamus and travels to the adrenal cortex in a closed portal system. It binds to receptors in the adrenal cortex causing the release of ACTH and β-lipotropin.

**CORTISOL:** Hydrocortisone; a glucocorticoid steroid hormone synthesized by the adrenal gland in response to binding of ACTH. Cortisol binds to cytosolic or nuclear receptors that act as transcription factors for glucocorticoid-responsive genes. In general, cortisol is a catabolic hormone that promotes the breakdown of proteins.

**CORTICOSTEROID:** A class of steroid hormones that include the glucocorticoids (eg, cortisol) and mineralocorticoids (eg, aldosterone). Glucocorticoids are involved in the maintenance of normal blood glucose levels, whereas mineralocorticoids are involved in mineral balance.

**HYPOADRENOCORTICISM:** A failure of the adrenal cortex to produce glucocorticoid (and in some cases mineralocorticoid) hormones.

**PROOPIOMELANOCORTIN:** A precursor protein synthesized in the anterior pituitary from which are generated several polypeptide hormones. It gives rise to ACTH, β-lipotropin, γ-lipotropin, α-MSH, γ-MSH, corticotropin-like intermediary peptide (CLIP), and β-endorphin (and potentially enkephalins and β-MSH).

## DISCUSSION

Cortisol is a member of the glucocorticoid steroid hormone family. It acts on almost every organ and tissue in the body in carrying out its vital role in the body's response to stress. Among its crucial functions, it helps maintain blood pressure and cardiovascular function; acts as an antiinflammatory; modulates insulin effects on glucose utilization; and regulates metabolism of protein, carbohydrates, and lipids. In all of its actions, **cortisol interacts with intracellular receptors** to trigger their binding to specific response elements in the **promoters of target genes** to influence **transcription of their messenger RNAs.**

Cortisol is produced by the adrenal gland under the precise control of the hypothalamus and pituitary. The hypothalamus secretes CRH in response to stress. CRH acts on plasma membrane receptors in corticotrophic cells in the anterior pituitary to stimulate their release of ACTH. Secretion is also under circadian regulation. Vasopressin and angiotensin II augment this positive response but by themselves do

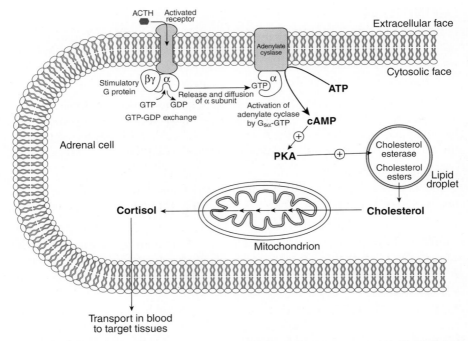

**Figure 49-1.** The sequence of events leading to the release of cortisol from the adrenal gland. Binding of ACTH to cell surface receptors activates adenylate cyclase to produce cAMP, which in turn activates protein kinase A. This causes phosphorylation events to occur that cause cholesterol to be released from cholesterol ester droplets in the cell. This initiates the conversion of cholesterol to cortisol, which is then released into the bloodstream.

not initiate it. ACTH is derived from the precursor polypeptide proopiomelanocortin after cleavage in the pituitary to release ACTH plus β-lipotropin, an endorphin precursor with melanocyte-stimulating activity. **ACTH binds to plasma membrane receptors in the adrenal gland to stimulate production of cortisol, a signaling response mediated by adenylate cyclase** (Figure 49-1). Increased blood cortisol levels exert feedback inhibition of ACTH secretion, a feedback loop acting at multiple levels including the hypothalamus, the pituitary and the central nervous system. Under separate positive control by norepinephrine, the intermediate pituitary converts ACTH to melanocyte-stimulating hormone (β-MSH) plus CLIP.

**Most cases of Addison disease are a result of idiopathic atrophy of the adrenal cortex induced by autoimmune responses,** although a number of other causes of adrenal cortex destruction have been described. Hypoadrenocorticism results in decreased production of cortisol and, in some cases, also results in decreased production of aldosterone, the other principal steroid hormone produced by this gland. If aldosterone levels are insufficient, characteristic electrolyte abnormalities are evident owing to **increased excretion of $Na^+$ and decreased excretion of $K^+$** chiefly in urine but also in sweat, saliva, and the GI tract. This condition leads to isotonic urine and **decreased blood levels of $Na^+$ and $Cl^-$ with increased levels of $K^+$.**

Left untreated, **aldosterone insufficiency** produces **severe dehydration, plasma hypertonicity, acidosis, decreased circulatory volume, hypotension, and circulatory collapse.**

Cortisol deficiency impacts carbohydrate, fat, and protein metabolism and produces severe insulin sensitivity. Gluconeogenesis and liver glycogen formation are impaired, and hypoglycemia results. As a consequence, hypotension, muscle weakness, fatigue, vulnerability to infection, and stress are early symptoms. A characteristic hyperpigmentation on both exposed and unexposed parts of the body is evident. Decreased blood levels of cortisol in Addison disease lead to increased blood levels of both ACTH and β-lipotropin reflecting decreased feedback inhibition by cortisol of their synthesis. β-Lipotropin has melanocyte-stimulating activity accounting for the increased pigmentation. The disease is progressive, with the risk of a potentially fatal adrenal crisis triggered by infection or other trauma.

Secondary adrenal insufficiency may result from lesions in the hypothalamus or pituitary, leading to impaired release of ACTH. This condition does not exhibit hyperpigmentation because release of feedback inhibition of ACTH production by low cortisol levels cannot overcome the primary defect in ACTH production. Usually, aldosterone secretion is normal.

By contrast, Cushing syndrome results from cortisol overproduction and most commonly is caused by a tumor in either the adrenal gland or pituitary.

## COMPREHENSION QUESTIONS

49.1  A 29-year-old woman exhibited a rounded face, hirsutism, upper body obesity, easily bruised skin, severe fatigue, muscle weakness, and anxiety. She also complained of irregular periods. As a woman with long-term asthma, she had been prescribed prednisone for the last 2 years. Findings on examination revealed high fasting blood glucose levels and high blood pressure. Cortisol levels were below normal.

Which one of the following is the most likely explanation to account for the patient's symptoms?

A.  Decreased levels of insulin

B.  Increased levels of testosterone

C.  Decreased secretion of ACTH

D.  Excess exogenous glucocorticoid hormone

E.  Increased hepatic metabolism of steroid hormones

49.2 A patient suffering from weakness, fatigue, nausea, and vomiting was found to have low blood concentrations of $Na^+$ and $Cl^-$ and high levels of serum $K^+$. Physical examination revealed a deep tanning of both exposed and unexposed parts of the body and dark pigmentation inside the mouth. The hyperpigmentation in this patient most likely resulted from which of the following?

A. Increased secretion of ACTH

B. Prolonged exposure of the patient to ultraviolet radiation

C. Excessive ingestion of β-carotene–containing foods

D. Activation of melanocytes caused by medication adverse events

E. Inhibition of plasma membrane $Na^+$, $K^+$-ATPase

49.3 Metyrapone is used to block the mitochondrial 11β-hydroxylase in the corticosteroid synthetic pathway and is administered to evaluate hypothalamic-pituitary-adrenal axis function. Which of the following results is most likely from this overnight diagnostic test in a healthy individual?

A. Feedback inhibition of cortisol biosynthesis

B. Increase in the levels of cortisol precursors

C. Decrease in ACTH levels

D. Inhibition of adenylate cyclase activity in adrenal cortical cells

E. Inhibition of pituitary function

## ANSWERS

49.1 **D.** Prednisone acts as a glucocorticoid hormone analog, giving rise to Cushing syndrome symptoms after prolonged administration.

49.2 **A.** Hyperpigmentation is a feature of Addison disease, the diagnosis in this case. Decreased plasma cortisol because of adrenal insufficiency releases feedback inhibition of ACTH secretion by the pituitary, resulting in elevation of ACTH biosynthesis. The ACTH precursor peptide is cleaved to also yield MSH, the factor responsible for hyperpigmentation even in areas not exposed to sunlight.

49.3 **B.** Inhibition of this step in cortisol biosynthesis relieves feedback inhibition of its biosynthetic enzymes, leading to accumulation of cortisol precursors, particularly 11-deoxycortisol. Normal patients will also have a compensatory increase in the secretion of ACTH.

## BIOCHEMISTRY PEARLS

▶ Most cases of Addison disease are because of idiopathic atrophy of the adrenal cortex induced by autoimmune responses.

▶ Cortisol interacts with intracellular receptors to trigger their binding to specific response elements in the promoters of target genes to influence transcription of their messenger RNAs.

▶ Under separate positive control by norepinephrine, the intermediate pituitary converts ACTH to MSH, which accounts for the "well tanned" appearance.

▶ Aldosterone insufficiency produces severe dehydration, plasma hypertonicity, acidosis, decreased circulatory volume, hypotension, and circulatory collapse.

## REFERENCES

Bowen RA, Austgen L, Rouge M. *Pathophysiology of the Endocrine System.* Colorado State University, 2006. http://arbl.cvmbs.colostate.edu/hbooks/pathphys/endocrine/.

Litwack G, Schmidt TJ. Biochemistry of hormones I: polypeptide hormones. In: Devlin TM, ed. *Textbook of Biochemistry with Clinical Correlations.* 7th ed. New York: Wiley-Liss; 2010.

A 32-year-old woman presents to her obstetrician/gynecologist with complaints of irregular periods, hirsutism, and mood swings. She also reports weight gain and easy bruising. On examination, she is found to have truncal obesity, a round "moon" face, hypertension, ecchymoses, and abdominal striae. The patient is given a dexamethasone suppression test that reveals an elevated level of cortisol.

▶ What is the likely diagnosis?
▶ What would an elevated adrenocorticotropic hormone (ACTH) level indicate?

# ANSWERS TO CASE 50:

## Cushing Syndrome

*Summary:* A 32-year-old woman with irregular menses, hirsutism, mood swings, weight gain, truncal obesity, hypertension, abdominal striae, ecchymoses, and elevated cortisol levels.

- **Diagnosis:** Cushing syndrome
- **Elevated ACTH level:** Likely cause of adrenal hyperplasia from ACTH-producing tumor

## CLINICAL CORRELATION

This patient presents with many of the classic findings of Cushing syndrome. Adrenal hyperplasia can be caused by excessive stimulation from ACTH (pituitary or ectopic production) or from a primary adrenal problem such as adenomas/carcinomas. In addition to above symptoms, patients with Cushing syndrome are also at risk for osteoporosis and diabetes mellitus (DM). The diagnosis is confirmed with elevated cortisol levels after a dexamethasone suppression test. Treatment depends on the underlying etiology and is often surgical.

# APPROACH TO:

## Cushing Syndrome

### OBJECTIVES

1. Describe the biosynthesis of steroids in the adrenal gland.
2. Explain from a biochemical standpoint why hypertension is a common consequence of Cushing syndrome.

### DEFINITIONS

**ABDOMINAL STRIAE:** Stretch marks of the abdominal region.

**ADRENOCORTICOTROPIC HORMONE (ACTH) OR CORTICOTROPIN:** Hormone produced in the anterior pituitary, which stimulates adrenal production of cortisol.

**ADENOMA:** Any benign tumor of glandular origin, typically found in the adrenal, pituitary, and thyroid glands (note: once an adenoma has progressed to malignancy, it is referred to as adenocarcinoma).

**CORTICOTROPIN-RELEASING HORMONE (CRH):** Hormone produced in the hypothalamus, which stimulates release of ACTH from the anterior pituitary.

**CUSHING DISEASE:** A specific form of Cushing syndrome, which is caused by an ACTH-secreting pituitary adenoma; represents approximately 66% of all cases of Cushing syndrome. Because of structural similarities with melanocyte-stimulating hormone (MSH), excess ACTH from pituitary adenomas can induce dermal hyperpigmentation.

**DEXAMETHASONE SUPPRESSION TEST:** An overnight test used to screen patients for Cushing syndrome by administering dexamethasone to a patient. Positive results for this test are indicated by a patient's inability to reduce cortisol levels after dexamethasone treatment—usually because the patient's feedback loop mechanism is ineffective at inhibiting cortisol release.

**ECCHYMOSIS:** Bruise or contusion; normally comes from damage to the capillaries at the site of injury, allowing blood to seep out into the surrounding tissue, presenting initially as a blue or purple color.

**ECTOPIC ACTH SYNDROME:** Form of Cushing syndrome in which benign or malignant tumors arise in places other than the pituitary, leading to excessive release of ACTH and subsequently, cortisol into the bloodstream; represents approximately 10% to 15% of cases of Cushing syndrome.

**HIRSUTISM:** Increased presence of hair in women on body regions where hair does not normally grow.

**HYPERCORTISOLISM:** A condition in which the body is exposed to an excess of cortisol for an extended period of time.

**IATROGENIC CUSHING SYNDROME:** Condition in which all symptoms of Cushing syndrome are brought on by administration of synthetic forms of cortisol, such as prednisone and dexamethasone. *Iatrogenic* originates from Greek and literally translates to "born from" the "healer."

**PSEUDO-CUSHING SYNDROME:** Condition in which alcohol induces symptoms of Cushing syndrome without the tumor that leads to increased cortisol levels.

## DISCUSSION

Cortisol is a stress hormone released in response to trauma—physical and emotional—that leads to several physiologic changes aimed at reducing the stress associated with this trauma. This process is helpful to the body because the activity of cortisol can limit the harmful effects of stress. However, if too much cortisol is secreted (hypercortisolism) symptoms of Cushing syndrome may appear.

Cortisol is secreted from the adrenal glands of the kidneys ("adrenal" literally means near or at the kidney). All steroid hormones are synthesized from cholesterol, with the rate-limiting step in steroid biosynthesis being the cleavage of the cholesterol side chain. This is done by several enzymes that make up the cytochrome P450 side-chain cleavage complex. High levels of $Ca^{2+}$ and protein phosphorylation—due to increased cAMP in the cytosol—increase the rate of cholesterol side-chain cleavage in the mitochondria. First, cholesterol is mobilized into the mitochondria of the adrenal cortex cells, where its side chain is cleaved by the cytochrome P450 cleavage complex (*CYP11A1*) to yield pregnenolone (Figure 50-1). Pregnenolone is oxidized by 3β-hydroxysteroid dehydrogenase to form progesterone, which is then converted into cortisol by the action of 3 cytochrome P450 enzymes, *CYP17*, *CYP21A2*, and *CYP11B1*. After synthesis is complete, cortisol is released from the zona fasciculata

**Figure 50-1.** Biosynthesis of cortisol. Cholesterol is the starting material for all steroid synthesis. Cortisol synthesis involves a series of oxidation reactions catalyzed by cytochrome P450 enzymes. (1) The cleavage of cholesterol's 6-carbon side chain is catalyzed by *CYP11A1*— the rate-limiting step in steroid synthesis. (2) This is followed by dehydrogenation of the hydroxyl group in pregnenolone, which is catalyzed by 3-β-hydroxysteroid dehydrogenase. (3) This molecule is then oxygenated at carbons 17, 21, and 11 by *CYP17*, *CYP21A2*, and *CYP11B1*, respectively, to yield cortisol. All structure modifications are indicated by dashed lines.

in the adrenal cortex via free diffusion into the blood stream for distribution to its target organs, such as liver and kidney.

The adrenal gland produces cortisol in response to intermediate hormones, called **ACTH** and **CRH** via the humoral stress pathway, which extends from the brain to the adrenals (Figure 50-2). Once the body has received an environmental stress signal, it is detected by neurons in the cerebral cortex and transmitted to the hypothalamus. The hypothalamus then releases CRH via the classic secretory pathway into the anterior pituitary. CRH stimulates release of ACTH, which then moves into the blood and down to the adrenal glands. Once in the zona fasciculata of the adrenal cortex, ACTH binds membrane receptors stimulating transfer of cholesterol to the mitochondria for cleavage events leading to synthesis and release of cortisol. After diffusing out of the cell into the blood stream, cortisol binds CBG, also known as transcortin. Cortisol then moves to receptors back in the pituitary to signal reduction of ACTH and CRH production, thus regulating cortisol synthesis by a negative feedback mechanism.

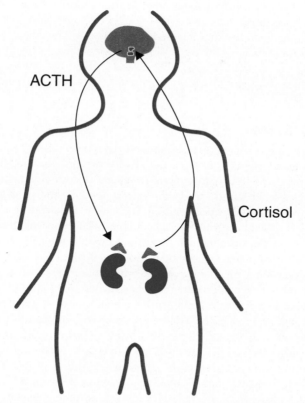

**Figure 50-2.** Induction of the humoral stress pathway. Once an environmental stress is detected by the central nervous system, this signals the hypothalamus to release CRH into the anterior pituitary. ACTH is then released from the pituitary into the blood and eventually binds membrane receptors in cells of the adrenal cortex. Cortisol is synthesized and leaves the cell via free diffusion into the blood and is eventually distributed to the hypothalamus and pituitary to inhibit release of CRH and ACTH, respectively, through a negative feedback loop.

As the major stress hormone, cortisol has many functions. For example, in trabecular bone, cortisol inhibits synthesis of new bone by osteoblasts and decreases absorption of $Ca^{2+}$ in the gastrointestinal tract, leading to osteopenia. However, the 2 principal influences of cortisol are on metabolism and the immune system.

## METABOLISM

Cortisol is catabolic and carries out lipolysis and muscle tissue degradation. Muscle catabolism provides a source of amino acids used by the liver to fuel gluconeogenesis and increases blood glucose levels. Proteolysis of collagen can lead to skin fragility, easy bruising, and striae. Lipolysis, or lipid degradation, generates free fatty acids in the blood, which when degraded by β-oxidation in the liver provide an alternative energy source, decreasing the demand for glucose. Increased lipolysis in Cushing syndrome is also thought to cause the redirection of fat deposition away from the limbs toward the trunk, leading to symptoms, such as "buffalo hump" and "moon face." In addition to increasing blood glucose levels, too much cortisol can inhibit insulin activity and exacerbate diabetic complications. Cortisol and cAMP induce 2 enzymes phosphoenolpyruvate carboxykinase (PEPCK) and glucose-6-phosphatase (G6Pase), both of which lead to increased glucose levels. The effect of cortisol is to induce PEPCK and G6Pase gene expression through a glucocorticoid response element (GRE) upstream of each gene. PEPCK and G6Pase both increase the rate of gluconeogenesis and antagonize insulin response activity, leading to increased levels of blood glucose.

## IMMUNE SYSTEM

Cortisol also has immunosuppressive effects and can reduce inflammation. For example, other synthetic forms of cortisol, such as hydrocortisone, are used medicinally to reduce inflammation. The immunosuppressive effects of cortisol are partly a result of its ability to sequester lymphocytes in the spleen, thymus, and bone marrow. Most other immunosuppressive effects come from the ability of cortisol to modulate gene transcription. Cortisol diffuses into the cell and binds glucocorticoid receptors, which disaggregate into single, or monomer, proteins. Now that the activated receptor, or transcription factor, has a free DNA-binding domain, it will translocate to the nucleus to alter gene expression. This activity induces transcription of several immunosuppressive genes that inhibit expression of target genes, such as that for interleukin 2 (IL-2).

Cushing syndrome is a rare condition in which elevated levels of cortisol are present in the patient for an extended period of time (hypercortisolism). Typically, it affects those between the ages of 20 and 50 years. On rare occasions, this disease may result from an inherited condition, which leads to growth of adenomas in endocrine glands, such as the adrenal, parathyroid, pancreas or pituitary glands. Benign tumors in the pituitary or adrenal glands can lead to excess release of ACTH or cortisol into the blood, causing the symptoms of Cushing syndrome. Typically, excess levels of endogenous cortisol—not synthetic forms of cortisol—can cause hypertension, most likely because of its weak binding capacity with mineralocorticoid receptors (ie, aldosterone receptors).

Typically, hypercortisolism comes from: (1) A pituitary adenoma, which secretes excess ACTH, thus causing release of cortisol from the adrenals, (2) an adrenal adenoma, which secretes excess cortisol, (3) a lung tumor, which secretes excess ACTH, or (4) administration of synthetic forms of cortisol (eg, dexamethasone, prednisone) due to previously diagnosed diseases, such as rheumatoid arthritis. In the case of a pituitary adenoma, the location of the adenoma makes the pituitary gland insensitive to the negative feedback mechanism brought on by excess cortisol in the blood. Sixty-six percent of all cases of Cushing syndrome are derived from pituitary adenomas. When hypercortisolism is due to exogenous administration of steroids it is referred to as **iatrogenic Cushing syndrome.**

In addition, because cortisol is a stress hormone, people who experience a great deal of stress, such as athletes, those who abuse alcohol, and pregnant women may have high blood cortisol levels and exhibit symptoms of Cushing syndrome (also known as **pseudo-Cushing syndrome**).

Treatment of Cushing syndrome is intended to return cortisol levels back to normal and usually occurs through surgery. In some cases medications, such as mitotane, which can lower blood and urine cortisol levels, can be used alone or in combination with radiation therapy.

## COMPREHENSION QUESTIONS

50.1  A 45-year-old woman presents with hirsutism, striae, bruising, acne, and hyperpigmentation of the skin. After a thorough physical examination the physician notes that she also has hypertension and shows signs of a "buffalo hump" on her back between the shoulders. Cushing syndrome is suspected and after laboratory tests show elevated blood cortisol levels she is given a dexamethasone suppression test. Her results are positive.

Following administration of dexamethasone, this patient exhibits elevated cortisol levels (a positive result) because of which of the following?

A.  The humoral stress pathway can no longer regulate cortisol levels via a negative feedback loop.

B.  There is a deficiency in the enzyme that breaks down dexamethasone, leading to excess amounts of glucocorticoid in the blood.

C.  The anterior pituitary is nonresponsive to excess cortisol and is aberrantly producing excess CRH.

D.  A CRH-secreting tumor of the adrenal glands is stimulating cortisol synthesis and is no longer responding to the negative feedback loop.

50.2  The hirsutism observed in question 50.1 is best explained by which of the following?

A.  ACTH stimulating synthesis of adrenal androgens

B.  CRH stimulating synthesis of adrenal androgens

C.  Cortisol activating aldosterone receptors

D.  Cortisol stimulating expression of adrenal androgen biosynthetic enzymes

50.3 The characteristic accumulation of adipose tissue in the facial, truncal, and cervical regions of the body in patients with Cushing syndrome is best explained by which of the following?

A. Excess adrenal androgens due to adrenal tumor

B. Excess cortisol over long periods of time

C. Cross stimulation of mineralocorticoid receptors by cortisol

D. Increased production of MSH

E. Increased proteolysis

50.4 The most common cause of hypercortisolism is which of the following?

A. Adrenal tumor that secretes excess cortisol and mineralocorticoid hormones

B. Lung tumor that secretes excess ACTH that leads to excess cortisol in the blood

C. Administration of synthetic cortisol by physician

D. Pituitary adenoma that secretes excess ACTH, leading to excess cortisol in the blood

## ANSWERS

50.1 **A.** The body's humoral stress pathway can no longer regulate cortisol levels via a negative feedback loop. By administering a synthetic form of cortisol (dexamethasone), the physician is testing the body's natural ability to reduce cortisol production. However, a patient with Cushing syndrome produces excess cortisol from one of several major sources, such as an ACTH-secreting pituitary adenoma, an ACTH-secreting lung tumor, or a cortisol-secreting adrenal tumor. Either one of these sources will be unaffected by the dexamethasone suppression test, thus exhibiting no change in blood cortisol levels. If the stress humoral pathway is intact, then the test will show a drop in cortisol levels.

50.2 **A.** Androgenic phenotypes are commonly seen in Cushing syndrome because ACTH, frequently in excess, stimulates synthesis of adrenal androgens in addition to cortisol.

50.3 **B.** Although the exact mechanism is not known, excess cortisol over long periods of time mobilizes lipids and redirects fat deposition away from the peripheral regions to the truncal region creating a "buffalo hump" appearance between the shoulders and a "moon face."

50.4 **D.** Although all of the choices can lead to hypercortisolism, about two-thirds of all cases are due to a pituitary adenoma that secretes excess ACTH, leading to excess cortisol in the blood.

BIOCHEMISTRY PEARLS

▶ All steroid hormones are synthesized from cholesterol, with the rate-limiting step in steroid biosynthesis being the cleavage of the cholesterol side chain.

▶ Cortisol is catabolic and carries out lipolysis and muscle tissue degradation.

▶ Cushing syndrome occurs from hypercortisolism over a long period of time.

▶ Cortisol has numerous effects on the body, and in excess, can cause hypertension, lipolysis, "buffalo hump," "moon faces," easy bruising of the skin, and truncal obesity.

## REFERENCES

Boron WF, Boulpaep EL, eds. *Medical Physiology: A Cellular and Molecular Approach.* 2nd ed. Philadelphia, PA: W.B. Saunders; 2011.

Lin B, Morris DW, Chou JY. Hepatocyte nuclear factor 1alpha is an accessory factor required for activation of glucose-6-phosphatase gene transcription by glucocorticoids. *DNA Cell Biol.* 1998;17(11):967-974.

Mahmoud-Ahmed AS, Suh JH. Radiation therapy for Cushing's disease: a review. *Pituitary.* 2002;5(3): 175-180.

Muller OA, von Werder K. Ectopic production of ACTH and corticotropin-releasing hormone (CRH). *J Steroid Biochem Mol Biol.* 1992;43(5):403-408.

Petersen DD, Magnuson MA, Granner DK. Location and characterization of 2 widely separated glucocorticoid response elements in the phosphoenolpyruvate carboxykinase gene. *Mol Cell Biol.* 1988;8(1):96-104.

Phillips PJ, Weightman W. Skin and Cushing syndrome. *Aust Fam Physician.* 2007;36(7):545-547.

A 42-year-old woman presents to the clinic with complaints of vague abdominal discomfort, weakness, fatigue, and bone pain. The patient gives no personal or family history of medical problems. The patient did remember that she has had frequent urinary tract infections and has had several episodes of kidney stones. Her physical examination was within normal limits. The patient had a normal complete blood count, and electrolytes revealed a significantly elevated calcium level and low phosphorus level.

▶ What is the most likely diagnosis?
▶ What is the biochemical secondary messenger activated in this disorder?

# ANSWERS TO CASE 51:

## Hyperparathyroidism

*Summary:* A 42-year-old woman with a history of frequent urinary tract infections and kidney stones is found to have vague abdominal pain and weakness, hypercalcemia, and decreased phosphorus levels.

- **Diagnosis:** Hyperparathyroidism, leading to hypercalcemia and hyperphosphatemia.

- **Biochemical mechanism:** Elevated parathyroid hormone level acts by binding its 7-helix plasma membrane receptor to activate the adenylate cyclase/protein kinase A signaling system.

## CLINICAL CORRELATION

This patient presents with kidney stones, which causes severe flank pain. The most common causes of hypercalcemia include malignancies or hyperparathyroidism. Other causes include granulomatous disorders such as sarcoid and tuberculosis, and less commonly, hypercalcemia may be the presentation of intoxication with vitamins A or D, or calcium-containing antacids, or occur as a side effect of drug therapies like lithium or thiazide diuretics. Genetic conditions like familial hypocalciuric hypercalcemia and hyperparathyroidism as part of a multiple endocrine neoplasia syndrome are also uncommon. **Primary hyperparathyroidism,** usually because of a **solitary parathyroid adenoma,** is the most likely cause when hypercalcemia is discovered in an otherwise **asymptomatic** patient on routine laboratory screening. Most patients have no symptoms with mild hypercalcemia below 12.0 mg/dL, except perhaps some polyuria and dehydration. With levels above 13 mg/dL, patients begin developing increasingly severe symptoms. These include central nervous system symptoms (lethargy, stupor, coma, mental status changes, psychosis), gastrointestinal symptoms (anorexia, nausea, constipation, peptic ulcer disease), kidney problems (polyuria, nephrolithiasis), and musculoskeletal complaints (arthralgias, myalgias, weakness). The **symptoms of hyperparathyroidism** can be remembered as: **stones** (kidney), **moans** (abdominal pain), **groans** (myalgias), **bones** (bone pain), and **psychiatric overtones.** Diagnosis can be established by finding hypercalcemia and hypophosphatemia, with inappropriately elevated parathyroid hormone (PTH) levels. Symptomatic patients can be treated with parathyroidectomy.

## APPROACH TO:
## Calcium Metabolism

### OBJECTIVES

1. Describe calcium metabolism.

2. Describe the regulation of serum calcium including the roles of PTH and calcitonin.

### DEFINITIONS

**CALCITONIN:** A polypeptide hormone of 32-amino acid residues that is synthesized in the parafollicular cells (C cells) of the thyroid gland. Calcitonin is secreted in response to elevated blood $Ca^{2+}$ levels.

**IP3:** Inositol 1,4,5-trisphosphate (inositol trisphosphate); a second messenger released by the action of phospholipase C on phosphatidylinositol 4,5-bisphosphate ($PIP_2$). $IP_3$ will bind to receptors on the endoplasmic reticulum (ER) to cause the rapid efflux of $Ca^{2+}$ from the ER into the cytoplasm.

**PHOSPHOINOSITIDE CASCADE:** The sequence of events that follow the binding of a hormone to a receptor that acts via a Gq-protein. Hormone binding to the Gq-coupled receptor activates phospholipase C, which cleaves $PIP_2$ to $IP_3$ and diacylglycerol, both of which are second messengers.

**PTH:** Parathyroid hormone; an 84-amino acid polypeptide hormone that is synthesized in the parathyroid gland and is secreted in response to low blood $Ca^{2+}$ levels. PTH acts to increase the $Ca^{2+}$ concentration in the blood by stimulating osteoclast formation and activity, thus releasing bone calcium and phosphate into the blood.

**VITAMIN D:** Vitamin $D_3$, a secosteroid (a steroid in which one of the rings has been opened) formed by the action of UV light on 7-dehydrocholesterol. The active form of vitamin D is the hormone 1, 25-dihydroxycholecalciferol (calcitriol), formed in the kidney in response to elevated PTH levels. It binds to nuclear receptors in intestine, bone, and kidney to activate the expression of calcium-binding proteins.

### DISCUSSION

Owing to the critical importance of calcium ion in a wide range of physiologic processes, blood calcium ion concentrations are tightly regulated. **Hypocalcemia rapidly leads to muscle spasm, tetany, cardiac dysfunction, and numerous other symptoms.** About half of the calcium ions in blood are bound to protein, and one-half are in the unbound state. Blood calcium ion concentrations are close to 1 mM, a value 10,000 times higher than free calcium ion concentrations in the cytoplasm. Normal calcium and phosphate concentrations in blood are near their solubility limit. Thus, elevation in these levels leads to precipitate formation and organ damage.

Intracellular calcium ion is largely sequestered within mitochondria and the lumen of the endoplasmic reticulum. Inositol trisphosphate ($IP_3$)—a second messenger of hormones that acts via stimulation of the phosphoinositide cascade (Figure 51-1)—binds its receptor on the endoplasmic reticulum membrane, triggering a rapid efflux of calcium ion from this intracellular store into the cytoplasm. The calcium-binding protein calmodulin senses fluctuations in intracellular calcium ion concentration by altering its conformation, thus influencing activities of its numerous enzyme ligands, including the calcium ATPase. This spike in intracellular calcium concentration is restored to the resting level by the activity of calcium transporters including the calcium ATPase and the sodium/calcium exchanger.

PTH plays a crucial role in regulating concentrations of calcium and phosphorus in the extracellular fluid. The major signal for parathyroid hormone release is low

Figure 51-1. The phosphoinositide cascade. Binding of hormone to the Gq-coupled receptor leads to the activation of phospholipase C, which hydrolyzes $PIP_2$ in the membrane to release the 2-second messengers, DAG and $IP_3$.

extracellular levels of free calcium ion. PTH acts on 3 major targets—small intestine, kidney, and bone—to restore calcium ion concentrations in the extracellular fluid to the normal range if they fall too low.

**PTH acts by binding its 7-helix plasma membrane receptor to activate the adenylate cyclase/protein kinase A signaling system.** In some tissues, receptor binding is also coupled to the phosphoinositide signaling system to activate protein kinase C.

PTH is synthesized as a 115-amino acid preprohormone in the chief cells of the parathyroid gland, where it is processed by proteolysis to an active 84-amino acid polypeptide and packaged in secretory vesicles. When **blood calcium ion levels fall** below normal, the active **hormone is secreted by exocytosis** into the blood. The parathyroid cell monitors calcium ion levels by means of a calcium-sensing receptor in the plasma membrane. Phosphate ion is a much less significant regulator of PTH secretion and does so by an indirect mechanism. Within seconds of calcium binding its receptor on the chief cells of the parathyroid gland, PTH secretion is decreased. Within a matter of hours, transcription of the preprohormone messenger RNA diminishes. If hypocalcemia persists over days and months, then the parathyroid gland enlarges in an effort to increase PTH production.

Bone serves as a vast reservoir of calcium in the body. Approximately 1% of calcium in bone can rapidly exchange with extracellular calcium ion. **PTH stimulates demineralization of bone and release of calcium and phosphate into the blood by stimulating osteoclast** formation and activity. This process is synergistically enhanced by vitamin D.

**PTH** also acts to **increase absorption of calcium ion by the small intestine.** It does this indirectly by promoting the formation of active vitamin D in the kidney. PTH acts on the final, rate-limiting step in vitamin D synthesis, the formation of 1, 25-dihydroxycholecalciferol in the kidney. If PTH is low, then formation of the inactive derivative, 24, 25-dihydroxycholecalciferol, is stimulated instead. Vitamin D acts on intracellular receptors in the small intestine to increase transcription of genes encoding calcium uptake systems, to upregulate their expression.

The kidney plays a critical role in calcium homeostasis. **PTH acts directly on the kidney to suppress calcium ion excretion in the urine** by maximizing tubular calcium reabsorption. It increases phosphate ion excretion in the kidney (phosphaturic effect) to prevent excessive accumulation of this anion released during bone demineralization.

Hyperparathyroidism results from oversecretion of PTH. This condition leads to excessive bone turnover and demineralization and must be treated by removal of the parathyroid gland. The disorder is classified into primary, secondary, and tertiary hyperparathyroidism. Sporadic primary hyperparathyroidism is the third most common endocrine disorder, after diabetes and hyperthyroidism. It is most common in women older than 55 years of age and the leading cause is a single adenoma, which secretes the hormone constitutively, without regulation. Symptoms can include osteopenia and bone fractures, renal stones (resulting from hypercalciuria), peptic ulcer disease, and pancreatitis. In milder cases, patients are asymptomatic or have only muscle weakness, fatigue, and/or depression.

Secondary hyperparathyroidism arises from chronic hypocalcemia. This condition can result from renal failure leading to poor reabsorption of calcium from the urinary filtrate. It can also arise from poor nutrition or malabsorption of vitamin D by the intestine. In response, parathyroid glands increase their secretion of PTH. This condition also leads to decalcification of bone. Tertiary hyperparathyroidism is often seen after renal transplantation. In these patients, the parathyroid gland secretes the hormone independently of blood calcium levels.

Paradoxically, although **chronic exposure to high PTH levels leads to bone decalcification,** administration in **pulses, as a once-a-day injection, stimulates an increase in bone mass.** This treatment is now used as an effective therapy for osteoporosis. **Calcitonin,** secreted by the parafollicular C cells of the thyroid gland, **opposes effects of PTH.** Calcitonin is secreted when blood levels of calcium are too high, and it acts to suppress reabsorption of calcium in the kidney and inhibit bone demineralization. However, in humans, it plays a minor role in regulating blood levels of calcium ion.

## COMPREHENSION QUESTIONS

51.1  A 54-year-old patient complained of muscle weakness, fatigue, and depression. She had a recent episode of renal stones and a bone scan revealed osteopenia. She had not yet entered menopause. She has taken a daily multivitamin tablet plus an additional 500 mg of calcium citrate for the last 20 years. Results from blood chemistry analysis indicated elevated levels of serum calcium ion. Urinalysis indicated phosphaturia. The patient's symptoms are most likely caused by which of the following?

A.  Excessive intake of vitamin D

B.  Excess synthesis of parathyroid hormone

C.  Excessive intake of calcium

D.  Excess synthesis of calcitonin

E.  Excess intake of phosphate

51.2  Before the introduction of vitamin D-fortified milk, children who spent most of their time indoors often developed rickets. In these vitamin D-deficient children, the most likely explanation for their bone malformations is which of the following?

A.  Excessive renal excretion of calcium

B.  Excessive renal excretion of phosphate ion

C.  Inadequate uptake of calcium in the intestine

D.  Lack of weight-bearing exercise

E.  Excessive renal tubular reabsorption of calcium

51.3 Why can excessive ingestion of a phosphate-containing soft drink in otherwise well-nourished individuals lead to decreased bone density?

A. Increased levels of blood phosphate ion interact with sensors on the membrane of parathyroid cells to stimulate parathyroid hormone release.

B. Phosphate ion binds the active site on calcium transporters in the intestine, thus inhibiting their ability to transport calcium.

C. Phosphate ion depletes cellular levels of ATP, thus resulting in inhibition of $Ca^{2+}$–ATPase calcium transporters.

D. Phosphate ion spontaneously forms an insoluble precipitate with calcium ion, thus decreasing its absorption in the intestine.

E. Phosphate ion is excessively incorporated into bone, thus weakening its structure.

## ANSWERS

51.1  **B.** Hyperparathyroidism is the likely cause of all of the patient's symptoms. Increased parathyroid hormone leads to bone demineralization, increased calcium uptake from the intestine, increased blood levels of calcium, decreased calcium ion excretion by the kidney, and increased phosphate excretion in the urine. Increased blood calcium levels caused renal stones, while bone demineralization progressed to osteopenia. The patient's intake of calcium and vitamin D are not excessive. Calcitonin acts to decrease bone demineralization. Muscle weakness and depression reflect the widespread role of calcium ion in many physiologic processes.

51.2  **C.** The major action of vitamin D is to increase absorption of calcium from the small intestine. Deficiency of the vitamin leads to low blood calcium levels, stimulation of parathyroid hormone secretion, and acting synergistically, promotion of bone demineralization. Renal excretion of calcium is decreased by hypocalcemia but elevated parathyroid hormone levels promote renal excretion of phosphate, to prevent excessive accumulation of this product of bone demineralization. Although lack of exercise decreases bone density, it does not lead to rickets if vitamin D is sufficient.

51.3  **D.** Precipitate formation effectively decreases available calcium ion. Because of widespread consumption of soft drinks rather than water by school age children aided by school vending machines, this consequence is of concern.

## BIOCHEMISTRY PEARLS

▶ Intracellular calcium ion is largely sequestered within mitochondria and the lumen of the endoplasmic reticulum.

▶ PTH acts on 3 major targets—small intestine, kidney, and bone—to restore calcium ion concentrations in the extracellular fluid to the normal range if they fall too low.

▶ Hyperparathyroidism causes elevated levels of calcium and phosphate.

▶ PTH acts by binding its 7-helix plasma membrane receptor to activate the adenylate cyclase/protein kinase A signaling system.

▶ PTH stimulates demineralization of bone and release of calcium and phosphate into the blood by stimulating osteoclast formation and activity, increases small bowel absorption of calcium ion, and acts directly on the kidney to suppress calcium ion excretion in the urine.

## REFERENCES

Chaney SG. Principles of nutrition II: micronutrients. In: Devlin TM, ed. *Textbook of Biochemistry with Clinical Correlations*. 7th ed. New York: Wiley-Liss; 2010.

Bowen RA, Austgen L, Rouge M. *Pathophysiology of the Endocrine System*. Colorado State University, 2006. http://arbl.cvmbs.colostate.edu/hbooks/pathphys/endocrine/.

Litwack G, Schmidt TJ. Biochemistry of hormones I: polypeptide hormones. In: Devlin TM, ed. *Textbook of Biochemistry with Clinical Correlations*. 7th ed. New York: Wiley-Liss; 2010.

A 35-year-old man presents with panic attacks, reporting that episodes of severe anxiety have been occurring for the last 4 months with increasing severity and duration. Along with the increased anxiety, he has experienced palpitations and headaches. Upon physical examination, he is found to be diaphoretic, his heart rate is 124 beats/minute, and blood pressure is 160/105 mm Hg. The heart rate is noted to be irregularly irregular. Electrocardiography (ECG) results show a rapid tachycardia without P waves. Elevated levels of catecholamines are present in the patient's blood sample and a suprarenal mass is detected on the abdominal computed tomography scan.

► What is the most likely diagnosis?
► What is the mechanism of the patient's symptoms?

# ANSWERS TO CASE 52:
## Pheochromocytoma

*Summary:* A 35-year-old man has anxiety, tachycardia, hypertension, elevated blood catecholamines and evidence of an adrenal mass. The examination and ECG findings reveal atrial fibrillation.

- **Most likely diagnosis:** Pheochromocytoma

- **Mechanism of symptoms:** Pheochromocytoma is a functional neoplasm arising from the adrenal medulla. It secretes the catecholamines epinephrine and norepinephrine in an unregulated manner. This increases the circulating levels of these hormones, which control heart rate, metabolism, and blood pressure. Symptoms are caused by the effects the increased hormone levels have on target tissues.

## CLINICAL CORRELATION

Pheochromocytoma is a rare functional tumor, usually of the adrenal medulla, that has periodically increases the production of catecholamine. These tumors can occur sporadically or in some familial genetic syndromes (multiple endocrine neoplasia [MEN] type 2 and von Hippel-Lindau [VHL] syndrome). The classic clinical triad is headaches, sweating, and tachycardia. However, some patients do not present with this triad. Paroxysmal hypertension (periodic) is the most common sign, which occurs in 50% of patients with pheochromocytomas. The diagnosis is confirmed with either elevated serum metanephrines or elevated 24-hour urine levels of catecholamines and metanephrines. Computed tomography or magnetic resonance imaging can be used to identify the neoplasm. Most tumors (90%) occur in the adrenal gland; however, extramedullary neoplasms can arise from the inferior para-aortic region, bladder, thorax, and head/neck. Surgical excision of neoplasm is the treatment of choice but is a very high-risk procedure that requires careful monitoring and preoperative medication preparation to prevent a hypertensive crisis. Most neoplasms are benign (90%). Long-term follow-up is essential, as some "benign" tumors can reoccur several years later with distant metastasis. Meanwhile, the patient has significant dangers to his cardiovascular health, such as atrial fibrillation with rapid ventricular response and hypertension. The priorities regarding treatment of the atrial fibrillation include sympathetic blocking agents and ventricular rate control. A short-acting β-blocking agent such as esmolol would be helpful. A-adrenergic blocking agent such as phentolamine is effective to treat the hypertensive crisis.

## APPROACH TO:
## Pheochromocytoma

### OBJECTIVES

1. Describe the normal regulation and secretion of catecholamines from the adrenal medulla.

2. Explain how catecholamines regulate metabolism, heart rate, and blood pressure.

3. Describe how the overproduction of catecholamines leads to the observed symptoms in the affected tissues and organs.

### DEFINITIONS

**AUTONOMIC NERVOUS SYSTEM:** A part of the nervous system that regulates key involuntary functions of the body, including the activity of the heart muscle, the smooth muscles, including the muscles of the intestinal tract, and the glands. The autonomic nervous system has 2 divisions: (1) the sympathetic nervous system, which accelerates the heart rate, constricts blood vessels, and raises blood pressure, and (2) the parasympathetic nervous system, which slows the heart rate, increases intestinal and gland activity, and relaxes the sphincter muscles.

**CATECHOLAMINES:** An amine derived from the amino acid tyrosine, including epinephrine (adrenaline), norepinephrine (noradrenaline), and dopamine, which act as hormones or neurotransmitters.

**FUNCTIONAL NEOPLASM:** A hormone-secreting tumor in an endocrine gland.

**GERMLINE MUTATION:** A gene change in a body's reproductive cell (egg or sperm) that becomes incorporated into the DNA of every cell in the body of the offspring. Germline mutations are passed on from parents to offspring.

**PREGANGLIONIC NEURONS:** A preganglionic neuron cell body is located within the central nervous system (brain stem or spinal cord). They send fibers out the ventral root and leave the spinal nerves through the white rami (myelin), entering the sympathetic trunk.

**SECOND MESSENGERS:** Molecules inside cells that act to transmit signals from a receptor to a downstream target.

### DISCUSSION

Pheochromocytomas are tumors of the adrenal gland, arising from chromaffin cells that synthesize, store, metabolize, and secrete catecholamines. The majority is benign with an incidence of malignancy commonly reported to be 10%, although they carry a high risk of morbidity and mortality from cardiovascular complications.

The normal age of presentation is early to mid-adulthood, although tumors may occur at any age. Normally, the adrenal medulla secretes hormones in response to stimulation by the sympathetic division of the autonomic nervous system. However, in the case of pheochromocytoma, catecholamine secretion becomes unregulated and excessive amounts are present in the blood stream. The resulting symptoms produced by such neoplasms directly relate to the effects of catecholamines on target tissues and include abdominal pain, chest pain, irritability, nervousness, pallor, palpitations, rapid heart rate, severe headaches, sweating, weight loss, hand tremor, high blood pressure, and difficulty sleeping.

Although most cases of pheochromocytoma are sporadic, a significant proportion have been linked to mutations in several genes known to cause various syndromes: VHL disease due to mutations of the *VHL* gene, MEN types 2A and 2B due to germline mutations of the *RET* gene, neurofibromatosis type 1 due to mutations of the *NF* gene, and pheochromocytoma syndromes caused by mutations of genes for members of the succinate dehydrogenase family (*SDHB*, *SDHC*, and *SDHD*). The proportion of pheochromocytoma cases due to these mutations has been reported to be as low as 10% and as high as 24%. Of these cases, germline mutations occurred most frequently in the *VHL* gene followed by *RET*, *SDHB*, and *SDHD* genes.

Normally, when the body is stressed, for example, during exercise or a fear response, nerve impulses from the hypothalamus stimulate sympathetic preganglionic neurons. The inner region (medulla) of the adrenal gland is a modified sympathetic ganglion of the autonomic nervous system. Although it arises from the same embryonic tissue as other sympathetic ganglia, its cells do not have axons and form clusters around blood vessels. When these cells (chromaffin cells) are stimulated by action potentials from sympathetic preganglionic neurons in the splanchnic nerve, they secrete the catecholamines epinephrine and norepinephrine. Catecholamines are synthesized from tyrosine, as depicted in Figure 52.1. These hormones augment the "fight-or-flight" response by increasing heart rate and the force of contraction, thereby increasing cardiac output and blood pressure. Simultaneously, the catecholamines dilate airways in the lungs, increase blood glucose and fatty acid concentrations to boost energy supplies, and increase blood flow to the heart, liver, skeletal muscles, and adipose tissue.

Epinephrine can exert its effect on target tissues by binding to two distinct types of G-protein coupled receptors, the $\beta$-adrenergic receptor or the $\alpha_2$-adrenergic receptor. These receptors are coupled to different intracellular G proteins. Both $\beta_1$- and $\beta_2$-adrenergic receptors are coupled to $G_s$ proteins, which activate adenylyl cyclase. In contrast, $\alpha_1$ and $\alpha_2$ receptors are coupled to two other G proteins, $G_q$ and $G_i$, respectively. $G_i$ inhibits adenylyl cyclase, and $G_q$ stimulates phospholipase C to generate inositol triphosphate and diacyl glycerol, which act as second messengers in intracellular signaling pathways.

During periods of physiologic stress, all tissues have an increased need for glucose and fatty acids. These fuels can be supplied to the blood in seconds by the rapid breakdown of glycogen in the liver (glycogenolysis) and of triacylglycerol in the adipose storage cells (lipolysis). Both adipocytes and hepatocytes contain $\beta$-adrenergic receptors that, when epinephrine binds, trigger the liberation of glucose and fatty acids through the above mentioned signaling pathways. Epinephrine also binds

**Figure 52-1.** Biosynthesis of the catecholamines norepinephrine and epinephrine from the amino acid tyrosine.

to similar β-adrenergic receptors on cardiac muscle cells to increase the contraction rate, thereby increasing blood supply to the tissues. Epinephrine bound to β-adrenergic receptors on smooth muscle cells of the intestine causes them to relax. The $\alpha_2$-adrenergic receptor is present on smooth muscle cells lining the blood vessels in the intestinal tract, skin, and kidneys. Epinephrine bound to $\alpha_2$ receptors causes the arteries to constrict, reducing circulation to these peripheral organs. Although the effects of epinephrine are diverse, they are each directed to supplying energy for the rapid movement of major locomotor muscles in response to bodily stress.

Pheochromocytoma treatment most often involves surgical removal of the tumor. In addition, blood pressure and pulse must be stabilized with medication before surgery.

When the tumor cannot be surgically removed, medication is utilized to manage the resulting symptoms. This is typically a combinatorial approach of medications to control the effects of the excessive amounts of circulating hormones. As most of the pheochromocytomas are benign, radiation therapy and chemotherapy have not been effective in curing this kind of tumor.

## COMPREHENSION QUESTIONS

52.1 Catecholamine secretion from a pheochromocytoma is considered unregulated. This is because the tumor:
   A. Lacks β-adrenergic receptors
   B. Contains defective transport molecules
   C. Is not innervated
   D. Lacks α-adrenergic receptors

52.2 Which of the following is not a tissue response of increased catecholamine secretion?
   A. Constriction of airways
   B. Hepatic conversion of glycogen to glucose
   C. Increased heart rate
   D. Dilation of blood vessels of skeletal muscle

52.3 Despite recommended preoperative preparation with α- and β-adrenergic blockers, severe hemodynamic instability may occur during operations to resect pheochromocytoma. Some preoperative protocols recommend the addition of the tyrosine hydroxylase inhibitor, metyrosine, in an attempt to better manage the hypertension of patients with pheochromocytoma undergoing surgical resection. What mechanism does this treatment utilize to control hemodynamic stability?
   A. Catecholamine metabolism
   B. Catecholamine synthesis
   C. Catecholamine-receptor binding
   D. Catecholamine secretion

## ANSWERS

52.1 **C.** Normally, catecholamine secretion is regulated by the hypothalamus through innervation of the adrenal medulla via sympathetic preganglionic neurons. A pheochromocytoma lacks this innervation and, thus, the normal regulatory mechanisms.

52.2 **A.** Catecholamine secretion enhances the "fight-or-flight response." Therefore, the complementary actions of target tissue are aimed at increasing blood flow, energy supplies in the form of glucose, and oxygen to skeletal muscles. The airways dilate rather than constrict to accomplish this goal.

52.3  **B.** Metyrosine is an inhibitor of the enzyme tyrosine 3-monooxygenase, and consequently of the synthesis of catecholamines. It is used to control the symptoms of excessive sympathetic stimulation in patients with pheochromocytoma.

## BIOCHEMISTRY PEARLS

▶ Pheochromocytomas are classified as functional neoplasms that secrete the catecholamines norepinephrine and epinephrine.

▶ Catecholamines function by signaling through G-protein coupled receptors on target tissues.

▶ Normal hypothalamic regulation of catecholamine release from the adrenal medulla is compromised by the hypersecretion of these hormones from the tumor.

## REFERENCES

Fishbein L, Nathanson KL. Pheochromocytoma and paraganglioma: understanding the complexities of the genetic background. *Cancer Genet.* 2012;205(1-2):1-11.

Goldstein RE, O'Neill JA Jr, et al, Clinical experience over 48 years with pheochromocytoma. 1999. *Ann Surg.* 1999;229:755-766.

Lodish H, Berk A, Zipursky SL, et al. G Protein–Coupled Receptors and Their Effectors. *Molecular Cell Biology.* 4th edition. New York: W. H. Freeman; 2000: Sec 20.3.

Tortura GJ and Derrickson B. The Endocrine System. *Principles of Anatomy and Physiology.* 11th edition. New Jersey: John Wiley & Sons; 2007: Chap 18.

Voet D, Voet JG. Signal transduction-hormones. *Biochemistry.* 3rd ed. Hoboken, NJ: John Wiley & Sons, Inc; 2004.

Young W, Kaplan N, Lacroix A, Martin K. Clinical presentation and diagnosis of pheochromocytoma. www.uptodate.com.

A 5-week-old boy is brought to the hospital emergency department following a 2-day bout of diarrhea, poor oral food intake, abdominal bloating, and an appearance of illness. The parents also indicate that the infant's complexion "looks darker than he normally looks." The boy is the product of an uncomplicated vaginal delivery at term. The child has been seen by his pediatrician for his first check-up and receives care during the day from his grandmother. The child is both nursed and bottle-fed. On physical examination, the infant is noted to appear ill with a dusky color and increased capillary refill time. Vital signs are pulse 150 beats/minute, blood pressure was 75/40 mm Hg, respiration 58 breaths/minute and shallow, and rectal temperature 100°F (37.8°C). Weight is 4.8 kg. The anterior fontanelle is sunken and mucous membranes are dry. Lungs are clear to auscultation, but breathing is labored. Heart sounds are normal. Extremities are poorly perfused. Laboratory results include a hematocrit level of 25.4%, white blood cell count of $28.6 \times 10^3/mm^3$, and a platelet count of $953 \times 10^3/mm^3$. Blood samples are noted to have a persistently darker, brownish color than normal infant samples. Arterial blood is found to have a pH of 7.18 (normal range: 7.35–7.45), a $pO_2$ of 190 mm Hg, and a $pCO_2$ of 24 mm Hg.

▶ What is the most likely cause of the infant's acidosis and abnormal signs on examination?

▶ What is the treatment for this condition?

## ANSWERS TO CASE 53:

## Pediatric Methemoglobinemia Following Diarrhea

*Summary:* A 5-week-old infant is found to have a dark complexion, shortness of breath, and acidosis on arterial blood gas. The blood is also noted to be darker than normal. The infant recently had what appears to have a gastrointestinal infection.

- **Most likely cause of infant's acidosis and examination findings:** Metabolic acidosis from recent gastroenteritis and likely congenital methemoglobinemia.

- **Treatment:** Methylene blue.

### CLINICAL CORRELATION

Methemoglobin is a form of hemoglobin in which the iron is found in the oxidative state (ferric). Ferric iron is not able to bind to oxygen leading to functional a functional anemia with reduced oxygen delivery to tissue. Affected individuals appear "cyanotic" and their blood is very dark in appearance. Cytochrome b5 reductase is important in the conversion of methemoglobin back to hemoglobin. Patients with a defect in cytochrome b5 reductase (congenital defect) are at risk of developing excessive amounts methemoglobin and anemia. In addition to congenital methemoglobinemia, there are other acquired causes (drug/chemicals) of this condition. Treatment is with methylene blue because it reduces the methemoglobin back to hemoglobin.

## APPROACH TO:

## Methemoglobinemia, Oxygen Binding, and Electrochemistry

### OBJECTIVES

1. Describe the molecular mechanisms for oxidation of hemoglobin to methemoglobin and how methemoglobin is reduced back to hemoglobin.

2. Explain why infants are susceptible to methemoglobinemia during the first few months of life.

### DEFINITIONS

**FETAL HEMOGLOBIN:** The fetal form of hemoglobin that contains 2 $\alpha$- and 2 $\gamma$-globin chains. In utero, $\gamma$ chains are the predominant $\beta$-type chain in hemoglobin. The adult form of hemoglobin in which the $\gamma$ chains are replaced by $\beta$ chains starts to increase in concentration about the 36th week of gestation; most fetal hemoglobin is replaced by adult hemoglobin by about 12 to 15 weeks following birth. Fetal hemoglobin has a higher affinity for oxygen than adult hemoglobin.

**LEUCOMETHYLENE BLUE:** The reduced form of methylene blue. Unlike the oxidized form, it is colorless.

**METHEMOGLOBIN:** Hemoglobin in which the iron ions of the heme prosthetic groups have been oxidized to the ferric ($Fe^{3+}$) oxidation state. Methemoglobin cannot bind oxygen.

**METHEMOGLOBINEMIA:** It is a disorder in which the red blood cells contain an excess of methemoglobin. Methemoglobin is normally kept at concentrations below 1%; when it exceeds this level, decreased levels of oxygen are delivered to the tissues.

**METHYLENE BLUE:** A heterocyclic, aromatic dye that contains both sulfur and nitrogen atoms. The oxidized form has a distinctive blue color when in aqueous solution; it can accept electrons to yield the reduced form, leucomethylene blue.

**OXIDATION:** The loss of electrons

**REDUCTION:** The gain of electrons

## DISCUSSION

Hemoglobin is the protein in the erythrocyte that is responsible for carrying oxygen from the lungs to the tissues that utilize it for production of ATP via mitochondrial oxidative phosphorylation. It is a multi-subunit protein consisting of 2 $\alpha$ chains and 2 $\beta$ chains, each of which has a recurring structure consisting of 6 $\alpha$-helices arranged in a 3-dimensional structure that is commonly called the **globin fold**. The $\alpha$ and $\beta$ chains function as 2 ($\alpha\beta$) dimers. Each of the $\alpha$ and $\beta$ chains has a hydrophobic pocket that contains the iron-containing prosthetic group heme. Heme is protoporphyrin IX with an iron ion bound in coordinate covalent bonds to the N-atoms of the 4 pyrrole rings. The iron ion binds a histidine residue of the protein in its fifth coordination site; oxygen binds at the sixth coordination site. Oxygen can only bind to the heme-iron when it is in the reduced, ferrous ($Fe^{2+}$) oxidation state. When the iron ion is oxidized to the ferric ($Fe^{3+}$) oxidation state, oxygen cannot be bound and hemoglobin becomes methemoglobin.

Oxygen is a very electronegative molecule, and hemoglobin will react with it to form methemoglobin and the superoxide anion:

$$Hb(Fe^{2+})-O_2 \leftrightarrow Hb(Fe^{3+}) + O_2^-$$

Because the heme prosthetic groups being positioned in hydrophobic pockets of the globin chains, the release of the superoxide anion very slowly occurs and the electron can return to the iron ion before oxygen release. Thus, the formation of methemoglobin slowly occurs; the rate of methemoglobin formation can be increased with increased oxidative load from exposure to a variety of xenobiotics, chemicals or drugs. Normally, the steady-state levels of methemoglobin in the red blood cell are kept to a minimum (< 1% of total hemoglobin) by the cytochrome $b_5$ reductase (NADH methemoglobin reductase) system of the erythrocyte, using NADH produced by glycolysis as the source of reducing equivalents (Figure 53-1). A minor system for reducing methemoglobin uses a cytochrome $b_5$ reductase that

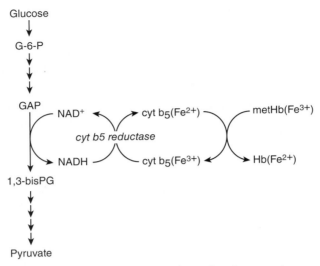

**Figure 53-1.** Reduction of methemoglobin by the cytochrome $b_5$ reductase system.

obtains its reducing equivalents from NADPH produced by the pentose phosphate pathway.

Methemoglobinemia is a condition in which the levels of methemoglobin exceed 1% of total hemoglobin. Hereditary methemoglobinemia is rare and occurs when there is a deficiency in the erythrocyte of either cytochrome $b_5$ reductase or cytochrome $b_5$ or when the patient has Hemoglobin M (wherein hemoglobin has been mutated to change an amino acid near the heme iron to make it more susceptible to oxidation). Acquired methemoglobinemia is much more common and can occur when oxidative stress exceeds the ability of red blood cells to re-reduce methemoglobin to hemoglobin. This can happen with the administration of certain pharmaceuticals (eg, benzocaine, dapsone, sulfonamides), use of recreational drugs such as amyl nitrate, or by exposure to pesticides or herbicides.

Infants, as in the case above, are particularly susceptible to episodes of methemoglobinemia because the cytochrome $b_5$ reductase is not expressed to adult levels until the infant has reached 2 to 6 months of age. In addition, the transition from fetal hemoglobin ($\alpha_2\gamma_2$), which is more susceptible to oxidation, to adult hemoglobin ($\alpha_2\beta_2$) is not complete until 2 or 3 months of age. The infant in the scenario has experienced acute gastroenteritis and diarrhea that resulted in acidosis, probably due to excessive loss of bicarbonate in the stool. The decreased pH of the blood further impairs the already low levels of cytochrome $b_5$ reductase. As a consequence, methemoglobin accumulates, thus decreasing the amount of oxygen that can be delivered to peripheral tissues. The respiration rate increases in an attempt to compensate for the decreased oxygen deposition. The increased concentration of methemoglobin will give blood samples a brownish color.

**Figure 53-2.** Treatment of methemoglobinemia with the dye methylene blue. The NADPH-dependent form of cytochrome $b_5$ reductase reduces methylene blue to leucomethylene blue, which transfers its electrons to methemoglobin, thus reducing the ferric ion to the ferrous form.

Acute infantile methemoglobinemia can be treated by administering methylene blue, which is a heterocyclic aromatic dye (Figure 53-2). When oxidized, the dye is blue, as its name suggests, but it is colorless when reduced. Methylene blue has been shown to increase the activity of the NADPH-dependent form of cytochrome $b_5$ reductase (NADPH methemoglobin reductase), which usually does not participate in reduction of methemoglobin. The enzyme reduces methylene blue to leucomethylene blue using reducing equivalents from NADPH. The reduced form of methylene blue then transfers its electrons to methemoglobin ($Fe^{3+}$), thereby regenerating hemoglobin ($Fe^{2+}$). The NADPH utilized by the reductase is produced by the oxidation reactions of the pentose phosphate pathway. Thus, this treatment will be ineffective if the patient has a deficiency in glucose 6-phosphate dehydrogenase. It also will be ineffective if there is a deficiency in the NADPH-dependent cytochrome $b_5$ reductase.

## COMPREHENSION QUESTIONS

53.1  When oxygen is bound to hemoglobin, the ferrous ion ($Fe^{2+}$) can be oxidized to the ferric ion ($Fe^{3+}$), which no longer binds oxygen. This results in production of the superoxide anion radical and methemoglobin. Methemoglobin levels are normally kept at a minimum by the action of which enzyme?

A.  Glucose 6-phosphate dehydrogenase

B.  Malic enzyme

C.  NADH-cytochrome $b_5$ reductase

D.  NADH dehydrogenase

E.  NADPH-cytochrome $b_5$ reductase

454 CASE FILES: BIOCHEMISTRY

53.2 A young Caucasian girl is brought to the pediatric clinic by her parents because they are concerned that she has a bluish hue to her skin. The physician suspects that the child has a congenital form of methemoglobinemia. However, an extract of her blood is able to convert added methemoglobin to hemoglobin. It is likely that the girl has which abnormal hemoglobin variant?

A. Hemoglobin $A_{1C}$

B. Hemoglobin C

C. Hemoglobin F

D. Hemoglobin M

E. Hemoglobin S

53.3 A 2-month-old male infant presents to the emergency department following a 2-day bout with diarrhea and poor oral food intake. The infant is lethargic, has a dusky color, and signs of dehydration. Lungs are clear to auscultation but his breathing is labored. In addition to dehydration, the child is diagnosed with methemoglobinemia. To treat the methemoglobinemia, the child is administered methylene blue. Methylene blue reduces methemoglobin by utilizing reducing equivalents (electrons) drawn from which of the following?

A. Tricarboxylic acid cycle

B. Pentose phosphate pathway

C. Oxidation of glutamate to $\alpha$-ketoglutarate

D. Glycolysis

E. $\beta$-Oxidation pathway

## ANSWERS

53.1 **C.** The levels of methemoglobin are normally kept below 1% by NADH-cytochrome $b_5$ reductase, which uses reducing equivalents from cytosolic NADH to reduce the ferric ion in methemoglobin to the ferrous ion in hemoglobin. The NADH primarily originates from the conversion of glyceraldehyde 3-phosphate to 1,3-bisphosphoglycerate in the glycolytic pathway. Glucose 6-phosphate dehydrogenase oxidizes glucose 6-phosphate to 6-phosphogluconolactone and converts $NADP^+$ to NADPH. The malic enzyme also produces NADPH when it oxidatively decarboxylates malate to yield pyruvate. NADH dehydrogenase is the first enzyme in the mitochondrial electron transport pathway. NADPH-cytochrome $b_5$ reductase plays a minor role in converting methemoglobin to hemoglobin but can play an important role in the treatment of methemoglobinemia.

53.2  **D.** Congenital methemoglobinemia can be due to a deficiency in cytochrome $b_5$ reductase activity, which would decrease the rate at which methemoglobin could be reduced to hemoglobin. Another cause is the abnormal hemoglobin variant hemoglobin M. Hemoglobin M is the term applied to a group of abnormal hemoglobins in which a single amino acid substitution in the hydrophobic pocket that binds the heme results in the heme iron being easily oxidized to the ferric state. An example is hemoglobin M Saskatoon, in which His at position E7 is mutated to a Tyr residue. Hemoglobin $A_{1C}$ results from glycosylation of normal hemoglobin at elevated blood glucose levels; it is used as measure of long-term blood glucose levels. Hemoglobin C is the result of a point mutation that converts a Glu residue to a Lys residue at position 6 of the β-chain. It results in loss of plasticity of red blood cells and a mild hemolytic anemia. Hemoglobin F is the fetal form of hemoglobin. Hemoglobin S is the hemoglobin variant that results in sickle cell anemia.

53.3  **B.** Treatment of methemoglobinemia with methylene blue requires a source of cytosolic NADPH and NADPH-cytochrome $b_5$ reductase. The cytosolic NADPH is primarily derived from the pentose phosphate pathway, although some can be obtained from the malic enzyme oxidation of malate to pyruvate. The TCA cycle is mitochondrial, as are the glutamate dehydrogenase reaction and the β-oxidative pathways; these also produce NADH. Glycolysis is cytosolic, but it produces NADH, not NADPH.

## BIOCHEMISTRY PEARLS

▶ Cytochrome b5 reductase allows the reduction of methemoglobin back to hemoglobin. Inherited conditions that affect this enzyme are at risk for the development of hemoglobinemia.

▶ Methemoglobin with iron in the oxidized state (Ferric) is unable to carry oxygen.

▶ Methylene blue allows reduction of the methemoglobin back to hemoglobin.

## REFERENCES

Ash-Bernal R, Wise R, Wright SM. Acquired methemoglobinemia: a retrospective series of 138 cases at 2 teaching hospitals. *Medicine.* 2004;83(5):265-273.

Jolly BT, Monico EP, McDevitt B. Methemoglobinemia in and infant: case report and review of the literature. *Pediatr Emer Care.* 1995;11(5):294-297.

Prchal J, Schrier S, Mahoney D, Landaw S, Hoppin A. Clinical features, diagnosis, and treatment of methemoglobinemia. www.uptodate.com.

Verive MJ. Pediatric methemoglobinemia. http://emedicine.medscape.com/article/956528-overview#showall.

# Listing of Cases

## Listing by Case Number

## Listing by Disorder (Alphabetical)

*Note:* Page numbers followed by *f* or *t* indicate figures or tables, respectively.

Coenzyme Q (ubiquinone), 143, 144, 147, 239, 241
Colchicine, 371, 372
Cold intolerance, in hypothyroidism, 387–388
Colipase, 168, 305
Coma, hepatic, 173–174
Common bile duct, 167
Complementary DNA (cDNA), 77
Confusion, in thiamine deficiency, 133–134
Congenital erythropoietic porphyria, 382f
Constipation
  in hypothyroidism, 387–388
  in irritable bowel syndrome, 219–220
Convicine, 289, 291f
Cooley anemia, 110
Coombs test, 204
Copper ions, 146
Coproporphyrinogen, 381f
Coproporphyrinogen oxidase (CPO), 379, 380
Cori cycle, 187
Cori disease, 180
Coronary heart disease
  hypercholesterolemia and, 264
  myocardial infarction and, 238
Corpus luteum, 411, 412f
Corticosteroid-binding globulin (CBG), 427
Corticosteroid(s), 68, 417
Corticotropin-like intermediary peptide (CLIP), 418
Corticotropin-releasing hormone (CRH), 417–419, 424, 427, 427f
Cortisol (hydrocortisone)
  in Addison disease, 416–419
  in Cushing syndrome, 423–424, 428–429
  functions, 417, 428
  release, 417–419, 418f
  synthesis, 425–427, 426f
Coupled oxidative phosphorylation, 143
Coupled respiration, 144
Coxibs (cyclooxygenase-2 inhibitors), 280–281, 282, 284, 284f
Creatine, 342
Creatine kinase, 239
Creatine phosphokinase (CPK), 184–185, 296
CRH (corticotropin-releasing hormone), 417–419, 424, 427, 427f
Cushing disease, 425
Cushing syndrome, 419, 423–431
Cyanide ion, 146t, 147
Cyanide poisoning, 141–150, 147f
Cyclic adenosine monophosphate.
    See cAMP
Cyclin-dependent kinases (CDKs), 29
Cyclins, 29

Cyclooxygenase-1 (COX-1) inhibitors, 280–281, 284, 284f
Cyclooxygenase-2 (COX-2) inhibitors, 280–281, 284, 284f
Cysteine, 358t
Cystic fibrosis, 75–82
Cystic fibrosis transmembrane conductance regulator (CFTR), 76–78
Cystinosis, 251
Cytochrome b5 reductase, 449–453, 452f, 453f
Cytochrome c, 143
Cytochrome c reductase, 143
Cytochrome P450 enzyme system, 296, 298, 348, 352–353, 352f
Cytochrome(s), 143, 144–146, 146f, 296
Cytosine, 27t

**D**
DAG (diacylglycerol), 70, 398, 435
Dantrolene, for malignant hyperthermia, 160, 162–163, 162f
Debranching enzyme, 175, 176
Decarboxylation, 135
Deer tick, Lyme disease and, 84
Dehydration
  in Addison disease, 419
  in diabetes insipidus, 397
  rhabdomyolysis and, 184–185
7-Dehydrocholesterol, 298, 299f
Dehydrogenase (definition), 135
Dehydrogenate complex, 136
3-Dehydrosphinganine, 249, 250f
Delavirdine, 50
Deletion, 119, 121
Dementia, thiamine deficiency and, 134
Denaturation, 57, 58, 59f
Deoxyadenosine, 19–20, 20f, 22
Deoxycholic acid, 274f, 276
Deoxyribose, 27t
Deoxyribose nucleic acid. See DNA
Deoxythymidine 5'-monophosphate (dTMP), 37–38
Deoxythymidylate (dTMP), 27, 29, 30f
Deoxyuridine 5-monophosphate (dUMP), 37
Dermatan sulfate, 258t
Desmopressin acetate, 396
Developmental delay, in phenylketonuria, 329–330
Dexamethasone suppression test, 423–425
DHAP (Dihydroxyacetone phosphate), 154, 239, 240f, 243f
DHF (dihydrofolate), 29, 30f, 39
DHFR (dihydrofolate reductase), 26, 27, 29, 37, 39
Diabetes insipidus, 395–400

Erythropoiesis, 111
Erythropoietic porphyria, 382f
Erythrose 4-phosphate, 137
Esmolol, 442
Esophagitis, candida, 45–46
Essential amino acids, 355–360, 358t. *See also* Amino acids
Essential fructosuria, 212, 214
Estradiol, 410, 411
Estrogen(s), 68
  in ovarian cycle, 409–413, 412f
  synthesis, 298f
Ethidium bromide staining, 78
ETS. *See* Electron transport system
Eukaryotes, protein synthesis and, 86–87, 87t
Exoglycosidase, 256
Exons, 47, 48

**F**
Fabry disease, 252t
Facilitative diffusion, glucose transporters and, 213
FAD (flavine adenine dinucleotide), 136, 136f, 144
  in fatty acid oxidation, 315
  in glycerol 3-phosphate shuttle, 242, 240f
  in tricarboxylic acid cycle, 127–129, 128f
Familial hypercholesterolemia, 267
Farber disease, 252t
Fasting state, 313–316, 315f–317f
Fatigue
  in Addison disease, 415–416, 419
  in folic acid deficiency, 36
  in G6PD deficiency, 287–288
  in HIV infection, 46
  in hypothyroidism, 387–388
  in megaloblastic anemia, 361–362
  in rhabdomyolysis, 184–185
Fatty acids
  acute fatty liver in pregnancy and, 175–179
  gluconeogenesis and, 231, 231f
  metabolism and mobilization, 313–318, 314f–318f
  pancreatic lipase and, 168
  uncoupling proteins and, 162
Fatty acyl-CoA dehydrogenase, 403, 404f
Fava beans, 289, 290–291
Ferrochelatase, 379, 380
Fertilization, 412
Fetal hemoglobin, 14–15, 111, 112f, 450, 452
Fetus
  inborn error in fatty acid metabolism, 175, 179
  neural tube defects, 36, 44

Fever
  in Lyme disease, 84
  in septic shock, 125–126
Fiber, dietary, 221–223, 221f
Flavin adenine dinucleotide. *See* FAD
Flavin cofactor, 144
Flavin mononucleotide (FMN), 144
Flurbiprofen, 284
FMN (flavin mononucleotide), 144
*FMR1* gene, 121–122
Foci, 105
Folic acid. *See also* Tetrahydrofolate
  absorption, 40–41, 40f
  deficiency, 35–43
  metabolism, 40–41, 365, 365f
  methotrexate and, 25–27
  sources, 39–40
Formyl-methionine-tRNA, 48
Formyl tetrahydrofolate, 30f, 32, 39, 39f
Founder mutation, 95
Fragile X mental retardation (FMR) protein, 118, 121–122
Fragile X syndrome, 117–124
Frameshift mutation, 111, 121, 121t
Free fatty acids, 305, 306f
Fructokinase, 213, 214, 214f
Fructose 1,6-bisphosphatase, 198
Fructose 1,6-bisphosphate, 187, 187f, 194f, 198f, 239, 240f, 243f
Fructose 2,6-bisphosphate, 193, 197, 198
Fructose 1,6-bisphosphate aldolase, 239, 240f, 243f
Fructose 1-phosphate, 214–215, 214f
Fructose 6-phosphate, 137, 197f, 205, 240f, 243f
Fructose intolerance, 211–217
Fructose metabolism, 213–214, 214f
FSH (follicle-stimulating hormone), 409–412
Fucose, 221, 222
Full mutation, 118, 121
Fumarase, 128f, 129
Fumarate, 129, 324, 325f
Functional neoplasm, 443

**G**
G protein–coupled receptor, 70, 390, 444
G protein(s), 67, 68–70, 69t
$G_0$ phase, cell cycle, 28
$G_1$ phase, cell cycle, 28, 28f
$G_2$ phase, cell cycle, 28, 28f
*Gag* gene, 50
Galactose, 213, 221, 222
α-Galactosidase A, 252t
Gallstones, 165–170, 271–278

Kidney. *See also* Renal failure
 in calcium regulation, 437
 stones, in hyperparathyroidism, 434
 vasopressin and, 397–398
Kinase, 95
Krebs cycle. *See* Tricarboxylic acid
  (TCA) cycle
Kwashiorkor, 312

**L**

Lactate, 129–130, 129*f*
 in anaerobic glycolysis, 243*f*
 in ischemia, 243
 in malignant hyperthermia, 162
 rhabdomyolysis and, 184–189
Lactate dehydrogenase, 129, 129*f*, 186*f*, 243*f*
Lactic acid dehydrogenase, 239
Lactic acidemia, 187
Lactic acidosis, 130
Lactose, 213
Lamivudine, 50
Lanugo hair, in anorexia nervosa, 338
LCHAD (long chain 3-hydroxyacyl-coenzyme A
  dehydrogenase), 174, 179
Lecithin-cholesterol acyl transferase (LCAT),
  265
Lesch-Nyhan syndrome, 371, 372
Lethargy
 in cirrhosis, 322
 in fructose intolerance, 211–212
Leucine, 343, 356, 358*t*
Leucomethylene blue, 451, 453*f*
Leucovorin, 32
Leukotrienes, 281
LH (luteinizing hormone), 411–413
Lignins, 221, 222, 223*f*
α-Limit dextrin, 168
Limit dextrins, 213
Lincosamides, 87–88
Lipase, 167–168
Lipemia retinalis, in hypertriglyceridemia,
  304, 308
Lipoamide, 136
Lipoprotein lipase (LPL), 304, 305, 306*f*,
  307–308
Lipoproteins, 265–267, 266*t*
Liposomes, 80
Lithocholic acid, 274*f*
Liver
 acetaminophen overdose and, 351–352
 acute fatty, in pregnancy, 173–181
 bile salt synthesis in, 273–276, 274*f*
 cholesterol synthesis in, 265
 failure, in fructose intolerance, 211–212
 in fed state, 313, 314*f*

 glucose metabolism in, 175–179, 176*f*, 178*f*,
   197, 198*f*, 229–233, 230*f*
 in postfeeding fast, 313–316, 315*f*–316*f*
 in starvation, 316–318, 318*f*
Locus control region, 111
Long chain 3-hydroxyacyl-coenzyme A dehydro-
  genase (LCHAD), 174, 179
Long-chain fatty acids, 403
Long terminal repeat (LTR), of HIV, 49–50
Lovastatin. *See* HMG-CoA reductase inhibitors
Low-density lipoprotein (LDL), 265–267, 266*t*,
   299, 306, 307*f*
Luteinizing hormone (LH), 411–413
Lyme disease, 83–90
Lymphadenopathy, in Lyme disease, 84
Lymphocytes, 341–342
Lysine, 356, 358*t*
Lysosomal storage disorders, 249, 251, 252*t*

**M**

M phase, cell cycle. *See* Mitosis
Macrocytic anemia, 35–43
Macrolide antibiotics, 88
Malaise
 in acute fatty liver of pregnancy, 173–174,
   175
 in cirrhosis, 322
 in folic acid deficiency, 35–36
Malate, 129, 186, 186*f*
Malate-aspartate shuttle, 129, 238–243, 239*f*
Malate dehydrogenase, 128*f*, 129, 186, 242, 239*f*
Malignant hyperthermia, 159–164, 161*f*
Malnutrition, 311–320, 314*f*–318*f*
Maltose, 213, 222, 222*f*
Mannose, 221, 222
Maple syrup urine disease (MSUD), 93–99
 causes, 95–97
 classification, 97
 mutations in, 97
 treatment, 97
Marasmus, 312
Marathon running, rhabdomyolysis and,
   184–189
MCAD (medium chain acyl-coenzyme A
  dehydrogenase), 179
McArdle disease, 181
Medium chain acyl-coenzyme A dehydrogenase
  (MCAD), 179, 401–407
Medium-chain fatty acids, 403
Megaloblastic anemia, 32, 37, 361–363
α-Melanocyte-stimulating hormone (α-MSH),
   417
Melanocyte(s), 333, 333*f*
Melatonin, 343
Menopause, 409–414